V 42437

THE LAW LORDS

OXFORD SOCIO-LEGAL STUDIES

General Editors: J. Maxwell Atkinson, Donald R. Harris, R. M. Hartwell

Oxford Socio-Legal Studies is a series of books published by the Centre for Socio-Legal Studies, Wolfson College, Oxford (a research unit of the Social Science Research Council). The series is concerned generally with the relationship between law and society, and is designed to reflect the increasing interest in this field of lawyers, social scientists and historians.

THE LAW LORDS

Alan Paterson
Lecturer in Law
University of Edinburgh

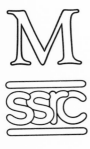

© Alan Paterson 1982

First published 1982 by
THE MACMILLAN PRESS LTD
London and Basingstoke
Companies and representatives
throughout the world

ISBN 0 333 23886 9

Printed in Great Britain by
THE PITMAN PRESS
Bath

Contents

Preface and Acknowledgements

The gestation period of this book has far exceeded that of an elephant. Its conception can be traced to 1970 when the author as a neophyte doctoral student at Oxford was required to settle on the specific content to be given to his hitherto generous thesis title. If the labour has been long and arduous, the trial of my wife's and friends' patience considerable, it has been for the most part a labour of love. Whether the product be mouse or mammoth is for the reader to judge. Its aim is to describe and, in part, to explain, in terms that I hope will be intelligible to lawyer, layman and social scientist, how decisions are made in the House of Lords, and to outline developments in the role of the Law Lord in the past thirty years. In particular it focuses on the remarkable contribution of the late Lord Reid of Drem to the work of the House during this period. It is to his memory and example that this work is dedicated.

Many individuals have contributed to the writing of this book. I owe an immense debt to my former supervisors Philip Lewis and Neil MacCormick for their encouragement and guidance over the years. To the Law Lords and counsel who were the subjects of the research, my debt is equally incalculable. Without their help, their candour and, not least, their generosity with their time there would have been little new for me to write and nothing for the reader to read. In this connection I gratefully acknowledge the assistance of Lord Bridge, Lord Cross, Lord Denning, Lord Devlin, Lord Elwyn-Jones, Lord Gardiner, Lord Guest, Lord Hailsham, Lord Kilbrandon, Lord MacDermott, Lord Pearce, Lord Pearson, Viscount Radcliffe (whose premature demise deprived him of the opportunity of finally revising the passages from his interview which appear in the book), Lord Reid, Lord Roskill, Lord Russell of Killowen, Lord Salmon, Lord Scarman,

Lord Simon of Glaisdale, Lord Wilberforce, Sir Desmond Ackner, Sir John Donaldson, Sir John Megaw, Sir Sydney Templeman, Sir James Comyn, Sir Douglas Falconer, Sir Neville Faulks, Sir Morris Finer, Sir Irvine Goulding, Sir Michael Kerr, Sir Neil Lawson, Sir Anthony Lloyd, Sir Peter Pain, Sir Roger Parker, Sir Gordon Slynn, Sir Haydn Tudor-Evans, Lord Thomson, Judge Everett QC, Michael Albery QC, Robert Alexander QC, Andrew Bateson QC, Louis Blom-Cooper QC, Alan Campbell QC, Colin Duncan QC, Sir Dingle Foot QC, Sir John Foster QC, David Hirst QC, Joseph Jackson QC, Raymond Kidwell QC, Mark Littman QC, John Lloyd-Eley QC, Douglas Lowe QC, Robert MacCrindle QC, Patrick Neill QC, Sir Ashton Roskill QC, Bryan Anns, Leon Brittan QC MP and Margaret Puxon. Sincere thanks are also due to Mr Richard Cave, formerly Principal Clerk of the Judicial Office of the House of Lords, Mr Ernest Mills, Registrar of the Privy Council, and Dr Francis Mann for assistance rendered to me in my researches.

The support of the Oxford Centre for Socio-Legal Studies, where I was a Research Associate in 1972-3, and of its Director, Don Harris, have been invaluable to me, both at the fieldwork and publication stages. Without their help this project would undoubtedly have been stillborn. I am grateful also for the grants which I received from Oxford and Edinburgh Universities in order to defray some of the minor expenses connected with my research. My task as a researcher was greatly eased by the publication of Robert Stevens' *Law and Politics* and Louis Blom-Cooper and Gavin Drewry's *Final Appeal*. I am particularly indebted to the authors of the latter work for permitting me to examine a copy of it while it was still at the proof stage.

Special mention must also be made of Neil MacCormick, who tirelessly bore the burden of commenting on my successive drafts, and of Don Harris and Keith Hawkins, who provided much-needed editorial assistance. I benefited greatly from the comments and advice of John Goldthorpe, Kit Carson and David Nelken at different stages in the research and writing up. Thanks are also due to all those who assisted with proof-reading and to the secretaries, Isobel Roberts, Pat Gibb, Lydia Lawson, Helen Dignan and Janis Eckford, who struggled, often against seemingly impossible deadlines, to produce a final typescript. Lastly, I should state that an abbreviated version of Chapter 7 first appeared in the *Oxford Journal of Legal Studies*.

One final point: in a work such as this, where so many of the participants in the research have been identified, it is peculiarly incumbent on the author to stress that he, and he alone, is responsible for the material presented. The theme, content and conclusion, warts and all, of the book, are mine. I am profoundly grateful to all who have contributed in one way or another to this work, but none of them must be taken to agree with all or any of the arguments which follow.

Edinburgh   Alan Paterson
March 1981

1 Introduction

> [N]one of us can offer anything better than hunches about the role of law and judges at various levels in the operation of a technological society. ... Without more detailed study there is little we can say profitably ... about the legislative role of the courts in Britain.
>
> W. J. M. Mackenzie, *Politics and Social Science*[1]

> [W]e ought to try and obtain a closer understanding of just what goes into a particular judicial decision. ... We must ask some unforgivable questions. What conversations go on, for example, after argument and before judgement? Everybody now knows that in *Donoghue* v. *Stevenson* Lord Atkin talked the majority round. It is now generally known that in *Rookes* v. *Barnard* in 1964 Lord Devlin did much the same. Surely this should be part of our material. It ought not to be shrouded in secrecy.
>
> K. W. Wedderburn, 'Law as a Social Science'[2]

The genesis of this book owed more to curiosity than to the utilitarian or historical concerns of others who have written on the House of Lords in the recent past.[3] Curiosity, first, as to the process by which appeals are decided in the Lords. Traditionally, academic discussions of judicial decisions and decision-making in the United Kingdom have taken as their starting points the judgements of the courts.[4] But do the wider legal community, solicitors, counsel, even academics themselves, not contribute to the development of the law in decisions of the courts? In appellate cases, how much depends on the interaction between the Bar and the Bench or that between the judges themselves? Is appellate decision-making a group activity, or as traditional analyses imply, merely several individuals at work? To restrict one's inquiry to the judgements of the courts, the end products of the decision-making

1

process, rather than scrutinising the dynamics of the process itself, is in some senses no more intellectually satisfying than attributing Christmas presents to Santa Claus, or babies to storks.[5] This work, then, is a first attempt to look at the process by which judicial decisions are arrived at in the House of Lords.

Curiosity, secondly, as to the judicial role in the development of the common law in the Lords. This is an important aspect of decision-making in the Lords. As Otto Kahn-Freund once observed:

> However much scholars have elucidated the principle of precedent no one has ever succeeded in lifting the dark veil that surrounds the relation between law finding and law making in the common law.[6]

What is the role of a Law Lord when confronted with an appeal where there is legitimate room for debate between the parties as to the existence, scope and applicability of one or more common law rules or principles? In such 'hard'[7] cases, how do the Law Lords demarcate their province from that of the legislature when it comes to 'developing' the common law? In the words of Brian Abel-Smith and Robert Stevens,

> [W]e must ask when and how far the appeal courts should deliberately seek to change the law, and how far they should clearly articulate their creative functions.[8]

Such questions, already pertinent in view of the creation of the Law Commissions in 1965 and the publication of the Practice Statement on Precedent in the House of Lords in 1966,[9] were made even more so by John Griffith's recent accusation in *The Politics of the Judiciary*[10] that there is no clear and consistent relationship between the general statements of the higher judiciary in Britain on 'judicial creativity' and what they do in court.

Many of these issues have, of course, been discussed at length by jurists - indeed the third attraction of 'judicial law-making' as a research area was precisely that it was an issue over which scholars such as Herbert Hart, Ronald Dworkin and Karl Llewellyn were fiercely divided.[11] Like others,[12] however, I felt that these jurists were often 'actually posing empirical questions[13] that [could not] be answered by a definition'.[14] Accordingly, I embarked on an empirical investigation of the area, drawing particularly on the perceptions of the Law Lords and the Bar. The approach adopted was role analysis, located within a broad interactionist[15] framework, which enabled me to focus on the role and performance of Law Lords in 'hard' cases. The value of the concept of 'role' for studies of the judicial process has been referred to by jurists such as Karl Llewellyn,[16] Julius Stone,[17] and William Twining,[18] and role studies of judges in the United States are not uncommon (see Appendix). Thus, one of the aims of this work is to highlight the contribution which role analysis can make in increasing our understanding of the decision-making process in the highest court in the United Kingdom.* Nevertheless, in the interests of readability, I have tried to avoid the use of unnecessary jargon. For similar reasons the detailed account of the version of role analysis which was used in the research appears in the Appendix rather than the body of the text. However, some explanation of the role-related terminology which is used in the text is required at this stage.

TERMINOLOGY

In this book, a person's *role* consists of the conduct that is expected of him in the particular social position which he occupies. Put another way, it is the cluster of normative expectations which exist at any given time as to the behaviour and attributes required of a person who holds a particular status or position. The actual behaviour of a person while 'on duty' in his position is sometimes referred to as his *role performance*.

The expectations which constitute a role are not simply derived from other relevant persons (reference groups) but also from the position incumbent's own expectations and perceptions as to the proper behaviour of an individual in his social position. *Role*, therefore, has a dynamic aspect in that a role and its performance are, to a greater or lesser degree, open to 'negotiation' between the incumbent and his audience. It is also dynamic because with the passage of time the expectations which constitute a particular role

*In this field it seems to me that the concept of 'role' is of importance, for it provides the middle range level of analysis linking social structure and individual action which is so conspicuous by its absence in much of present-day sociology of law.[19]

are likely to change.

Not only is *role* a dynamic concept, it is also a dimensional one. First, the dimension of *legitimacy*.[20] Incumbents of social positions regard some expectations, and some sources of expectations, as to their behaviour, as more legitimate than others. Secondly, the dimension of weight or *functional importance*. The expectations which constitute a role can also be classified according to their centrality or importance to the role. Least important are those that are 'peripheral' to the role, so that compliance with them might be considered optional; next are those that are sufficiently 'relevant' to the role that their absence, variation or abrogation leaves it imperfect or incomplete; finally 'pivotal' expectations are those that are so central to the role that they are fundamental to its character or existence.

Because 'role' is both dynamic and dimensional there is considerable scope for conflict between expectations held by different reference groups, or by different members of the same reference group, or between these externally derived expectations and the position incumbent's own expectations for his conduct. Research has shown (see Appendix) that position incumbents respond to such *role conflicts* in a number of recognised ways.

RESEARCH METHODS[21]

The research focused primarily on the English common law[22] 'hard' cases heard in the Lords between 1957 and 1973, although I have not hesitated to draw on other relevant cases and material from within and without this period. Although my data was primarily gathered from interviews, a number of other sources and research methods were also used.[23] The principal documentary sources were the official law reports (the Appeal Cases) during the chosen period. Use was also made of judicial biographies, extra-judicial writings and of a number of printed Cases (the written material in a case which counsel provides to the Judicial Office in advance of the oral hearing) as well as numerous other books and articles. The fieldwork had four elements.

First, observation of the interaction between the Law Lords and counsel in a variety of appeals in the years 1972 and 1973. Secondly, interviews with strategic or other well-informed individuals concerning the Law Lords and their role. These included the Principal Clerk of the Judicial Office, his deputy, the Registrar of the Privy Council, the Chairman of the Law Commission and the Lord Chancellor's Permanent Secretary. The third and fourth parts involved in-depth interviews with the Law Lords and counsel who had argued 'hard' cases before them, in an attempt to ascertain their role perceptions. Occasionally, it was possible for me to combine several of these methods in relation to one appeal. Thus in *Cassell & Co. Ltd* v. *Broome* and *Heatons Transport Ltd* v. *TGWU* I was able to attend the hearings and to read the printed Cases, interview several of the counsel involved and also one of the sitting Law Lords during or shortly after the hearing of the appeals.

The primary research subjects were the Law Lords, that is, those judges eligible to sit in the Lords,[24] who were active[25] in 1972. Interviews were also sought with Law Lords who had sat regularly in the Lords between 1957 and 1973 but who were no longer active judges in the House. The secondary subjects were the members of the Bar who had most frequently appeared in 'hard' cases decided in the Lords during the chosen period. The sample selected was the thirty counsel who had argued three or more 'hard' cases in the Lords in that time. Finally, I approached a further group of barristers who had appeared in certain key 'hard' cases during my period.

Considerable problems have been encountered by various researchers who have endeavoured to conduct interviews with British judges and counsel.[26] It is only fair to record that I did not encounter such difficulties. Courtesy and forbearance were extended to me, almost without exception, by those whom I interviewed. Of the fifteen active Law Lords, nine agreed to a tape-recorded interview[27] (including Lords Cross, Gardiner, Guest, Kilbrandon, Pearson, Reid, Salmon and Wilberforce), one (Lord MacDermott) was prepared to be interviewed but not recorded and Lord Hailsham LC answered in writing the open-ended questions contained in the questionnaire which formed the framework of the other interviews. Four (Lords Dilhorne, Diplock, Hodson and Morris) declined to participate in the research. All four 'inactive' Law Lords approached (Lords Denning, Devlin, Pearce and Radcliffe) agreed to a taped interview. By 1972/3, when the bulk of my fieldwork was undertaken, the status of many of the 'counsel' contained in my samples from the Bar had changed, and there have been further changes since. In the text these individuals will be given their status at the time of their interview, although for the purposes of this work they are in fact 'appearing as counsel'. Of the thirty counsel in the primary sample from the Bar, twenty-three agreed to an interview. These included Mr Justices Ackner, Donaldson, Faulks, Goulding and Lawson; Judge Everett QC; eleven Queen's Counsel (Louis Blom-Cooper, James Comyn, Colin Duncan, Sir Elwyn-Jones, Sir John Foster, David Hirst, Mark Littman, Anthony Lloyd, Robert MacCrindle, Peter Pain and Roger Parker); and Mr Gordon Slynn. The secondary sample of counsel all agreed to an interview. They included Lord Justice Russell; Mr Justices Bridge and Scarman; twelve Queen's Counsel (Michael Albery, Andrew Bateson, Alan Campbell, Douglas Falconer, Morris Finer, Sir Dingle Foot, Joseph Jackson, Raymond Kidwell, John Lloyd-Eley, Douglas Lowe, Patrick Neill and Sydney Templeman); and Mr Robert Alexander. In all, twenty-eight judges, twenty-six Queen's Counsel and seven juniors were interviewed.

Although the interviews were partially structured by my checklist of questions,[28] in accordance with standard practice in elite interviewing[29] almost all of the questions were open-ended and the checklist was not administered in an inflexible fashion. The frequency with which the respondents anticipated my questions and the variations in the time which they allotted to me for the interviews (the Law Lords' interviews ranged from thirty minutes to two and a half hours), meant that it was often necessary to vary the sequence of my questions or to drop some of them altogether.

The accuracy of interview responses is always a problem. In elite interviews if time is at a premium it is both wasteful and potentially dangerous to introduce questions designed merely to cross-check on those which have gone before. Inevitably there were apparent inconsistencies in some of the interviews and on one or two occasions subsequent events gave me reason to question the accuracy of an answer which I had received. But, as we shall see, I found a remarkably high consistency between the respondents' answers and their performance in decided cases. Furthermore, over a third of my questions related to matters of fact which could potentially be corroborated from the answers of other respondents. On these matters the interviews were highly consistent, internally, as between one another, and over time. The

Law Lords were each given the opportunity to revise their interview transcripts both at the end of the fieldwork and in 1979/80 prior to the publication of this book. Counsel were also given the opportunity to revise any quotations or other material derived from their interviews which have been used in this work. Once issues of confidentiality had been dealt with,[30] very few amendments of any substance were made. The great majority of those interviewed, agreed, on this second approach, to the publication of extracts from the interviews and to the ascription of the extracts to them by name, although I have not always taken advantage of the licence granted to me in this respect. Quotations in the text which are not otherwise attributed are derived from the interviews.

The book is divided into eight chapters, with an appendix. Chapter 2 attempts to identify the individuals or groups whose views influence the role and role perceptions of a Law Lord - particularly in 'hard' cases. Chapters 3, 4 and 5 highlight the crucial significance of the interchanges which take place between counsel and the Law Lords and between the Law Lords themselves, for the outcome of appeals. Chapter 3 deals with these exchanges from the standpoint of counsel and Chapter 4 is written from the standpoint of the Law Lords. Chapter 5 provides the first published account of the 'behind the scenes' aspects of decision-making in the Lords.[31] Chapters 6 and 7 are devoted to the Law Lords' perceptions of their role and their decisions in 'hard' cases during my research period. They demonstrate how and why the role of the Law Lord as a decision-maker has changed in the past thirty years. They also contain the most complete account yet to be published on the background to the Practice Statement on Precedent in the House of Lords which was issued in 1966. A major theme in these chapters is the influence of Lord Reid on the role of the Law Lord during my research period. Chapter 8 consists of reflections on the jurisprudential and political science implications of my study. The Appendix provides a more extended account of role analysis as applied in my own and other research on judges.

In short, the thesis of this book is that decision-making in the House of Lords should be seen as a social process. I found that the wider legal community had a part to play in the process, and that counsel through their restrictive and persuasive arguments had a highly significant contribution to make to decisions. Decisions in the House are not the product of five individuals sitting in their own rooms painstakingly writing out their opinions. The printed speeches are but the end product of a complex series of exchanges between Bar and Bench and between the Law Lords themselves. This process is structured around the perceptions held by counsel and Law Lord alike as to the parameters of legitimate behaviour both for themselves and for each other, in particular contexts. Such role expectations, and the roles of counsel and Law Lord, are themselves the outcome of an interactive process. I discovered that the roles of counsel and Law Lord were in part subjectively defined, that inherent in the roles were certain unresolved conflicts, and that individuals in responding to these conflicts had contributed to changes in both of the roles in the past thirty years. In demonstrating the utility of a concept of role which has dynamic elements, this book also suggests a path for further developments in role analysis.

2 Who Influences Law Lords?

Quis custodiet ipsos custodes?

Decision-making in the Lords does not take place in a vacuum. A number of individuals and groups exist whose notions of acceptable behaviour for a judge when deciding appeals (*i.e.* of his role), potentially have an influence on a Law Lord. These potential or would-be reference groups* might include fellow Law Lords, other members of the Judiciary, Benchers, barristers, legal academics, litigants, solicitors, the legislature, the media and the general public. But which, if any, of these actually do influence the Law Lords when they are deciding appeals? Those whom the Law Lords have in mind as audiences when preparing their speeches, those with whom they most frequently discuss their decisions and those whose criticism the Law Lords pay most attention to, would seem to be the prime candidates.

AUDIENCES

Precisely which audiences appellate judges have in contemplation when writing their opinions is a topic which has recently attracted some attention from legal scholars. The work of Perelman on audiences,[1] an interest in the comparative style of judicial opinions and in the justification of judicial decisions have each been in part responsible for this attention. Little consensus has emerged. Wetter[2] and Heuston[3] consider that appellate opinions in England are primarily aimed at the legal advisers of the litigants. Goutal[4]

---

*'Reference group' is a term that has been used in a variety of ways by researchers. For my purposes, a person's reference group consists of those individuals or groups who hold and articulate normative expectations as to his behaviour, who act as a general audience for his role performances and who are used by him to evaluate his performances.

9

suggests that English appellate judges are teaching the legal profession (judges, barristers, solicitors and students) in their opinions. For Rudden[5] it is the litigants' advisers, the judge's colleagues and future judges; for Prott[6] it is the legal profession, the litigants and 'every concerned citizen'; while in Tunc's[7] eyes it is the parties, their advisers, the judge's erstwhile colleagues and his fellows in his Inn of Court.

Interviewing the Law Lords did not entirely clarify the matter. Of the fifteen active Law Lords, fewer than half appeared to have given any detailed consideration to the question of who their audiences were. In constitutional theory the answer is that the opinions of the various members of the Appellate Committee are speeches delivered in a debate in the Chamber of the House of Lords following a motion from the Woolsack 'That the Report of the Appellate Committee be now considered'.[8] When one considers that the speeches are no longer read out* and that a deceased Law Lord can now give a speech[9] it is not surprising that none of the Law Lords considered that their fellow Peers were their audience.

Perhaps more surprising was the disclaimer by one or two Law Lords that their speeches were in any way directed at their fellow Law Lords. Yet from their response to other questions some Law Lords would seem to write their judgements with an eye to persuading one or more of their colleagues to adopt their position. Only two Law Lords referred specifically to the judiciary in the lower courts but from other answers and from speeches such as Lord Hailsham's in *Cassell* v. *Broome*[10] it appears that a majority of the Law Lords perceive their speeches as, where the occasion demands, either correcting mistakes of lower courts or providing guidance to them. Not a single Law Lord said that he wrote with academics in mind. Lord Guest specifically stated that he did not write for the law journals or for posterity, though two other Law Lords asserted that they did write with an eye to their successors. Three more (Lords Reid, MacDermott and Pearson), indicated that where possible the judgements should be intelligible to the man in the street.[11] In a few cases, where a Law Lord considers the law to be in an unsatisfactory state but feels unable to rectify matters, he may 'aim' his speech at Parliament or a particular

---

*The practice was abandoned in 1963 after it had been computed that the time taken to read out all the judgements issued in a single year exceeded 24 hours.

government department.

In fact, over a third of the Law Lords denied that their opinions were written with anyone in particular in mind.* This somewhat Olympian stance was mitigated by the fact that most of the Law Lords qualified their denials with the assertion that they had a general audience in mind, namely, other lawyers. Viscount Radcliffe's response encapsulates this general view,

> Well, that I think, is a very good question, and I don't know whether there's a really good answer to it ... Probably there's no single answer. They were not written, obviously, to the world at large. They were not written to one's immediate colleagues, because one tried to avoid bickering in that sense, so that I would have thought probably you were aiming at the middle distance, which was the court whose judgements you were dealing with, including the first court ... and to some extent the Bar.

SANCTIONABILITY

The elevated status of Law Lords and the doctrine of the separation of powers combine to make them peculiarly immune from sanctions for alleged 'deviance'. I am not aware of any attempt to remove a Law Lord being made in the past 100 years, on such grounds.[12] They have usually reached the peak of their careers and so cannot have their chances of promotion blighted. The main sanction available to the Lord Chancellor lies in his power to decide in which cases a particular Law Lord will take part and whether he will sit in the Privy Council or the House of Lords. The first Lord Hailsham, when Lord Chancellor, used this power for the very purpose of curtailing Lord Atkin's 'deviance' in being too much of a reformer,[13] but there is little evidence of such 'court-packing' manoeuvres in more recent times.

This relative immunity to sanction entails that those who wish to influence the Law Lords have to rely on persuasion and criticism rather than stronger and more coercive sanctions. This is usually attempted by indirect means, e.g. textbooks, journals or

---

*At least one Law Lord implied that to write with an audience in mind might be in conflict with the judicial obligation to act without fear or favour.

the media, for few of them have opportunities of interacting directly with the Law Lords.

INTERACTION

The interviews revealed that direct interaction between the Law Lords and potential reference groups was indeed very limited. In some ways the Law Lords lead even more cloistered lives than judges lower down the hierarchy.

The Lords of Appeal and other Law Lords sitting on a case, spend their working days in the Palace of Westminster or No. 1 Downing Street and generally lunch together in the peers' dining room. Only on Fridays, weekends and in the evenings do they regularly go to their clubs or to the Inns of Court. Whether or not Law Lords regard themselves as bound by the Lord Chancellor's directive that judges should not give interviews to the media without first consulting him, they rarely discuss cases or the judicial role in the media.[14] Of course Law Lords read newspapers, listen to the radio and watch television, but comment and criticism of their decisions, except in the most superficial form, is uncommon in the media. Similarly, criticism of decisions of the House of Lords is an infrequent occurrence in Parliament, although, as we shall see, the fear that they may be accused of usurping the function of Parliament appears to influence some of the Law Lords, on occasion.[15]

On the question of whom the Law Lords discussed their decisions with (once judgement had been delivered), two things emerged from the interviews. First, that most Law Lords had no objection to discussing their cases with anyone and, secondly, that the persons with whom they most frequently discussed them were fellow Benchers. This is probably due to the fact that fellow Benchers are the only persons with whom they directly interact on a regular basis (apart from their families) who are interested in discussing their decisions. For a variety of reasons most Law Lords do not interact on a regular basis with the group who might be thought most interested in discussing their decisions - legal academics. Friendships between Law Lords and academic lawyers who are not honorary Benchers or fellows at the Law Lords' Oxbridge college are rare.[16] Only a handful of academics (almost invariably of professorial rank) ever achieve the status of honorary

Benchers.[17] It is not surprising therefore that only two of the active Law Lords indicated that they had ever consulted or written to an academic when in doubt in a case.[18] (Lest it be thought that the other Law Lords had not answered this question with candour it should be said that at least three of them saw nothing reprehensible in such consultations.)

Would-be reference groups may therefore be forced to resort to other, less direct, methods of interaction. Although Justices in the US Supreme Court not infrequently receive letters following the publication of the Court's decisions,[19] nothing in the interviews with the Law Lords indicated that this occurred frequently to them. None of the Law Lords mentioned receiving such letters and I have seen no evidence to suggest that they are a common event.[20] Academic friends and judges lower down the hierarchy have been known to write to Law Lords but such letters are usually sympathetic rather than critical and thus operate in reinforcement of role perceptions already held by the Law Lord concerned.[21]

Judges and barristers have made sufficient flattering, if slightly tongue-in-cheek, statements in the recent past to the effect that legal academics in general or writers in the *Law Quarterly Review* in particular, now constitute the Final Court of Appeal in England,[22] for academics to conclude that they can make up for their lack of direct contact with the Law Lords by publication in the learned journals. As we shall see shortly, the Law Lords' responses did not entirely bear this out.

In any event, interaction with the Law Lords is only the first step.[23] Would-be reference groups must also articulate their expectations and assessments of the Law Lords' performances. Whilst academics in their writings usually meet this requirement (though not always - the comments must be role specific), the same cannot be said of others who, when they meet a Law Lord, often feel too respectful or too inhibited to voice any criticisms which they might have. Thus the great majority of the counsel whom I interviewed did not feel able to criticise the Law Lords' decisions to their faces. Such conduct would, they implied, be both impolite and impolitic.

But even if a group succeeds in communicating its expectations to the Law Lords, this is still not enough. The latter's relative immunity from sanctions entails that, by and large, groups will act as reference groups for the Law Lords only if they are perceived to be such by the judges. That is, if the Law Lords consider that the expectations which the groups hold for the behaviour of the Law Lords are at least in part legitimate and worthy of serious consideration. With this in mind I asked the Law Lords to identify the sources of criticism to which they paid most attention.

The source which the Law Lords mentioned most frequently was fellow Law Lords (although Lord Cross indicated that he found his colleagues' comments too polite to be of assistance). Three Law Lords (including Lords Cross and Guest) mentioned Benchers, including the judges in the courts below, or counsel who had argued the case in the Lords. But as in the case of another three (Lords Kilbrandon, MacDermott and Reid) who made some reference to academics, it emerged that much would depend on which particular counsel or academic was endeavouring to influence them. (Professors Cross and Goodhart were particularly highly respected.) Finally, there were occasions when the Law Lords in deciding 'hard' cases took account of views which they attributed to Parliament or the general public* - whether or not either of them actually held these, or any other, views of the role of the Law Lord in the circumstances in question.[24]

LAW LORDS AND ACADEMICS

Let us turn to consider in greater detail the three main groups mentioned by the Law Lords, but in reverse order. First, legal academics. As we have seen, few of them have the opportunity to interact on a direct basis with the Law Lords. But what of the academic comment and criticism in the legal journals - does this not reach the Law Lords? Not necessarily, is the answer. Of the nineteen Law Lords in the sample, four (including Lords Kilbrandon and Diplock[25]) regularly read the prestige law journals, e.g. the Law Quarterly Review and the Modern Law Review, in depth; five (Lords Hailsham, MacDermott, Reid, Salmon and Pearce) regularly glanced at them; three (Lords Gardiner,

*Although there is no empirical data it is likely that the findings of surveys in the United States in relation to the Supreme Court and the general public, would be replicated in the United Kingdom. These are that the public has little awareness of judicial decisions and judicial behaviour in the highest court in the land. For a summary of these surveys, see Sarat, 'Studying American Legal Culture', 11 Law and Soc. Rev. (1977) 427, and Caldeira, 11 Law and Soc. Rev. (1977) 851.

Denning and Devlin) only read them occasionally and four (Lords Pearson, Cross, Guest and Radcliffe) hardly ever read them.[26] Moreover, academic criticism tends to be fairly muted. When he was editor of the *Law Quarterly Review*, Professor Goodhart is reputed to have had a policy of preventing stringent comment on the performances of the Law Lords on the grounds that it would offend the Law Lords, most of whom read the journal. My findings do not entirely support Goodhart's thesis. It seems that the general editor of the *Modern Law Review* in 1950 was summoned by the Law Lords and solemnly reproved for publishing an article by Professor Gower that included a criticism of the judicial attitude to academics.[27] But whatever may have been the case twenty years before, the Law Lords in 1972 were not particularly sensitive to, or likely to be influenced by, academic comment. One Law Lord indicated that he very seldom found the law journals of any assistance in their comments or criticisms because they were not critical enough. He went on,

> I'd much sooner have a much more detailed criticism than what one gets - the sort of notes which are couched in very respectful language, are not particularly helpful, to us at any rate. I would much sooner have a more robust thing of much greater length.

Some Law Lords indicated that they did not pay much attention to academic comment in any event. This is not surprising in the case of the four who never read the journals, but others who did read them also voiced such an opinion, *e.g.* Lord Kilbrandon, who said, 'I think that sometimes in a jocular way you'll say ... "I don't think Professor X will like that very much" ... but it might not influence you very much in your judgement.'

It might thus appear that academics, unless they are Benchers, have very little influence as a reference group for the Law Lords. Such a view is lent credence by the relatively low status ascribed to legal academics in England as compared to those in some continental countries and in the United States.[28] Nevertheless, the academics could achieve the status of a reference group to the Law Lords by indirect means. First, by influencing future generations of Law Lords in their lectures and writings. Secondly, by helping to create a groundswell of professional opinion on matters relevant to the role and performance of the Law Lords in hard cases. Thirdly, by influencing the Bar and in particular, counsel who appear most frequently before the Lords, and through their arguments, influencing the Law Lords.

This third form of influence has increased in importance in the past twenty years largely because, paralleling the trend in the United States and Canada,[29] there has been a relaxation of the rule against citation from the works of living academic writers. Although the barristers whom I interviewed revealed that it was rare for them to consult an academic in the preparation of their arguments for a case in the Lords, and although barristers who are also academics do not commonly take part in such appeals, even as a junior, most barristers felt it incumbent upon them to look at any relevant academic material they could find in the preparation of their arguments. In the 1950s barristers by and large seem to have felt unable to breach the non-citation rule in arguments before the Lords.[30] An examination of the English appeals reported in 1955 Appeal Cases reveals that there were seven references by counsel to textbooks whose authors were alive and two references to articles. In all the Law Lords' speeches reported in that year in English appeals there were only six references to textbooks and none to articles. Viscount Simonds did on the other hand state at the end of his speech in *Benmax* v. *Austin Motor Co. Ltd* that he was indebted to certain writings of Professor Goodhart in the preparation of his speech.[31]

Even as late as 1961 the position had only marginally changed.[32] Counsel cited textbooks by living authors on only eleven occasions in the English appeals reported in 1961 Appeal Cases. However, gradually the tide had begun to turn. The evasive tactic of counsel 'adopting as their argument' academic writings had appeared[33] and soon became the commonplace that it now is in the House of Lords. A study of the English appeals reported in 1971 Appeal Cases reveals not only a threefold increase (as compared with the 1955 figures) in the number of references by counsel to living authors but also a similar increase in the references contained in the Law Lords' speeches. In some recent cases in the House of Lords the welter of academic references on both sides of the Bar has reached floodlike proportions which would have astounded their counterparts of twenty years ago.[34] The vital influence exercised by an academic article on the Law Lords' decision in *Oppenheimer* v. *Cattermole* would make many a continental academic writer envious. The article[35] led not only to two re-hearings before the House and a referral back to the commissioners but also to a majority of the House deciding the appeal contrary to the way they would have done had the article not come to their attention.

The changed attitudes which have led to such a transformation, albeit gradual and unplanned, have recently been articulated by Lords Reid and Diplock. The former, commenting on the problems of interchange between academics and judges, said,

> But I think we are making some progress ... In the House of Lords at least we turn a blind eye to the old rule that an academic writer is not an authority until he is dead, because then he can no longer change his mind.[36]

The latter in a tribute to A. L. Goodhart said,

> In contrast to the judicial attitude in my early days at the Bar, judges no longer think that the sources of judicial wisdom are confined to judgements in decided cases and, exceptionally, some pronouncement of the illustrious dead. In appellate courts, at any rate, when confronted with a doubtful point of law we want to know what living academic jurists have said about it, and we consider that counsel have not done their homework unless they come equipped to tell us about it.[37]

The bulk of the barristers with experience of arguing in the Lords over a period of years, agreed in their interviews that the Law Lords had grown more receptive to the citation of academic writings during the 1960s.

However, the increased citation of academic writings does not necessarily mean that academics as a group exercise a significant influence on the Law Lords. First, some Law Lords have dissented against the change. In *Palmer* v. *The Queen* Lord Avonside refused to allow Professor Gordon's treatise on *The Criminal Law of Scotland* to be cited in the Privy Council on the grounds that it was 'not authority'.* In the course of my interview with Lord Salmon the latter remarked,

---

*This may simply reflect the fact that the relaxation of the non-citation rule has not gone so far in Scotland as it has in England. But there is a certain irony in that barely one month before *Palmer* was argued, Professor Gordon's book was cited without objection in the House of Lords in *Treacy* v. *DPP* at p. 546. Lord Morris was present on both occasions but seems to have felt some difficulty in challenging Lord Avonside's assertions.

Writings of academic lawyers, however brilliant, are not
authority but counsel often cites them in order to make them
part of his own argument, and we listen to them all with great
attention,[38]

and Lord Wilberforce in a note published in 1978, reaffirmed the
existence of the non-citation rule.[39]

The second caveat relates to the present status of such academic
writings as are cited to their Lordships. Do the Law Lords even
treat them as persuasive[40] sources of law? A survey of three recent
hard cases, Knuller v. DPP, R. v. Hyam, and DPP v. Majewski, is of
some assistance here. In each of these cases the Law Lords were
being asked to reconsider a previous decision of the House of
Lords which had been subjected to considerable criticism by
academics.[41] In each, the articles critical of the previous decisions
were cited to the Law Lords. In Knuller counsel for the respondents
even felt it incumbent upon him to devote a section of his
argument to replying to some of the articles cited by the
appellants. Law Lords in each of these cases indicated, in their
speeches, their awareness of the substantial academic criticism of
the earlier cases. These Law Lords further accepted that such
criticism was worthy of respect.[42] But their Lordships by and large
experienced very little difficulty in rejecting the academic criticism
as being misdirected (Knuller),* excessively logical (Majewski) or
not in point (Hyam). Moreover in situations where one might
expect to find Law Lords citing the academic writings to reinforce
propositions which the Law Lords favoured, e.g. the dissents of
Lords Diplock and Kilbrandon in Hyam or in the speeches in
Conway v. Rimmer overruling Duncan v. Cammell Laird, very little
attempt was made to cite academic writings for support. On the
other hand, Lord Denning once accounted for the rejection of
Candler v. Crane, Christmas & Co. in Hedley Byrne v. Heller by saying,
'The commentators helped a lot. They made useful criticisms.
Those things do influence even the House of Lords.'[43] Even so
there seems little evidence that the Law Lords regard
pronouncements of living academic writers (as a group) as having
even persuasive authority. Their practice seems to be to accord

---

*In view of my findings as to the high standing of Professor Goodhart it is
interesting to note that although only one academic article favouring the
decision in Shaw v. DPP was cited by counsel in Knuller (and ten were cited
criticising Shaw), that one article was by Professor Goodhart.

such writings merely 'permissive' status.[44] Intriguingly, there is evidence to suggest that appellate court decisions in the United States and particularly in the Commonwealth,[45] which are also more frequently cited in the House of Lords than was the case twenty years ago,[46] are treated by some of the Law Lords as having persuasive authority. But, as with the academics, the Law Lords have experienced little or no difficulty in rejecting or ignoring the consensus of these other countries when they prefer to retain their own line.[47]

The third caveat is that for academic criticism to operate as a reference group activity it must meet the tests mentioned earlier. Its content must relate to the Law Lords' role. Whilst the comments of academics on the 1966 Practice Statement and the Law Lords' interpretation of it, or on judicial 'activism' in general are clearly role related, bald statements of the law in a standard textbook do not pass the test so easily. Again, though the relaxation of the non-citation rule has increased the opportunities for the communication of expectations held by academics to the Law Lords there are still several hurdles to overcome. First, the academic's own reticence at expressing his criticism in a forceful manner lest it be perceived as disrespectful; secondly, the censorship of the editors of the prestigious journals; thirdly, the reluctance of barristers to cite articles which are strongly critical of incumbent Law Lords;[48] and lastly, persuading the Law Lords to take account of the criticism.

I adverted earlier to the fact that few academics other than the handful who have attained Bencher status ever have the opportunity of interacting with Law Lords over an extended period. Similarly it appeared from my interviews and from the citations which are reported in the Appeal Cases that certain distinguished academics are regarded with a respect and are quoted with a frequency denied to their lesser brethren. A revealing indication of this was to be seen in the oral argument of *Morgans* v. *Launchbury*[49] when counsel read a passage from the *Law Quarterly Review*. Lord Wilberforce then asked, 'Is it by any particular authority? By A. L. Goodhart or Professor Cross?' And Lord Reid when discussing academic criticism of the Law Lords observed to me,

If Professor Goodhart or someone like him is criticising you in the *Law Quarterly Review* then you sit up and take note, if it is

somebody you've never heard of, perhaps you don't take so
much notice.

In the light of such statements it could be argued that these select
individuals act as a small but significant reference group within a
wider less significant group or even that they act as reference
individuals to the Law Lords. As we have seen, it is probable that
Professor Goodhart performed such a function during the period
of my study.[50] Lord Diplock in a tribute to Goodhart attributed
the relaxation of the non-citation rule very largely to the latter's
influence, observing that he possessed two attributes which are
vital to one who wishes to alter the judicial role, community
acceptance and endurance.

> ... in what tends to be an inward-looking community, the Inns
> of Court where judges and leading members of the Bar meet
> together and 'everyone knows everyone else', the impetus for
> change depends upon the personal persuasion of someone who
> is accepted as a member of the community ... He who sets out
> to alter the habits of mind of judges must be possessed of
> stamina and patience and, if he hopes to see some positive
> results, blessed with longevity.[51]

Thus, certain academics can lay claim to the accolade of being a
reference group to the Law Lords in their role as decision-makers,
even if a question mark must remain over the size of the group and
its influence. Whether these academics influence the Law Lords
by the authority of their reasoning or by reason of their authority,
is equally unclear.

LAW LORDS AND COUNSEL

What influence did the counsel who appeared most frequently
before the Law Lords exercise upon them in hard cases? Were
they a significant reference group for the Law Lords? The Law
Lords' interviews did not resolve these issues. Certainly, the
counsel interviewed all held fairly clear normative expectations for
the behaviour and attributes of the Law Lords in hard cases.[52]
These ranged from the expectation that Law Lords should restrict
the propositions of law in their speeches to matters covered by

counsel in argument (held by a majority of counsel), to the situations in which (and the frequency with which) it would be proper for the Law Lords to overrule earlier decisions of the House of Lords or for them to develop the law to meet changing circumstances rather than to leave it to Parliament. Again, counsel in the main had little difficulty in deciding whether the Law Lords ought to settle for less than ideal justice in return for certainty in the law, or to seek to do justice even at the expense of certainty. But were these expectations communicated to the Law Lords? And how did counsel perceive their role in arguing before the House?

Counsel and Law Lords encounter each other most frequently in the committee rooms of the House of Lords, where appeals are argued, and in the Inns of Court. The interchange between them in the committee rooms, as we shall see, is the central element in the whole decisional process. Nor is there any doubt that the arguments used by counsel in such appeals frequently relate to the role of the Law Lord. Perhaps the most obvious examples concern the 1966 Practice Statement on Precedent (permitting the House to depart from one of its own precedents). In most of the twenty-nine or so cases in which the Practice Statement has been raised in oral argument before the House since 1966, counsel have made assertions as to the conditions under which the Law Lords should feel it right to overrule an earlier decision in the House.[53]

Similar assertions were made as to the 'creative' role of the House in cases where the Law Lords were being asked by one side to extend existing principles of law into new areas, *e.g. Hedley Byrne* v. *Heller, National Provincial Bank* v. *Ainsworth, Home Office* v. *Dorset Yacht Co.* and *Morgans* v. *Launchbury*. Again, one of the arguments based on parliamentary inactivity (Parliament has had an opportunity of dealing with this matter recently and has not done so, therefore we should assume that they are satisfied with the existing law) which both counsel and Law Lords invoke from time to time[54] contains an implicit role expectation. This is that the House of Lords should not usurp the law-making functions of the legislature. The same expectation is sometimes voiced explicitly by counsel, *e.g. Shaw* v. *DPP, Williams* v. *Williams*[55] and *Morgans* v. *Launchbury*.[56] Even counsel's increased citation of academic writings by living authors carries with it the implication that the Law Lords ought to pay attention to such writers in making their decisions.

It might seem legitimate to conclude from the foregoing that counsel who appear before the Lords are acting as a reference group to them in the oral argument. In practice it is far from clear that this is the case. The flaw in the argument is the implicit assumption that the counsel will limit their submissions to the Law Lords to their perception of what it is legitimate for a Law Lord to do. They do not. Counsel certainly observe limits in their arguments to the Law Lords *e.g. R.* v. *Miah*[57] where the appellant's counsel said that he 'had been unable to find any argument which he thought he could properly submit to the House', or the appellant's counsel in *Knuller* v. *DPP* [58] where he admits that he is unable to argue that the case is distinguishable from *Shaw*'s case. Again, even in the years immediately preceding the 1966 Practice Statement no counsel felt able to argue that the Law Lords were not bound by their own precedents.*

But it became clear as the research progressed that the limits which counsel observed in the forensic struggle were not related to their own perceptions of the legitimate conduct of a Law Lord in a hard case. Thus Roger Parker QC, who in *Anisminic* v. *Foreign Compensation Commission* and in the *Jones'* case had requested that the 1966 Practice Statement be invoked, was to be found hinting a few months later in *Cassell* v. *Broome* that the Practice Statement was possibly invalid.[59] Parker was not alone, for although the overwhelming majority of counsel interviewed considered that the Statement should be invoked very sparingly, the frequency with which the Law Lords have been asked to overrule a previous decision of the House has been startling. In no fewer than six of the twenty-nine cases reported in 1972 Appeal Cases counsel endeavoured to invoke the statement.

THE ROLE OF COUNSEL ARGUING BEFORE THE HOUSE

I asked counsel whether they experienced any difficulty in putting forward an argument which, if accepted, would involve the Law Lords in acting in a manner which the counsel considered

---

*There was one exception. It is not generally known that not long before the Practice Statement, Mark Littman QC, the respondent's counsel in *West & Son* v. *Shephard* was asked by Lord Reid (the presiding Law Lord) to address the House on whether it was bound by its own previous decisions. The cases he cited (although not the interaction) are recorded on p. 337.

illegitimate. None of them had.

Michael Albery QC said,

> One's function as counsel, subject to quite a number of overriding considerations, is to win the case for one's client, who after all pays one to do it. There are certain things you can't do in trying to promote that end. You can't deceive the Court, you may have, in certain cases, to draw the attention of the Court to authorities that are clearly in point and that are against your case. But subject to those kind of things, it's your job to win the case and the only test as to whether you should put an argument or not is whether it's likely to persuade your tribunal or not.[60]

Another lawyer told me, 'It's not counsel's job to say to the House, "You can't do that" ... Counsel's paid to represent and win for his client.' And a Lord Justice agreed with him, 'As an advocate I don't think you should mess up one's client's case with any personal idealism.'

When I asked a Chancery judge who was very strongly opposed to 'judicial legislation' if this would ever have prevented him from arguing a point, when he was counsel, he said,

> Not in the least. If it's in the interest of my client to attack certainty of law it wouldn't upset my conscience at all to put the argument. As an advocate one is paid to put one's client's case as well as one can within the bounds of honesty. One is not concerned with the results as a matter of policy. It's for the judges to know that.

and Lord Evershed MR once wrote that subject to counsel's duty to the court,

> Your whole duty is to your client. Fight for your client as hard as you can. You must allow no personal reasons to enter in ... no consideration of private inclination. This does not mean that you have to talk nonsense. There is almost always a lot of sense to be said for both sides.[61]

One QC was even prepared to assert that,

There are really no limits, I mean, you can say whatever you can get away with, the court by and large is very patient ... you should temper your arguments to meet anything that will help you to win your case. Your job is to win your case - playing according to the rules.

Mr Justice Donaldson on the other hand seemed to be an exception, for he said, 'One's only object is to win one's case for one's client. But, if possible, one should try to avoid the law going wrong in the process.' Yet his rationale for this was not based on his conception of counsel's duty to the court but that owed to his clients. As a commercial specialist, he felt that when he represented one shipowner he should try if possible to safeguard the interests of all shipowners. If he was representing a shipowner, however, he felt no duty to charterers and *vice versa*.

Despite such statements, we have already seen that advocates do clearly perceive some limits to exist to the arguments which they feel able to submit to the House. Thus Sydney Templeman QC, having argued initially that 'there are no limits, you merely try and pick out arguments whether of policy or construction which suit you and which you feel will be convincing', subsequently qualified this by adding, 'There are limits ... You know how far a particular House of Lords is likely to go ... In a good many cases you wouldn't put forward the argument because you know it wouldn't be acceptable.'

These limits, which are, in effect, counsel's perceptions of their own role as counsel, seem to be derived as much from pragmatic considerations - what one can get away with - as from normative considerations. There was, for example, a fairly high consensus amongst the counsel interviewed that arguments based on the 'floodgates' thesis,[62] or on 'parliamentary inactivity' were all legitimate but rarely of great persuasive value in the House of Lords. As Louis Blom-Cooper QC remarked in relation to the 'floodgates' argument,

It doesn't carry very much weight with them ... It's the sort of argument that's liable to crumble in the advocate's hands ... it doesn't have anything to support it, at least so long as you don't adopt a sort of Brandeis brief technique.

In fact, in any given appeal counsel may have perceptions of the role of the Law Lords (*i.e.* what he thinks is legitimate for them to do), perceptions of his own role (what he thinks it is legitimate for him to ask the Law Lords to do) and perceptions about where the legal and moral merits of the case actually lie. Sometimes it has been asserted that counsel do not get involved in what are called the merits of their clients' cases, since their duties to the profession and to the court ensure detachment. My researches did not bear this out. By the time counsel had argued the same case in two or three courts he had frequently lost the semblance of detachment. Mr Justice Ackner remarked,

> I think if you have a firm belief in the validity of your argument your submissions carry a ring of sincerity which is an enormous advantage to an advocate. If you think that what you are saying is a lot of rubbish then the tongue in cheek becomes almost perceptible, which is thoroughly bad.

One of his colleagues added,

> I didn't try and put an argument unless I believed it was a reasonably sound argument. ... You're unlikely to be in the Lords unless you believed you had a chance of winning. ... You have got to have a certain amount of conviction as to the validity of your arguments, otherwise you'd find it extremely difficult to put them in a convincing way.

Anthony Lloyd QC was of the same opinion,

> I think by the time one advances the argument one always believes in the validity of it. I don't think one could advance an argument unless one believed in it ... not that it will actually win - you accept that there may be a better argument for the other side.

and Mark Littman QC observed in similar vein, 'You do become party to one's own cause - one is not objective.'

Again, Michael Albery QC, in discussing a related theme, told me,

> One always likes to win cases - obviously one hates losing - at least I do and I think everybody does. I think once one begins to

cease to mind whether you win or lose cases, you're probably no good at the Bar.[63]

Even one of the dissentients, James Comyn QC, saw some advantages in a lack of objective detachment, for he said,

Basically it is completely wrong for counsel ever to come to the point of believing in their client or their claim. To have too much faith in what you are arguing can be just as much of a handicap as the opposite extreme because counsel can have pet points which they are more convinced of than the court. On the other hand it helps any argument to really have your heart in it, of course.

Each of the three varieties of perception held by counsel may have an effect on the types of argument counsel feels able to make to the Law Lords, but the influences will sometimes pull in different directions. Such divergences produce a situation of self-role conflict, *i.e.* the personal feelings and opinions of the actor are in opposition to the behaviour required of him by his role. This type of conflict has long been recognised at the Bar and the standard solution to it was put forward by Dr Johnson where he said,

[Y]ou do not know ... [a cause] ... to be good or bad till the judge determines it. ... An argument which does not convince yourself may convince the judge to whom you urge it; and if it does convince him, why, then, ... you are wrong and he is right. ... A lawyer is to do for his client all that his client might fairly do for himself if he could.[64]

The American Bar Association Code of Professional Ethics[65] reaches the same conclusion,

The advocate may urge permissible construction of the law favourable to his client, without regard to his professional opinion as to the likelihood that the construction will ultimately prevail. His conduct is within the bounds of the law, and therefore permissible, if the position taken is supported by the law or is supportable by a good faith argument for an extension, modification, or reversal of the law. However, a lawyer is not justified in asserting a position in litigation that is frivolous.

And in a subsequent ABA Opinion[66] it was asserted that,

> The lawyer ... is not an umpire, but an advocate. He is under no duty to refrain from making every proper argument in support of any legal point because he is not convinced of its inherent soundness. ... His personal belief in the soundness of his cause or of the authorities supporting it, is irrelevant.

Traditionally, counsel have resolved this conflict by ranking their obligation to act as a mouthpiece for their client above their personal conceptions of the law,[67] of justice or of the role of courts as law-makers in a democracy. As a consequence, counsel in arguing a hard case before the House, tend to settle for pragmatic limits to their arguments, *i.e.* as far as their client's interest requires them to go if they are to win the case (provided that there is no violation of their duty to the court), rather than following their conceptions of the bounds of legitimate law-making by the Lords. One significant conclusion to be drawn from this is that counsel in the Lords - the apotheosis of the adversary system - consider that they have no responsibility for the proper development of the law. On this score they are not after all, it would appear, any different from their counterparts in inquisitorial systems - indeed, institutionalised arrangements whereby certain lawyers are required to take account of the proper development of the law have taken a stronger hold in inquisitorial systems than in the United Kingdom. Here the Attorney-General, the Lord Advocate, or the Official Solicitor rarely intervene as *amicus curiae*, yet in France and Russia[68] the Procurator-General is active and an Advocate-General appears in every case before the European Court of Justice.

The orthodox response of counsel to the self-role conflict just outlined has, however, sometimes come under attack. In March 1976 Melford Stevenson J attacked certain of the defence counsel in the London bomb trials for 'subservience to what are called the client's instructions'. The judge went on to assert his expectations for the conduct of counsel, stating that they ought to be 'something more than a mere loudspeaker to a maladjusted set'. He concluded by endeavouring to sanction the 'deviance' of these counsel by suggesting that their legal aid costs be disallowed in part. Although the counsel were exonerated by the Court of Appeal, a practice direction was introduced in 1977 permitting judges in the Crown Court who disapproved of the way a defence case had been argued, to suggest to the appropriate authorities in a legally aided case that the counsel's expenses and fees be disallowed in part. Some members of the Bar, not surprisingly, see this as putting them in the position of pre-judging their clients' instructions or risking a cut in their fees.

In the United States the attacks have come from another quarter. Commentators have begun to suggest that an attorney is necessarily implicated in his client's conduct and that he should seek to a certain extent to influence or prevent actions by clients which are considered improper or contrary to the public interest.[69] Such arguments question the fundamental premises of the ideology of advocacy and if accepted would have a profound impact on the provision of legal services.[70] Whether such a development would be desirable is a topic which merits a book for itself - but the challenge thrown down by the critics is one which advocates of the orthodox response should take seriously. There may still be room for change in the role of the advocate.

If we return to the main thrust of this chapter, it might be argued that even if the limits imposed by counsel on their arguments are not those which are in accordance with their perceptions of legitimate judicial behaviour, the Law Lords could still perceive these pragmatic limits as expressions of role expectations by a reference group. Logically, it would be possible for the Law Lords to perceive counsel's arguments in this light. Counsel's submissions, however derived or restricted, are still couched in normative language. They assert either that a certain proposition is a sound statement of the law (with the normative consequences that flow from such a status) or that it is legitimate for the Law Lords to embark on a certain course of conduct. The fact that counsel does not personally believe in the validity of his arguments, or that he considers that the 'legitimate' course he is advocating the House to take is really 'illegitimate', will merely test his skill at dissemblance.

Nevertheless there are two further factors which cast doubt on the significance of counsel's arguments as reference group activity. First, in most cases, counsel will usually be seen by the Law Lords as performing a role the essence of which is persuasion, even in relation to normative standards, rather than acting as commentators asserting objectively that a particular submission is an accurate statement of the law. And if a Law Lord perceives counsel to be a hired advocate with little duty in relation to the sound and proper development of the law, then he will not perceive him as acting as part of a reference group - at least in that context. As one Law Lord remarked during my interview with him,

> We look at things in a much more, I hope, sophisticated way than counsel do. Counsel put the argument for their party in the best possible way. Their job is to win their case, our job is to lay down the law.

Secondly, we have to consider where the pragmatic limits to counsel's arguments - what he considers it is legitimate for him to ask the Law Lords to do - are derived from in the first place. In the main, it seems, they are derived from counsel's perceptions of what the Law Lords might consider a tenable argument. So, rather than counsel being a reference group for the Law Lords, counsel by accepting the Law Lords' views as to the boundary for tenable argument are treating the Law Lords as a crucial reference group for themselves. Moreover, the Law Lords take the view that counsel's obligation to the court has implications for the types of argument counsel may put forward. Thus in *Cassell* v. *Broome* (No. 2), the Law Lords considered that the respondent's counsel could have won the appeal by a quicker route, without arguing that the House should overrule one of its own decisions. The respondent was accordingly penalised in the award of costs, to the extent of the extra time 'wasted' by the 'unnecessary' argument. Again in *Norwich Pharmacal Co.* v. *Commissioners of Customs and Excise*, Lord Reid stated, 'Thereafter the appellants caused much extra expense by putting their case much too high. In the circumstances I would award no costs in the Court of Appeal or in this House.'[71] A fair conclusion as to the status of counsel (in court) as a reference group would seem to be that to the extent that counsel confine their submissions within the bounds which they think the Law Lords recognise as the limits of tenable argument, to that extent they are acting as a secondary reference group reinforcing the expectations of the basic primary reference group for the Law Lords, namely, the Law Lords themselves.

COUNSEL OUT OF COURT

Counsel also interact with the Law Lords outside the courts -
particularly in the Inns of Court. Could they act as a reference
group in this setting? The Law Lords do not necessarily perceive
counsel as carrying their role of advocacy beyond the environs of
the court. As one Law Lord put it,

> [W]e all go to our Inns and we meet other judges, perhaps those
> from whom the Appeal has come or counsel in the case and they
> will quite openly tell you how little they think of your decision
> occasionally ... it's a very good thing.

And, as we have seen, most of the Law Lords interviewed
expressed a willingness to discuss their decisions (once the
speeches had been delivered) with people they meet at their Inns.
In practice, however, the interviews with the Bar revealed that
even counsel who appeared with some frequency before the House
of Lords and the Privy Council rarely had an opportunity for such
discussion with Law Lords, unless they were Benchers of the Inns.
Those non-Benchers who had discussed a case with a Law Lord
had felt unable to criticise the decision, except occasionally by way
of a jocular remark. Even amongst the Benchers[72] who had the
opportunity of discussing cases with the Law Lords, very few felt
able to criticise them to their face. Several counsel indicated that
before they would initiate or respond critically to a serious
discussion of an appeal by a Law Lord they would have to know
him personally. P. C. Duncan QC remarked, 'I've never seriously
attacked a Law Lord for one of his decisions - that would be a little
embarrassing for both of us', and in the same context Sir Elwyn-
Jones QC said, 'No, that would not be right. I would not think of
doing that, and if it were done it would be very ill-regarded.'
   One High Court judge spoke for more than himself when he
commented, 'I didn't criticise them, it would have been a fruitless
activity.' Members of the Bar who felt less inhibited about directly
criticising a Law Lord face to face, without the Law Lord taking
the initiative, were very much in the minority.[73]
   The general tenor of my interviews with the Law Lords on this
matter also suggested that criticism from fellow Benchers is not an
everyday experience. Lord Cross told me that it was difficult to
know if counsel were critical since politeness prevented them from

saying very much. Benchers who are judges in the lower courts may feel less constrained than counsel, but there are still problems of interaction.[74] When I asked Lord Reid if he had ever discussed a case with a lower court judge once it was all over he replied,

> Oh, I expect I have in a general way, you know, but only in a general way. I've discussed cases occasionally with some of the Court of Appeal people who I know better perhaps, because I suppose half of the judges now I don't know at all. Time is going on, and there is no means of getting to know them, that's one of the troubles, nowadays. We're too isolated without enough opportunity to meet the others, you've got to go and wash up your dishes and you haven't got time to go and meet them.

In any event it is likely that, as with the counsel in my sample, the Law Lords form a more important and powerful reference group for lower court judges than the reverse. They have the sanction of overruling the lower court's decisions and on occasions may criticise their role performances in very explicit terms.[75]

We may conclude therefore that, by and large, counsel do not form an important reference group for the Law Lords. But this does not mean that they cannot influence the Law Lords in other ways. For example, Law Lords in deciding hard cases sometimes take cognisance of the 'climate of professional opinion' on the point in question. As Lord Guest commented,

> The climate of legal opinion percolates through to the Benchers, to the judges. I think they get the idea that there is a feeling amongst lawyers, barristers, solicitors and lower judges that something should be done, and that does percolate.

Similarly, Lord Kilbrandon felt that the climate of legal and academic opinion, if unanimous, would have some effect on the House's decisions and Lord Radcliffe thought it was a factor which would influence perhaps three out of the five Law Lords sitting on a particular appeal. Lord Justice Russell also felt that if a judge knew that there was a consensus on a point amongst the profession this was a relevant matter for him to take into account in reaching his decision. Lord Simon explicitly argued that professional opinion could have an influence on the Law Lords in

Jones v. *Secretary of State for Social Services*, where he stated that,[76]

> informed professional opinion is probably to the effect that your
> Lordships have no power to overrule decisions with prospective
> effect only; such opinion is itself a source of law; and your
> Lordships, sitting judicially, are bound by any rule of law
> arising extra-judicially.[77]

And Lord Diplock has argued that,[78]

> the way in which Courts in fact adapt themselves to the
> changing pattern of society is influenced less by conscious
> intention than by the training, practice and habits of thought of
> the legal profession as a whole.

Secondly, counsel who argue before the House have an
influence, which is considerably greater than has been commonly
recognised, on the Law Lords' decisions. This influence, which is
the subject of the next chapter, results from the interaction
between the counsel and the Law Lords during the oral argument.

LAW LORDS AND LAW LORDS

That the third main group mentioned by the Law Lords, namely,
their fellow Law Lords, should transpire to be the principal
reference group for most, if not all, the Law Lords, should not be
particularly surprising in the light of the foregoing discussion. For
this group meets all the criteria that a would-be reference group
has to meet. Their application can be briefly summarised.

Decisions of the House of Lords are highly visible to the Law
Lords. Even those who have not sat on a particular case
automatically receive a copy of the printed speeches in the case
once the decision has been handed down.[79]

We have seen that the Law Lords lead relatively cloistered lives
- at least in the sense of isolation from potential reference groups.
But the one group that a Law Lord interacts with, with the
greatest frequency, is his colleagues. The Law Lords may travel to
work together, they frequently lunch together (not all together but
in small groups) and they are constantly interacting at other times
during working hours. In these interchanges they discuss the case

in which they are involved - even with Law Lords who are not sitting in that particular case. As we shall see, Law Lords not infrequently attempt to persuade their colleagues to share their view of the facts and the law in an appeal, particularly if its outcome is finely balanced. Some Law Lords write their judgements specifically in an endeavour to win over a colleague who is in doubt. Where the case is a hard one, the Law Lord will often articulate expectations concerning judicial 'law-making', the exercise of the 1966 Practice Statement on Precedent, and the legitimate sources of the rules to be applied in this particular appeal. In all this he is likely (unless he is a staunchly independent judge such as Lord Atkin and Lord Denning), to be wary of flouting the expectations which his colleagues hold for him. For antagonism is rarely a helpful precondition for persuasion. With a small, relatively isolated, tightly-knit group we should not be taken aback if a member takes cognisance of the expectations of his colleagues even if he does not entirely share them. As we have seen, the Law Lords are particularly immune to sanctions from outside groups, indeed the separation of powers is intended to achieve this result. Yet Law Lords are human, and the desire for acceptance and esteem from their peer group may be hard to resist.

It is hardly surprising, therefore, that the source of critical evaluations mentioned most frequently by the Law Lords was their fellow Law Lords. Certainly, colleagues' comments are often so polite as to be of little assistance, yet on occasions critical comment intended as a sanction for 'deviance' will be expressed in print, *e.g.* Viscount Simonds in *Rahimtoola* v. *Nizam of Hyderabad* [80] and *Scruttons Ltd* v. *Midland Silicones Ltd* [81] criticising Lord Denning (expressly in the first case and impliedly in the second); Lord Reid's dissent in *Shaw* v. *DPP* [82]; and Lord Atkin's dissent in *Liversidge* v. *Anderson*. If further evidence of the primacy of the Law Lords in defining their role is required, reference need only be made to the 1966 Practice Statement on Precedent which clearly altered the role of a Law Lord in certain hard cases yet which was introduced by the Law Lords and not by the Legislature.

CONCLUSION

We may conclude, therefore, that although Benchers, and

particularly academics or lower court judges, do act as a reference group to the Law Lords, they do so only to a very limited extent. The most significant reference group for a Law Lord is likely to be his fellow Law Lords. Of course, each Law Lord's reference groups and reference individuals will differ slightly from those of his colleagues, but the formative processes for a Law Lord's role are largely the same in each case, namely, anticipatory socialisation and judicial interaction. In other words, a Law Lord will form his perceptions of his role by watching the performances of the Law Lords while he is still a barrister or a judge in a lower court, and from his interaction with his fellow Law Lords following his elevation to the Lords.

3 Courtroom Interaction: The Bar's Perspective

How many judges do you know whose analysis of the case and of the situation is a major fresh creation, a 'Let there be Light!', rather than that lesser type of building which consists in merely modifying the theory of one advocate or of the other?[1]

The function of an advocate is not to enlarge the intellectual horizon. His task is to seduce, to seize the mind for a predetermined end, not to explore paths to truths.[2]

INTRODUCTION

We saw in the last chapter that counsel do not greatly influence the role of the Law Lord or how it is perceived by the Law Lords. Nevertheless, in this chapter, I shall argue that counsel in their exchanges with the Law Lords in the committee rooms can have a very significant influence on the Law Lords' decisions. This will hardly be a novel proposition to students of the English legal system. Oral advocacy is central to the 'adversary' system. Yet numerous observations of the court in action have led me to the conclusion that the importance of these interchanges between Law Lords and counsel has been unjustly neglected by the commentators.[3]

The House, by comparison with the United States Supreme Court, devotes far more of its time to oral debate. Whilst the latter will only hear argument for half an hour from each side in a case[4] and restricts oral arguments to two weeks in every four (during term time), the former gives practically unlimited time to the parties[5] and hears arguments during most weeks in term time.[6] Justices of the Supreme Court in the past have not infrequently

35

stressed the importance of the 'Socratic dialogue between Justices and counsel' for the outcome of appeals.[7] Yet the severe time restrictions on oral argument and Chief Justice Burger's strictures on the standards of oral advocacy in the United States[8] would suggest that nowadays the Supreme Court relies mainly on the written briefs provided by counsel and on the research of the Justices' law clerks.[9] As Justice Marshall once remarked,

> ... it is the brief that does the final job, if for no other reason than that opinions are often written several weeks and sometimes months after the argument. The arguments, great as they may have been, are forgotten. In the seclusion of his chambers the judge has only his briefs and the law books. At that time your brief is your only spokesman.[10]

In fact the oral argument in the Supreme Court is tape recorded and the tapes are available to any Justice who wishes to hear the argument again in his chambers - though Justice Marshall's comments suggest that his brethren and he did not take advantage of this facility as often as they might.

The Law Lords, on the other hand, although they receive a printed Case which contains counsel's submissions for all the parties concerned and the judgements of the lower courts together with copies of the documentary evidence, rely far more on the oral interchange than the written material in deciding an appeal.[11] The members of the Bar whom I interviewed were overwhelmingly of the opinion that the oral argument and the interchange between them and the Law Lords were of greater significance for the determination of an appeal than the written matter. Despite this, the House, like the Supreme Court, cannot be neatly classified as a 'hot bench' (one which has read the briefs in advance) or a 'cold bench' (one which has not) since the work habits of the judges vary. In the past certain Law Lords[12] made a practice of never reading the Case in advance of the oral argument, and even in recent times several Law Lords, *e.g.* Lords Denning, Radcliffe, Reid and Devlin, only read the materials very casually in advance. As Lord Devlin put it, 'I never used to read the printed Case. I would have done if I hadn't known it was going to be said all over again in oral argument.' Conversely other Law Lords, including several of the present Law Lords, have had a practice of working hard on the papers in advance - though this is sometimes regarded as a mixed blessing by colleagues. Lord MacDermott, for instance, observed to me that he had, ' ... known some who've read their written material closely beforehand who have tended to push others into a line of thought too early.'

Counsel, too, have problems with a 'partially hot' bench particularly in hearings before an Appeal Committee (requesting leave to appeal to the House), where one at least of the three Law Lords (usually the presiding one) is expected to have read the papers thoroughly beforehand, and the scope for oral argument is considerably curtailed. Robert Megarry QC graphically described counsel's difficulties in this situation as,

> akin to those of trying to tell a long but funny story to an audience which has announced that it has already heard some, if not all, of it, but politely inquires whether you wish to make sure that they have seen the point.[13]

The point was made repeatedly to me in the interviews that the advantage of a predominantly oral approach lies in the flexibility it gives to the arguments. Counsel can, and are expected to, respond to the thoughts expressed by the Court and to adjust their arguments accordingly. Lord Reid asserted,

> [Counsel] have got to know their stuff and know it backwards and they have got to be a little bit, taking a hint, you know. A man who simply reads out his stuff from his notes and will not take a hint is not a good advocate.

Thus a case can change course in mid-stream as a result of a point thrown up in the debate. Lord Guest remarked on this in our interview,

> I have known cases in which when the case started I was convinced that the appellant was either right or wrong and during the course of the case a point made either by me or by one of my colleagues has completely changed one's view.

Written briefs, on the other hand, have difficulty in catering for such developments without becoming impossibly lengthy. At any rate, the Law Lords and counsel interviewed were strongly in favour of retaining the predominantly oral approach - only a handful wanted to move towards the American position - indeed, several of them were of the opinion that too much time and effort was expended by counsel in the compilation of the printed Case, as it was.

Oral argumentation would appear to have two consequences for the Law Lords' performances as law creators in hard cases. First, it has the effect of restricting the range of judicial creativity; second, it has a persuasive influence on the decision that is ultimately reached.

THE RESTRICTIVE POWER OF COUNSEL: LAW LORDS' OPINIONS AND COUNSEL'S SUBMISSIONS

Amongst the majority of the current Law Lords and counsel who appeared before them, I discovered that there was a shared expectation that a Law Lord in giving his reasons for deciding for or against the appeal 'ought to confine his propositions of law to matters covered by the arguments of counsel'.[14]

Alan Campbell QC made the point forcefully,

A judge judges on the arguments addressed to him, and each side is given an opportunity in fair discussion to meet the points, and if the judges are going to take advice outside the area of the courtroom, well it's fundamental that justice is in jeopardy - it cannot be seen to be done.

This view was shared by a clear majority of counsel interviewed, and in each case the justification given was that counsel ought to have an opportunity of considering any point or authority against him upon which the judge wishes to rely.[15] Although some judges have felt able to ignore the expectation in the past,[16] when Viscount Simonds was presiding Law Lord in an Appellate Committee such conduct was deprecated. In *Rahimtoola* v. *Nizam of Hyderabad* Lord Denning admitted at the close of his speech that he had considered some questions and authorities which were not mentioned by counsel. He had done so because he felt that the law on the subject was of great consequence but plainly in an unsatisfactory state, and that the House should seize the opportunity to put matters right.[17] Viscount Simonds on reading this added to the end of his speech the comment that he must not be taken as assenting to Lord Denning's views on these questions and authorities 'in regard to which the House has not had the benefit of the arguments of counsel or of the judgement of the courts below'.[18] Lords Reid, Cohen and Somerwell expressed their entire agreement with Viscount Simonds's concluding obserations. These remarks were intended, and were interpreted by the recipient,[19] as a rebuke.* As far as I can trace, this expectation was shared by most of the Law Lords at that time.[20] But by the time I came to do my survey a considerable difference of opinion existed between the Law Lords on the point.

On the one hand there was the group[21] which clearly saw the norm as a 'relevant' role expectation.

> Well if a judge is going to take some point that has not been dealt with, well then he ought to tell ... [counsel]. He certainly should not, I think, shoot off on one point that has not been argued. (Lord Gardiner)

> I think it is most unfair if a judge in the House of Lords puts forward a proposition of law which has never been advanced either in the courts below or in counsel's arguments. It is unfair to the courts below, it's unfair to counsel and it's most unsatisfactory, because very often if he had put forward this point to counsel, counsel would have had an answer and maybe would have cited a case which would have shown that he was wrong. It's a dangerous practice. (Lord Guest)

> [One should not rely on] ... cases which have not been cited, because there is an etiquette against bringing in extraneous matter ... (Lord Pearson)

*This episode highlights the difficulties experienced by a 'new boy' to a role, particularly where one's colleagues are the basic reference group. This was Lord Denning's first case in the Lords (as a Lord of Appeal) and he had come to the court with the perception that the House being the final court of appeal could and should take a broader approach to developing the law than the lower courts. He thus devoted the better part of a summer vacation (he has since asserted that he took more pains about the case than any other case in which he has taken part - see *Thai-Europe* v. *Government of Pakistan* at 966f) to research on points not raised by counsel only to have his knuckles rapped for an elementary error in the role performance of a Law Lord in a hard case. The fear of making similar role specific errors is frequently reflected in the cautious behaviour of a new Law Lord both in the oral debate and in written judgements.

I think by the time you get to the House of Lords, it is very unfortunate if that is not the situation ... In a way it is a criticism of yourself, you ought to have foreseen the point in the course of the argument, especially if it spreads over a couple of days, and put it to counsel ... I think that it is quite wrong. (Lord Cross)

On the other hand there was a second group who were more ambivalent on the issue.[22]

I wouldn't subscribe to that. I think that it will almost always happen that you do restrict your judgement to matters raised by counsel, but if counsel have omitted something then I think that the court is bound to take it up. Of course it is dangerous because the judge may be misinformed, he may have misinformed himself and counsel would have been able to put him right. But you couldn't make a formula out of this, I don't think you could lay down a rule.[23] (Lord Kilbrandon)

Usually, but not necessarily. The quality of counsel's argument varies and it is sometimes necessary to break new ground.[24] (Lord Hailsham)

... where a 'court does its own researches itself', as it often will and sometimes must, it should proceed with special caution since it is thereby acting without the benefit of adversary argument.[25] (Lord Simon)

Lord Wilberforce in his speech in *Saif Ali* v. *Sydney Mitchell & Co.*[26] seemed to cast doubt on the existence of the norm where he asserted in discussing certain *obiter dicta* in *Rondel* v. *Worsley* that,

It may be true that the counsel in the case did not present detailed arguments as to the [point] ... but I cannot agree that this invalidates or weakens judicial pronouncements. Judges are more than mere selectors between rival views: they are entitled to and do think for themselves.

But his pronouncements elsewhere are more equivocal. In 'La Chambre des Lords'[27] he indicated that a Law Lord generally hesitates to use arguments in his speech which have not been debated during the hearing of the appeal. In *Abbott* v. *The Queen*[28] he and Lord Edmund-Davies[29] criticised the three Law Lords in the majority for advancing a point for the first time in their judgement 'upon which appellant's counsel has not been heard'. Again in *Federal Commerce and Navigation Ltd* v. *Molena Alpha Inc.*[30] he declined to make a ruling on issues which were of concern to the commercial community, in part because counsel did not address arguments on them. Lord Diplock strenuously rejected the supposed norm in *Cassell* v. *Broome.*

> On matters of law no court is restricted in its decision to following the submissions made to it by counsel for one or other of the parties. After listening to a lengthy argument which embraced a full examination of a large and representative selection of the relevant previous authorities this House was fully entitled to come to a conclusion of law and legal policy different from that which any individual counsel had propounded.[31]

Yet, he seemed by implication to give the norm some weight in *Trapp* v. *Mackie*[32] and *Cookson* v. *Knowles.*[33]

Nevertheless there was clearly disagreement between these two groups (and possibly amongst them) on the issue. For some Law Lords it was a relevant role expectation,[34] for others it was merely a peripheral one - for most its weight depended on the circumstances. This dissensus amongst the current Law Lords was attributable, at least in part, to the conflict between the Bar's expectation that the Law Lords' speeches should not contain propositions which have not been submitted by or put to counsel during the hearing (an expectation shared by the Law Lords to varying degrees), and the expectation that Law Lords also hold that particularly in the final appeal court, decisions should be reached in the light of all the relevant authorities whether discussed by counsel or not.* Robert Megarry QC suggested a way in which this role conflict could be resolved in his Hamlyn Lectures in 1962:

---

*The *per incuriam* doctrine is based on precisely such a failure to pay heed to relevant authority. It is worth recalling that Lord Denning MR and his colleagues in the Court of Appeal endeavoured to attack Lord Devlin's exegesis on exemplary damages in *Rookes* v. *Barnard* on exactly these grounds in *Broome* v. *Cassell.*

Doubtless the counsel of perfection is to notify counsel of the uncited cases and restore the case for further argument, if need be, on these cases. If the cases indeed bear on the essence of the decision, then this, indeed, seems to be the only really satisfactory course to adopt. ... If, on the other hand, the cases are only marginal in their bearing, then it may be best to omit any reference to them from the judgement, or at all events to make it explicit that, although no argument on them had been heard, they could not affect the result of the case in any way.[35]

This solution to the dilemma involves ranking the expectations according to their perceived weight and legitimacy. Megarry's answer is that in most cases the Bar's expectation should prevail.

The actual practice of the Law Lords has varied. In several cases a hearing has been reconvened because the Law Lords wish to hear counsel's arguments on a point which was not raised at the first hearing or on material which a Law Lord has discovered subsequent to the first hearing. They include *Regis Property Co.* v. *Dudley*, *Rookes* v. *Barnard*, *Oppenheimer* v. *Cattermole* and possibly *Thomson* v. *Moyse*. On the other hand in three recent cases the Law Lords have revealed their differences on the issue. In *R.* v. *Hyam*, Lord Diplock and Viscount Dilhorne had no hesitation in dealing with (and differing on) the question whether *R.* v. *Vickers* had been rightly decided. Lord Cross, however, indicated that he was

not prepared to decide between them without having heard the fullest possible argument on the point from counsel on both sides - especially as a decision that it was wrongly decided might have serious repercussions since the direction approved in that case must have been given in many homicide cases in the last 17 years.[36]

In *Miliangos* v. *George Frank Ltd*, Lord Simon said,

where a 'court does its own researches itself' ... [and] such research throws up an authority or argument which is material (even if only to be finally distinguised or rejected), it is better that it should be mentioned in the judgement, for the benefit of those who have subsequently to consider the judgement.[37]

and Lord Fraser cited an early Scottish appeal to the Lords in his speech which was not cited by counsel in argument.[38]

Finally, in *DPP* v. *Humphrys*, Lords Salmon and Edmund-Davies in their opinions raised a question as to the powers of a court to quash an indictment, which was not argued by counsel. This provoked Viscount Dilhorne to dissent from their views even though he did not consider it necessary to decide on the point to dispose of the appeal.[39] Lord Fraser however, reasserted the old orthodoxy by observing, 'The question of whether a court in England can decline to allow a prosecution to proceed ... was not argued in this case and I reserve my opinion on it.'[40]

In sum, although the position at present is more fluid than twenty years ago, the expectation holds a strong sway, as it did throughout the period of my research.[41] This undoubtedly means that counsel, even though they do not form a significant reference group for the Law Lords, have been, and continue to be, able to impose considerable limitations[42] on the creative performance of Law Lords in hard cases.* We can see this in the tone of regret and on occasion irritation, which tinges a Law Lord's comments when he feels unable to make a ruling on a particular point or to decide an appeal on a particular basis because counsel refuses to take the point.[43]

In *Federal Commerce and Navigation Ltd* v. *Molena Alpha Inc.* Lord Wilberforce observed,

> Counsel at the bar ... did not address arguments on [the deduction issues]. While therefore I recognise the interest which the commercial community may have in a decision of them ... I must reluctantly agree to decline this task on the present occasion.

and Viscount Dilhorne added, 'It is indeed unfortunate that determination of [the deduction issues] ... must be left to another

---

*Counsel may have a variety of reasons for wanting to impose these restrictions. His clients may wish a ruling on a particular point of law in a case which the Law Lords feel can be decided on other grounds. Counsel may therefore not take the alternative points or he may concede them: see *British Railways Board* v. *Liptrot*. Again, counsel may wish to force a decision from the Law Lords on a point of law which he suspects the House will endeavour to avoid deciding if it possibly can. He will accordingly plan the case with this in mind. See D. N. Pritt's account of his tactics in *Liversidge* v. *Anderson* in *Law, Class and Society*, Book 2 (London: Lawrence and Wishart, 1971) p. 106.

occasion.'[44] Again, in *British Airways Board* v. *Taylor*, Lord Wilberforce and Viscount Dilhorne appear to have considered that the case might have been disposed of on the basis of a particular approach. However as the former remarked,

> ... counsel for the Board disclaimed any such contention and both sides agreed that the appeal should be decided on the basis that, in both respects, the charge had been correctly framed.[45]

Counsel can also hamstring the Law Lords by conceding points at an earlier stage in the case. The case of *Bank N.V.* v. *Administrator of Hungarian Property* was fought in the Lords on the basis of a concession made by the Crown while the case was before Devlin J. The Law Lords were clearly irritated that they had to decide the case on the artificial basis created by the concession which counsel could not or would not retract.

But perhaps the most open display of judicial annoyance to have occurred in recent times in this connection, relates to counsel's refusal to argue that the Divisional Court decision of *Scott* v. *Baker* was wrongly decided. The matter first arose in *DPP* v. *Carey* where it appears that the Law Lords expressly invited appellants' counsel to argue that the *Scott* case was wrongly decided. Counsel declined to do so.[46] As a result each Law Lord mentions in his speech that the *Scott* case may have to be reconsidered but the lack of argument on the point by counsel restrains him from going further. The trailing of the judicial robes seemed to have borne fruit in the case of *Walker* v. *Lovell* when the Divisional Court framed their second certified question for the purposes of the appeal with 'the clear purpose of enabling [the] House to consider the much discussed and frequently criticised decision of the Court of Appeal in *Scott* v. *Baker*'.[47] (The essence of the criticism was that the courts by their rigid application of the doctrine laid down in *Scott* v. *Baker* were encouraging drivers to flout the laws against 'drinking and driving'.[48])

Yet, to the evident dismay of the Law Lords, counsel for the prosecution (the appellant) announced that he felt unable to question the correctness of the decision in *Scott*'s case and declined to argue against it. In the event, the Law Lords (though some with better grace than others) indicated that the failure of counsel to argue the point precluded them from expressing an opinion as to whether *Scott* v. *Baker* had been correctly decided.[49] Lord Edmund-

Davies summarised the feelings of the House when he said,

> ... I share the regret expressed by my Lords that learned counsel for the appellant did not see his way clear to present for the consideration of this House any submissions critical of ... [*Scott* v. *Baker*]. This is the second time that such a thing has occurred. ... Foiled though the House again is from considering the acceptability of the extended uses to which that decision is now frequently put, the day may yet dawn when we shall be free to do so.[50]

The Law Lords reiterated their dislike of *Scott* v. *Baker* in *Baker* v. *Foulkes*, but when at last the opportunity arose to reconsider *Scott* v. *Baker* in *Spicer* v. *Holt*, the Law Lords to their evident chagrin, found themselves unable to overrule it.

An equally irritating situation for a Law Lord arises when the judgements of the Court of Appeal in the instant case contain propositions of law which the Law Lord considers mistaken and misleading, yet neither counsel in the Lords relies on them or attacks them. Here the House is caught in a conflict between the expectation concerning counsel's arguments on the one hand and the expectation held by the Law Lords that they ought to provide guidance to the lower courts.

As we might expect the Law Lords when faced with this situation have tended to rank the functional importance of the latter expectation above that of the former. Certainly in several recent appeals the Law Lords appear not to have experienced any difficulty in rejecting propositions contained in the judgements in the Court of Appeal (mostly in Lord Denning's) which counsel have not relied on in the House.[51] Indeed in *Davis* v. *Johnson* where the Law Lords took strong exception to the Court of Appeal's arguments on whether it was bound by its own decisions they expressly directed counsel not to address them on the topic: 'The House would deal with that question itself.'[52]

THE RESTRICTIVE POWER OF COUNSEL: RAISING POINTS NOT ARGUED BELOW

According to Blom-Cooper and Drewry,

> It is an unwritten, but firm rule of the House not to consider arguments which have not been considered by the courts below. In only twelve cases ... [between 1952 and 1968] was this rule expressly waived.[53]

At first sight this 'rule'[54] appears to be more of a restriction imposed on counsel's arguments by the House than one imposed by counsel on the Law Lords. In a sense this is true, yet the 'rule' (which emanates in part from expectations of the Bar and litigants) when taken in conjunction with the expectation that a Law Lord should confine his propositions of law to matters covered by the arguments of counsel, inhibits the Law Lords from deciding an appeal on a point which they have put to counsel in the hearing, which has not been raised in the lower courts. To the extent that the 'rule' exists, the Law Lords' propositions of law should be confined to the arguments which counsel took at the lower levels.

Lord Kilbrandon, in my interview with him, agreed that the unwritten 'rule' existed, adding,

> ... I think this is in the interests of justice between litigants rather than in the interests of the orderly statement of the law. It isn't fair to decide a case on a point which wasn't taken against a man in the courts below; and also it's very difficult for a superior court to come to a reliable opinion if the court below hasn't dealt with the point.

Yet Lord Guest's formulation of the 'rule' was less absolute. He said,

> ... it is the practice of the House in normal circumstances not to consider an argument which has not been advanced in the courts below and which is not contained in the written Case. It is possible for counsel to put forward an argument in their Case which hasn't been considered in the court below, and the House will consider it. But if it's neither in the Case nor in the courts below, their practice is in normal circumstances to refuse to allow it. And I think that's right.

The procedural rules of the House also envisage that on occasion the 'rule' will not be applied.[55] Indeed, as repeated *dicta* from Law Lords and submissions of counsel in the past decade have made clear, the issue is one which is entirely at the discretion of the House. But as Blom-Cooper and Drewry indicate, the discretion is not exercised very frequently. The reason for this is that yet again the Law Lords are caught in a conflict. On the one hand, the Bar and litigants expect that the rules of pleading and fair notice (which are an integral part of the adversary system) will be adhered to - particularly if the failure to do so will deprive one side of the fruits of their litigation in the lower courts. On the other hand, the Law Lords consider that in the final court of appeal decisions should be reached in the light of all the relevant legal points.

Lord Cross outlined the typical response of the Law Lords when faced with this dilemma,

> It is completely a matter of discretion ... it rather depends on how good ... [the Law Lords] think ... [the point is]. If they think there is not much in the point anyway, they probably say 'Oh, we couldn't listen to that because it was not mentioned in the Case.' But if they think it is something that really goes to the root of the thing, if they think the whole thing would be rather a mess if they did not allow it to be argued, then they would probably allow it on terms as to costs.

Similarly Lord Reid observed in *Kaye* v. *Hosier & Dickinson*,

> It is entirely within your Lordships' discretion whether or not to allow a new point to be taken at [a] very late stage. ... When a point is taken at the proper time we have the advantage of having before us the considered opinion of the learned judges in the Court of Appeal and of hearing well prepared arguments of counsel. If I were satisfied that there could be no valid answer to the new point I would be prepared to forego those advantages and decide the case on the new point with a suitable order for costs against the employers. I am, however, not so satisfied ... [and therefore] this new point should not be taken or entertained by your Lordships.[56]

This pragmatic strategy involves ranking the expectations according to their perceived functional importance in the particular case. In a sense this role conflict arises from the ultimate incompatibility between the goal and the means of the adversary model of adjudication - the attempt to attain the truth or soundness in legal outcome on the one hand and the insistence that this should only be done by adherence to the rules of the game, on the other. It is a testimony to the strength of the adversary model in the House of Lords that the Law Lords so frequently favour the rules of fair play to the pursuit of soundness or comprehensiveness in the legal result.[57]

Certainly the instances when the Law Lords have deviated from the normal practice seem to bear out the accounts given by Lord Cross and Lord Reid. In *Rookes* v. *Barnard* the respondents had not taken the point at a lower stage that exemplary damages could not be awarded in the case and indeed did not attempt to put it forward until the rehearing before the Law Lords. Despite objections from the appellants the respondents were permitted to make their submissions on the matter, at some length, but were penalised in the award of costs.[58] Similarly in the *Suisse Atlantique* case the Law Lords permitted the appellant's counsel at the conclusion of his opening speech to put forward a new argument which he had not argued before, which for the first time introduced the doctrine of fundamental breach into the appeal. It was this point rather than the arguments considered in the Court of Appeal that occupied the bulk of the speeches of the Law Lords. In deference to the expectation of the Bar the Law Lords insisted on an adjournment followed by the filing of supplementary Cases by both sides. They also extracted an undertaking from the appellants to pay the additional costs. The same procedure was followed in *Padfield* v. *Minister of Agriculture, Fisheries and Food*, where the new point won the appeal for the appellants at the expense of a reduced award of costs. Again in *Liverpool City Council* v. *Irwin* although no supplementary Case was required, the success of the appellants' new argument was not rewarded with an award of costs.[59]

The Law Lords are more likely to permit a point to be taken late if the other side does not object.[60] And in some situations the House permits points to be raised before it for the first time because in the nature of things the argument could not be taken below, for example, where one side wishes to argue that a previous House of Lords decision was wrongly decided or where the basis of the Court of Appeal decision in the instant appeal has been overruled by a subsequent ruling in the House of Lords.

Finally the House has also proved willing, on occasion, to

permit a point to be taken before them which was conceded in a lower court but which counsel subsequently wishes to reopen. This may be prompted by a hint in the Court of Appeal judgements[61] or by a hint from the Law Lords themselves,[62] or it may simply be that counsel has thought better of it.[63] Almost every instance where the House has permitted concessions to be withdrawn is, however, consistent with the statements of Lords Cross and Reid.[64]

The United States Supreme Court is not so restrictive in its approach to counsel's arguments. Indeed Justice Jackson once observed in an opinion of the court that 'in this Court the parties changed positions as nimbly as if dancing a quadrille'.[65] Nevertheless it is rare for the oral arguments to depart significantly from the issues set out in the briefs or those raised in the lower courts. One important case where this did occur was *Mapp* v. *Ohio* which in the lower stages, in the appellant's brief and in the initial phase of oral argument in the Supreme Court, was fought as an obscenity case. Sensing that he was making little headway, counsel for Miss Mapp switched to a new line of argument on the suppression of evidence obtained by illegal search and seizure. This issue, which had appeared hitherto only as an aside in the majority opinion in the court below and as a tailpiece to the *amicus curiae*'s brief in the Supreme Court, was seized on by the majority of the court,[66] dominated the opinions delivered and is the one which made the case a constitutional landmark.

THE PERSUASIVE POWER OF COUNSEL

The second, and more important, aspect of counsel's arguments in relation to the role performance of the Law Lords lies in their persuasive influence. For the object of advocacy is persuasion. When advising his client, counsel, with an eye to negotiations or a settlement with the other side, will adopt the role of a judge - stating his view of the law as it is and what the courts might hold it to be. But when it comes to argument in court counsel resumes the role of the advocate. In this context, as we have seen, the counsel whom I interviewed perceived their role to be to persuade the Law Lords, by any legitimate means, to decide in favour of their clients. This was the case even if it involved going against counsel's own private views as to the state of the law and its desirable or legitimate development.

Viewed from an interactionist perspective this persuasive role of counsel is of particular interest. The 'symbolic environment' constituted by the legal world is not static. Within it social actors are frequently required to negotiate and renegotiate their definition of situations. From such interactions new meanings and symbols may emerge. Thus in the House of Lords, as in lower courts,[67] counsel compete with each other to establish their version of reality. In the adversary system the victor's reward is to have his version of reality established as 'true' or 'correct'. Accordingly, counsel's job is to negotiate with the court an account of the law and the facts which in that case will lead to a favourable decision for his client. Such a negotiation is not restricted to matters of law, even in a hard case, for in his presentation of the facts found in the lower courts counsel is arguing for a selective interpretation of past events - what Carlen calls 'a particular classificatory framework of legal relevancy'.[68] In achieving this goal, particularly in hard cases which by definition are concerned both with the parameters of the body of legal norms which comprise English Law, and the parameters of the judicial role *vis-à-vis* that of the legislator, counsel may also - perhaps inadvertently - have persuaded the Law Lords to redefine incrementally the judicial role in hard cases.

In contrast to courts of first instance,[69] the negotiation process in the Lords which I have just outlined takes place almost exclusively with the judiciary. It excludes the other side (except in cases where an agreement is reached between the opposing counsel to endeavour to obtain a ruling from the Law Lords on a particular point[70]), the public and the court officials. As Lord Kilbrandon put it, ' ... if you really want to know ... the debate is really much more between counsel and the Bench than it is between opposing counsel'. From this dialectic between Bench and Bar,[71] which resembles nothing so much as a 'conversation between gentlemen on a subject of mutual interest',[72] 'the judge is forced to come to terms, openly and explicitly, with the views of counsel; to present, in short, his own assessment of them and, where necessary, his counter-argument'.[73] The counsel whom I interviewed also perceived the oral interaction with the Law Lords to be a combative and challenging experience. Colin Duncan QC observed,

The secret is to modify your argument to the climate which is developing in the House. When you are standing up there at the rostrum what you want is an alert mind with nothing too fixed in advance ... There's a lot to be said for playing by ear when you get there.

Another QC, now a judge, described the dialogue between Bar and Bench as, ' ... like a football game: you only play as well as the opponents let you - and by opponents I mean the tribunal'.

This conclusion, that in some senses the principal opponent of counsel in the Lords is the Appellate Committee, has two implications. First, that the conventional model of the adversary system in which hired champions joust in the arena with the adjudicator sitting in an elevated position (in the hope that his view will not be obscured by the dust), does not adequately convey the realities of proceedings in an appellate court. The battle is not so much between the hired champions as between them and the Law Lords sequentially.[74] Perhaps as John Davis (a celebrated American advocate) once suggested,[75] the more appropriate analogy is to picture counsel as skilled anglers, with the Bench as the fish. Indeed one English 'fish' not long ago described counsel's submissions on one point as 'A most skilful presentation of a highly attractive fly.'[76] Moreover, as in fishing, the choice of fly (the argument to be run) depends on the conditions, the climate and the weather prevailing at the time in question.

Secondly, it means that the arguments put forward by counsel will be directed more at persuading the Law Lords than at attacking the propositions of the other side. Their goal is the presentation of a picture which will win the case for their clients,[77] not to engage in a blow by blow refutation of the submissions of their opponents. As a matter of tactics few counsel will take the risk of ignoring their opponents' strong points and in practice the effect of the rules of pleading so restrict counsel's room for manoeuvre that more often than not they will consider much the same points (albeit from different perspectives) as their opposite number. Furthermore, as we shall see, the Law Lords in their interaction with counsel are frequently requesting their views on a point raised by their opponents or indicating that they do not require to be addressed in reply on a point raised by the other side. In either event the Law Lords are drawing the attention of counsel to the importance they attach to opposing arguments on points of

difficulty. But because the primary focus is on convincing the Law
Lords, occasions do arise when the competing arguments run on
quite different lines. Thus in *St Aubyn* v. *Attorney-General* Lord
Simonds said,

> On this question counsel on either side agreed in saying that
> there was no direct authority and they agreed too that the
> reason for that was that the answer was clear. But unfortunately
> here harmony ended, for the clear answer given on the one side
> was the exact opposite to the clear answer given on the other.[78]

TECHNIQUES OF PERSUASION

Given that counsel is endeavouring to persuade the Law Lords to
accept his definition of the legal and factual realities involved in a
particular appeal, the question arises, how does he set about his
task? Comparatively little research has been done to date on the
psychology of persuasion in a legal setting[79] but there have been
some excellent writings on advocacy in appellate courts. Counsel
should begin with the statement of the facts.

> It is trite that it is in the statement of the facts that the advocate
> has his first, best, and most precious access to the court's
> attention. The court does not know the facts, and it wants to.[80]
> It is trite, among good advocates, that the statement of the facts
> can, and should, ... produce the conviction that there is only
> one sound outcome. (Karl Llewellyn)[81]

> [I]t cannot be too often emphasised that in an appellate court
> the statement of the facts is not merely a part of the argument, it
> is more often than not the argument itself. (John Davis)[82]

Some Law Lords are well aware of this. Viscount Radcliffe once
observed,

> Facts and law often interpenetrate each other more thoroughly
> than theory allows for. Indeed the presentation and arrange-
> ment of facts constitute half the art of exposition.[83]

Similarly Lord Atkin's daughter recorded that her father,

When he gave us the facts of a case and asked us what we thought about it, his way of presenting the problem was such that there was never any suggestion in our minds that the other side would have a leg to stand on.[84]

Thus in the Lords the fact that counsel who is opening the argument (the appellant) has the duty of expounding the facts giving rise to the appeal (as found proved in the lower courts), may convey a considerable advantage. Some counsel are very skilled at presenting a version of the facts which, while not demonstrably incorrect, manifestly favours the appellant. Although respondent's counsel has the right to add any points he may wish, sometimes it is too late and the damage has been done. Michael Albery QC told me,

Whoever opens the case presents all the facts and gives them just the comments and asides and the slants that he wants and the man who gets up afterwards can't go all over them again and re-present them as he wants. He has just to take them as he finds them and make comments.

Again it is Llewellyn who has stated this point most graphically.

He [the respondent] cannot rest on any properly done statement of facts by the appellant. Neither can he allow the court to settle back with a bored sigh: 'Do we have to listen to all this again!'[85]

You need your positive case, not only in the law; you need your positive case in the facts. ... If you start to say, 'The facts are different', or 'These are the facts', they'll go to sleep on you, or get mad at you. But if on the other hand you say, 'There is one point that I don't think my brother has developed quite as fully as he might', and pick up some fact or other you can build on, by the time you get done with that, you can swing into the recital of the whole.[86]

The second stage, which follows from but also underpins the statement of the facts is, the framing of the issue - the fitting of the edited version of the facts into a 'persuasive, even compelling legal frame'.[87] To quote Llewellyn once more,

... the first art is the framing of the issue so that if your framing
is accepted the case comes out your way ... Second, you have to
capture the issue, because your opponent will be framing an
issue very differently. ... and third, you have to build a
technique of phrasing your issue ... which will stick your
capture into the Court's head so that it can't forget it.[88]

The trick is to frame the issue so that it contains the answer which
you want the court to reach. Take, for example, the case arising
out of the crash of a Brazilian airliner on a domestic flight in
Brazil. Counsel for the defendants posed the issue as being,
'Should the plaintiff be given preferred status over other
passengers on the flight from Rio to Sao Paulo, solely because he is
a resident of New York?'[89]

Examples of the same art exist in the House of Lords. A little
known but very important instance occurred in *Derry* v. *Peek*.
Fletcher Moulton QC was appearing for the directors of the
tramway company who were being sued for damages resulting
from an untrue statement in the company's prospectus. Moulton
framed the issue by arguing that for the plaintiff to recover he
must prove fraud on the part of the directors. He then set about
persuading the Law Lords to accept his definition of reality. His
tactics were to stress the stigma attached to the word 'fraud' and to
paint a picture of his clients as Victorian gentlemen of honour who
had simply made a mistake. From there it was a short step to
saying,

Every one of us knows what fraud is. We know that it is not a
legal quibble, but a fact implying personal dishonesty. We
don't shake hands with a man who has been guilty of fraud.[90]

By this simple device Moulton was able to hamper the
development of the law of misrepresentation for several decades. A
similar form of advocacy by Buckmaster KC in *Boyd and Forrest* v.
Glasgow and South Western Railway Company seems to have had the
same effect on the Law Lords. Lord Macmillan records in his
autobiography[91] that the Lord Chancellor announced after the
second appeal, '[T]hose who make allegations of fraud which they
are unable to substantiate will receive in this House justice, bare
justice.'

Part of framing the issue is the selection of a legal classification or categorisation that favours the decision which the framer desires. While such classifications, once accepted, can often appear inevitable (a result which is reinforced by the work of textbook writers or headnote writers in the law reports), academic writers can sometimes overlook the problems that practitioners experience in locating which legal rules may or may not impinge on the facts of a case. One QC (now a High Court judge) told me,

Since law and decision-making are not exact processes, nearly all cases at appellate levels turn on the basic initial approach or smell by the tribunal; certainly if they have read the judgement below. Depending on the way in which they start looking at a case, you will get a different result.

Justice Jackson of the US Supreme Court made a similar point when he observed,

It may sound paradoxical, but most contentions of law are won or lost on the facts. ... A large part of the time of conference is given to discussion of facts, to determine under what rule of law they fall.[92]

Thus in *Hedley Byrne* v. *Heller* the appellants relied heavily on negligence and the general duty of care articulated by Lord Atkin in *Donoghue* v. *Stevenson* whilst the respondents tried to concentrate on the contractual or agency aspect of the case. The Law Lords accepted the appellant's classification in part but rejected the applicability of *Donoghue* v. *Stevenson* except by way of analogy.

In *Adams* v. *National Bank of Greece* the successful appellant argued that the issue should be classified as one of succession, whilst his opponents failed to convince the Law Lords that the case should be categorised as one of status. Similarly, the respondent's argument based on the assertion of an equity was rejected in favour of the appellant's submission based on common law rights in *National Provincial Bank* v. *Ainsworth*.

The third method counsel employs to try to win over the tribunal to accept his picture of the law and facts involved in a particular appeal is the insertion of plausible analogies in his submissions, which if accepted, reinforce the validity of the picture he is projecting. As examples of this technique, let us consider the cases of *Carmarthenshire County Council* v. *Lewis*, *White and Carter Ltd*

v. *McGregor* and *Attorney-General* v. *Times Newspapers*. In the first the appellants tried to argue that the law governing liability for damage caused by animals straying on the highway should be applied to liability for damage caused by small children straying on the highway. All five Law Lords rejected the analogy in their speeches and dismissed the appeal, but the argument was by no means untenable. In *White and Carter* the respondent argued that if the appellants' contention was upheld by the Lords, 'an expert employed by a large company to travel abroad for the purpose of drafting an elaborate report' would be able to waste thousands of pounds in preparing it despite the fact that the company had repudiated the contract before anything was done under it.[93] Lords Morton and Keith were obviously much taken by this hypothetical analogy which figures in both their dissenting speeches.[94] Lord Reid too was troubled by the analogy (which he discusses at length in two parts of his speech) and only by references to 'legitimate interest financial or otherwise, in performing the contract ...', 'the *de minimis* principle' and 'the general equitable jurisdiction of the court' does he feel able to distinguish the analogy from the facts of the appeal.[95] In the *Times Newspapers* case, the respondents raised two analogies;[96] one relating to press comment on local authority evictions of squatters, and one relating to the hypothesised comments of the 'Venetian Times' on the conduct of Shylock. Both analogies appear in the Law Lords' speeches although neither was upheld by a majority.[97]

TECHNIQUES OF PERSUASION: EVIDENCE FROM THE INTERVIEWS

The interviews provided empirical support under several heads for these arguments on the persuasive techniques and power of counsel. The first concerned the order of presentation of oral argument in an appeal. In the House of Lords the appellant speaks first and last. The respondent speaks only once, in reply to the appellant. Both counsel and Law Lords were asked whether they considered that the ordering of the arguments gave an advantage to the appellant. Research conducted by experimental psychologists in the United States simulating the presentation of evidence in a case at first instance (published while I was conducting my fieldwork) suggested the reverse, *i.e.* that it was an advantage to go second.[98] But almost every counsel whom I interviewed considered that the appellant did have an advantage from speaking first. Anthony Lloyd QC commented,

> Very often in an appeal you can make a terrific difference within the first half hour of argument. This is why the appellant always has an advantage because if he's good and makes use of his opportunity to start by putting it very clearly and attractively and simply, he can win the court round.

Louis Blom-Cooper QC observed in similar vein,

> I always like to be an appellant because you can shape the nature and tenor of the oral argument. The way the case is opened, the first two hours, particularly if the Law Lords have not read the Case, is crucial.

Counsel were clearly alive to the benefit to be had from 'setting the stage' or 'drawing up the scheme for the case in a way that is impalpably in favour'[99] of their clients. The Law Lords, however, were markedly divided on the question. Lords Devlin, MacDermott, Salmon and Kilbrandon considered that there was no advantage in being the appellant. Others were less sure.

> It depends on the judges sitting, some are pro-appellant, others favour the *status quo*. (Lord Radcliffe)

> No, but it's slightly easier to have the first word. (Lord Hailsham)

> I think it used to be, but now we can keep an open mind long enough to take in what the respondent says. (Lord Reid)

> It depends on the case. (Lord Guest)

A third group answered in the affirmative,

> Undoubtedly ... a good QC can win many cases in the first half hour. We all know this from experience. (Lord Wilberforce)

> Yes. I think it has a greater advantage with some judges. Sir

Wilfrid Greene, for example, was very much an appellants' judge. He had a very acute mind, and he always liked trying to think of how he would put the case himself and what points could be said against the judgements. Of course, other judges rather take the view, well, unless you can absolutely convince me the judge was wrong, I shall stick by what the judge said. But by and large, I think it is an advantage to be the appellant. (Lord Cross)

The advantage of opening is a well known theory at the Bar ... I suppose it is true. ... The appellant has the advantage because he can set out the facts and arguments from his point of view. He can thus set the lines of development of the case. (Lord Pearson)

Lords Denning and Gardiner agreed with this group. Intriguingly, there is a strong correlation between those Law Lords who pay more attention to the written materials and those Law Lords who consider that the appellant has an advantage from opening in the Lords. It is almost as though they have developed the habit of reading the printed Case in order to negative the advantage which they perceive the appellant to gain from opening the appeal.

In earlier days, however, appellants do not seem to have gained much advantage from opening. Indeed they often met with judicial hostility. Lord Haldane recounts in his autobiography how he endeavoured to turn this hostility to his advantage,

I have sometimes stated the point as it had been decided against my side in the court below before the tribunal could realise on which side I was arguing. I have done this when I saw that they were in an obstinate mood, with fairness, but with the result that they jumped from sheer combativeness against the proposition of law which I intended in the end to overthrow, and it was then that I gradually disclosed how it was that I was really there to argue the other way. The results were sometimes good.[100]

Even when the Law Lords were not actively hostile they might still be suspicious. Thus Lord Morton once recalled how when he was opening in an appeal in the House of Lords he was brought up short by a remark from one of the Law Lords, 'You are galloping along very smoothly now, but as you are for the appellant I suppose there is a water jump coming.'[101]

Further evidence on the persuasive power of counsel emerged from my questions on the qualities of 'good' advocacy in the Lords. One constant theme in American writings on appellate advocacy is the importance of 'going for the jugular',[102] *i.e.* getting to the heart of the case by selecting and arguing its one or two controlling issues, to the exclusion of the minor or subsidiary propositions. A simple and coherent presentation, it is argued, is the best way to 'capture the issue' and to 'stick that capture' into the minds of the judges.[103] This argument received support from both Law Lords and counsel.

I personally prefer the counsel who puts his best point and doesn't necessarily throw all his points at you. A good advocate uses discretion in his presentation. (Lord MacDermott)[104]

Counsel in the Lords should have a lively appreciation of the points that matter, and should not take a lot of bad points. (Lord Salmon)

You choose one or two key points and run them to see what reaction you get. There's always a quick response which tells you whether to press on or to abandon the points and try something else ... Your task is to clarify, distil and crystallise the main points in the case. (Mr Justice Lawson)

Advocacy ... calls for appreciation of when to go and when to stop. (Lord Rawlinson QC)[105]

But, as Sir Patrick Hastings KC shrewdly noted,[106] 'The ability to pick out the one real point of a case is not by itself enough; it is the courage required to seize upon that point to the exclusion of all others that is of real importance.'

It is recorded of Sir Walter Monckton QC that he had the ability and the daring when faced with twelve points to choose from, to pick the best one and abandon the other eleven to press it.[107] But lesser mortals are acutely aware of the risks involved in such a procedure, particularly when they know from experience that,

Sometimes an argument which appears to counsel not to be a particularly good one, appeals to the tribunal ... so that all the time one has to adjust one's sense of what are the strong arguments and what are the weak ones. (Louis Blom-Cooper QC)

Michael Albery QC explained to me that in the case of *Kammins Ballrooms Ltd* v. *Zenith Investments* he had had two points for the respondents. The first, on statutory construction, he considered to be far stronger than the second which related to waiver of rights. The respondents won on the first point all the way to the Lords and lost on the second. Against his own feelings about not holding on to bad points and against the suggestion of his junior he retained the waiver point in the Lords, 'for insurance purposes'. To his considerable surprise and dismay he sensed (correctly) in the Lords that he had lost the argument on statutory construction and so had to fight 'tooth and nail' on the 'weaker' second point to scrape home by a majority of three votes to two. As we have seen, a similar situation seems to have arisen in *Mapp* v. *Ohio*. The danger in such situations, as Albery was aware, is that if counsel misreads the response of the House he may find himself adding a bad point to good ones - an event which Albery likened to, 'the thirteenth chime of an unsound clock - it contaminates or detracts from all that has gone before'.

Counsel were divided on the proper line to take with their weak points. Some favoured camouflage or evasion. Others preferred to face up to their difficulties before the other side had an opportunity of exploiting them. But few if any of them would consider emulating the tactics occasionally adopted by Wilfrid Greene KC. In one appeal Greene, who considered Lord Dunedin to be rather conceited, decided to take advantage of this in his argument. In the course of his opening speech he made his argument weaker than it needed be: 'I don't know how I'm going to win this case, the point against me is very strong ... I don't know what the answer is ... ', at which Lord Dunedin, in order to show himself cleverer than Greene, said, 'But surely Mr Greene, the answer to the point against you is so and so ....'

At this Greene sat down quickly. His opponent got up and said, 'I think your Lordship has forgotten case X.' 'I forgot nothing of the sort.' Thus Greene succeeded in interposing the judge between his weakest point and his opponent and won the case.[108]

Similarly Lord Hailsham has written of an occasion when Greene had asked him,

> Suppose you had two bad points to argue before the House of Lords, and suppose one was slightly less bad than the other, which would you argue first?
>
> 'Well I suppose', I answered naively, 'the one which was less bad'.
>
> 'You would be wrong' said Wilfrid. 'In such circumstances I always argue my worst point first, and argue it as well as I can, and as they are very intelligent they always beat me. When they have done so I somewhat hesitantly say "There is a second point, My Lords. But here I am in some difficulty", and then I put the better point a little less well than it ought to be put. One of them always says to me, "But surely, Mr Greene, you could put it like this", and tempted by my error, he puts the argument correctly ... and I know that I am half-way to winning the case.'[109]

Lord Halsbury LC adverted to the same technique when he explained why he considered a little-known barrister was the best advocate he had ever heard, 'Well, he had the great gift of always making it appear that he had a first class case being hopelessly ruined by a third class advocate.'[110]

These anecdotes demonstrate how experienced counsel have exceptionally been able to take advantage of a group trait of the Law Lords, namely, their intelligence. My interviews with counsel revealed that the ability to tailor one's arguments to the individual traits of the Law Lords was also prized. All the Law Lords and counsel interviewed recognised that a certain proportion (although there was no consensus on the size of that proportion) of appeals turn on which five Law Lords actually sit on the Appellate Committee. Yet the counsel indicated that the problem of handling five separate minds at one time was sufficient to deter all but the most self-confident of advocates from trying to take advantage of the individual traits of the Law Lords. Counsel's difficulties in this area were not helped by the Judicial Office's policy[111] of refusing to reveal in advance which Law Lords would sit on a particular appeal.

Generally counsel seem to have settled for a shepherd and sheepdog approach. On the one hand they sought by gentle

persuasion to lead the court to their view, while on the other hand
they tried to keep the Law Lords together by striving to head off
the Law Lord(s) leading the hunt against them. Most would have
agreed with Walter Monckton's observation that,

> ... your job at the Bar is to persuade that old man sitting up
> there that you are right ... watch him like a lynx. Try to get
> inside his head and follow his train of thought. Deal with the
> points that are troubling him.[112]

Lord Devlin certainly did. He told me that the highest form of
advocacy,

> ... seems to be a sort of instinct of knowing what is going on in
> a particular judge's mind .... That's much more difficult to do
> when there are five people but the man who was best at it in my
> time was Walter Monckton. He had an uncanny facility for
> knowing what was troubling you almost before you knew it
> yourself.

But few counsel aspired to such heights when faced with a panel of
five judges. At most they would consider whether corporately the
five (or a majority of them) would be likely to be more receptive to
an appeal to the merits of the case - 'the fireside equities'[113] - or to
a narrow statement of principle. Only the bold advocates - those
confident enough to try 'managing the court'[114] - occasionally
adopted the tactic of attempting to win over one Law Lord in the
hope of setting him off against his colleagues and bringing them
round to his way of thinking. James Comyn QC was such an
advocate. He remarked,

> The ideal in any appeal is to get one judge who will be
> outspokenly on your side in argument, who will polish your
> arguments and as it were throw them back at you in a polished
> state and indeed get to the point of answering any of his
> colleagues who are critical of you.

It seems likely, however, that such tactics were more in evidence
in the early years of this century when it was possible to spend
most of one's practice in the Privy Council and the House of Lords
and thus to become acquainted with the idiosyncracies of each and

every Law Lord. Thus Lord Haldane records in his autobiography,

> I knew the Judges in the House of Lords and Privy Council so well that I could follow the working of their individual minds. If, for example, Lord Watson, who was by no means a silent judge but who was a man of immense power, started off by being against me, I would turn round to some colleague of his on whose opinion I knew he did not set much weight, and who would be sure merely to echo what Lord Watson had just said. By devoting myself to the judge who had merely repeated Lord Watson's point I well knew that I should speedily detach Lord Watson from it and bring him out of his entrenchments.[115]

Support for the persuasive power of counsel comes finally from the occasions when counsel's submissons are adopted (sometimes verbatim) by one or more Law Lords in their speeches. We have already seen two cases, *White and Carter Ltd* v. *McGregor* and *Attorney-General* v. *Times Newspapers* where counsel's analogies were taken up by the Law Lords in their speeches. Similarly, Law Lords during the period of my study on occasions openly acknowledged that a part of their judgement was derived from counsel's submissions. Thus in *Boardman* v. *Phipps* Lord Guest said,

> [T]he Court of Appeal ... decided the case in the respondent's favour on the basis that ... I prefer, however, to base my opinion on the broader ground which was epitomised by [counsel for the respondent] in his closing submission.[116]

In most cases where such 'borrowing' occurs, however, it is unacknowledged. For example, in *White and Carter Ltd* v. *McGregor* the appellant's junior is reported as arguing,[117] 'Equity will not rewrite contracts which may turn out to be improvident' and Lord Hodson in his speech says, 'It is trite that equity will not rewrite an improvident contract where there is no disability on either side.'[118] And in *Cassell* v. *Broome* the appellant's argument on innocent printers and single awards against joint tortfeasors was reproduced by Lord Reid.[119] Several counsel said they could recall discovering parts of their arguments repeated without acknowledgement by the Law Lords. But they were in no way taken aback at this. Some

went further, saying 'That's what counsel are there for.' As
Llewellyn argued in *The Common Law Tradition*,[120] every brief
should contain a 'proffered, phrased, opinion-kernel' - a point
echoed by Mr Justice Ackner[121] who observed to me,

> It depends - sometimes you find quite a lot. Every counsel's
> speech should if possible be so framed as to be capable of being
> incorporated into a judgement. What one is seeking to serve up
> to them is how they should write their judgement.

CONCLUSION

I have tried to show in this chapter that counsel in the Lords have
restrictive and persuasive powers which can in certain
circumstances exercise considerable influence over the Law Lords
and their performance in hard cases in the House of Lords. As
Lord Scarman recently observed,

> The judge, however wise, creative, and imaginative he may be,
> is 'cabin'd, cribb'd, confined, bound in' not, as was Macbeth,
> to his 'saucy doubts and fears' but by the evidence and
> arguments of the litigants. It is this limitation, inherent in the
> forensic process, which sets bounds to the scope of judicial law
> reform.[122]

The importance of this was seen by Wetter for he asserts in his
book, *The Styles of Appellate Judicial Opinions*, that,

> From a broad, jurisprudential point of view, the most notable
> effect of a court considering the primary function of its opinions
> to be the rendering of conclusive answers to the allegations of
> counsel ... is that of shifting the responsibility for judicial law-
> making from the courts to the Bar ...[123]

This conclusion, which flows directly from the premises of the
adversary system as it operates in the United Kingdom has, I
believe, been neglected in much of the recent jurisprudential
writing on judicial creativity.[124] It is also one that highlights the
significance of the finding, set forth in the previous chapter, that
counsel in the Lords consider that they have no responsibility for

the proper and orderly development of the law.

In part the dangers inherent in this situation are mitigated by the shared understandings or consensus[125] between Law Lords and counsel as to the acceptable limits of argument or at least by counsel's pragmatic acceptance of the Law Lords' notions of the boundary of tenable argument before the House.[126] Moreover, the discussion in this chapter has largely reflected the viewpoint of the Bar, and my arguments on the restrictive and persuasive power of counsel's submissions have been deliberately pitched at a high level, as a counter to the benign neglect by recent commentators of the part played by counsel in decision-making in the Lords. The next chapter is intended to restore the balance by approaching the interaction between Bench and Bar from the perspective of the Law Lords.

4 Courtroom Interaction: The Law Lords' Perspective

The House is a clinical environment. It's as though you had a sort of mortician's slab in the middle and five searchlights trained on it. Lord Reid once told me that the difference between advocacy in the Lords and any other court was that you couldn't so easily get away with prepared positions. In the House of Lords it's absolutely essential that the advocate should be able to think on his feet.

Mark Littman QC

Despite the impression which may have been conveyed in the previous chapter, the oral interaction between Bench and Bar in the Lords is not the one-sided affair that oral argument is in certain courts in Europe, where an intervention by a judge may be viewed as a sign of bias by his colleagues. Law Lords have not only restrictive and persuasive powers but interrogative powers as well and they do not hesitate to exercise them in getting to grips with counsel's argument.

THE POWER OF THE PRESIDING LAW LORD

The individual with potentially the greatest influence on the oral interchange is the presiding Law Lord.[1] This is because, as Lord Denning observed, ' ... in a way he conducts the argument'. It is to him that counsel's submissions appear to be made (even though counsel may be intending to win round a different member of the Committee), except where counsel is responding to a question from another Law Lord. Lord Guest, in our interview, suggested that,

66

... the tendency of the discussion is very largely governed by the presiding judge, because ... the tradition is that if you and the presiding judge start interrupting at the same time then you give way to him, and accordingly it is always he who has the say in asking questions.

However, from my own observations of the court and from the interviews it became clear that different presidents interpret their role in different ways. As Lord Cross remarked,

Some presiding judges are very fond of guiding counsel and sometimes of raising points which counsel does not think of raising himself and going off on all sorts of by-paths. Other presiding judges want to put an end to the discussion as early as possible. I suppose ideally one wants to be betwixt and between.

In part, the discrepant role performances are explicable in terms of the personal attributes of each presiding judge. Roger Parker QC observed with feeling,

All presiding Law Lords are different. The difficulty is if a particularly quick minded man is in the chair. He may grasp and accept your argument before the others. They want to hear you and he doesn't. He wants you to go on, but you've to bring them all with you.

Yet in part the differences in behaviour are also responses to the conflicting expectations experienced by presiding Law Lords. On the one hand, there are the expectations that judicial time should not be wasted, that public funds - and those of the litigants - should not be expended on the unnecessary prolongation of appeals and that reasonable expedition should prevail in order that the court schedule (and therefore other litigants' appeals) should not be thrown into disarray. On the other hand, there are the expectations of counsel that their submissions should be listened to courteously by the Law Lords and that their presentations should not be destroyed by frequent interruptions by the Law Lords, and also the expectation that in a final court of appeal the fundamental issues of law raised in appeals should be given unhurried and thorough consideration.

In earlier times presiding Law Lords do not seem to have been unduly troubled by this role conflict, perhaps because the latter cluster of expectations was less developed or because judicial tempers were shorter then. Thus in the late eighteenth century when counsel in a Scots appeal announced, 'I will noo, my Lords, proceed to my seevent pownt *(sic)'* the Lord Chancellor (Thurlow) riposted, 'I'll be damned if you do ... this House is adjourned till Monday next.'[2] By the early part of the twentieth century matters had hardly improved. (While in 1825, 86 appeals were heard by the House in 89 days, in 1908, 84 appeals took only 83 days to hear.) Presiding Law Lords still interrupted frequently either to curtail counsel's submissions or to take over the argument with a view to forcing it along lines favoured by the presiding judge. Thus D. N. Pritt QC in his autobiography[3] records one occasion when Lord Buckmaster endeavoured to 'smash' an appeal which Pritt was arguing. The particular case was a complex one but Buckmaster,

> began at once, with all the advantages of his quickness of thought,[4] with a long series of interruptions .... The warfare went on for a day or two, and then Lord Buckmaster said: 'Mr Pritt, their Lordships ... would like to know how long this nonsense is going to continue.' [Pritt] replied: 'About ten days, if interruptions continue on their present scale, and a few days less if they diminish.'

After further interruptions Pritt could endure it no longer and, slamming a book on the lectern before him, he shouted, 'Your Lordships are going to hear this case!' They did. Pritt won. On other days the Law Lords were quite capable of sustaining the argument of an appeal with only the occasional assistance of counsel.

But gradually the balance between the conflicting expectations began to change, and with it the role of the presiding Law Lord. (By the 1950s the average appeal was taking three days to hear and since then the average has remained between three and four days.) Lord Guest, when he became a Lord of Appeal in 1961, noticed a significant difference in the Lords from when he had appeared before them as counsel.

> ... my experience over the years extends fairly far back and I can remember Lord Dunedin, Lord Thankerton and Lord

Blanesburgh. I would say the climate of judicial behaviour has altered considerably since I first appeared. In those days the interruptions were constant, counsel was only allowed to say a few words before another judge would interrupt him. Generally speaking, judges are much more polite now to counsel than they used to be in the old days and give them more opportunity for developing their argument.

In fact, by 1954 when Lord Simonds returned from the Woolsack to preside in the House, the hallmark of the president's role was restraint: restraint on himself, restraint on unnecessary interruptions by his colleagues, and restraint on irrelevant argument by counsel. Lord Radcliffe, a great believer in the presiding Law Lord's role in 'concentrating the argument', recorded that,

> They [the Law Lords] are more considerate, they show more humane manners, and they exercise much more self-control in sticking resolutely to the real issues. A good presiding judge counts a lot here. ... There have been fine lawyers, for instance, such as Lord Blanesburgh and Lord Atkin, themselves the nicest of men, who seemed positively to prefer that a case should go on for ever to the possibility of an argument of which they disapproved remaining on its legs: whereas Lord Simonds, whom many think of (wrongly) as an obstinate and prejudiced judge, was a model in his conduct of a hearing, concise, courteously patient and resignedly fair.[5]

By the early 1970s the pendulum, if anything, had swung even further. Lord Gardiner, at least, believed this for he commented in our interview,

> It is the business of any judge not to let the case take longer than it need. I am afraid there is a modern tendency to be too courteous and let counsel talk too much [but] it is better than the other extreme. When I was called to the Bar they shut one up rather brutally, now they are much more courteous ... Viscount Simonds used to keep counsel shorter than the present lot do.[6]

Curiously a continuation of this trend would not be welcomed by counsel. Silent presidents such as Lords Radcliffe and Wilberforce place counsel in a quandary.[7] Lord Justice Russell remarked, 'It's frightfully difficult to argue against a brick wall of silence. I liked a point to be put to me so that I could see how that man's mind was working.' Similarly one QC observed that,

> ... an advocate faced with a silent tribunal may deceive himself into supposing that a particular point that he is making has been fully understood, or even fully accepted, by the Court.

Patrick Neill QC put the point forcefully: 'Silence is death in the House.' Counsel does not know whether to elaborate on his points or whether he is pushing at an open door. Sometimes he is being passively discouraged. Lord Kilbrandon, for instance, commented,

> The way to discourage counsel if you think they are talking nonsense is to remain completely silent. If you interrupt a man and say 'But Mr so-and-so, how can you say that' that simply means he says it all over again.

Yet my observations of the court in the 1970s suggested that if there was a silent president, as Lord Wilberforce tended to be, one of his colleagues, for example, Lord Dilhorne, would take over the interaction with counsel. Furthermore, there were occasions when one or two of the presiding Law Lords were considered by counsel not to be silent enough. In *Cassell* v. *Broome* on the first day there were 99 judicial interventions, 61 of which came from the central chair. Constant judicial interruptions are no more popular in the US Supreme Court. Counsel in particular may be upset since time taken by judicial questions is not automatically added to counsel's time allowance. It is at the Chief Justice's discretion. Thus unruly judges can ruin the oral argument in the Supreme Court. Frankfurter's frequent interrogation of counsel was unpopular not only with counsel but also with his colleagues. Professor Fred Rodell once related the tale of the

> ... large very rich corporation [which] had been guilty of breaking the antitrust laws and had carried its case to the Supreme Court, which had allotted a whole day for so important an argument. The corporation's lawyers then had a

brilliant idea. Aware that the Justices regularly whisper to each other on the bench during the course of argument, they smuggled two professional lip-readers into seats at their counsel's table to catch the drift of judicial comment. Would it be discouraging or hopeful? Should they change the thrust of their appeal for the afternoon session? At the lunch recess, as soon as the Justices trooped off, the lawyers leapt for the lip-readers who looked woebegone. 'Sorry' said one lip-reader finally, 'but all we got was when Justice Frankfurter kept asking that lawyer all those questions and Justice Douglas turned to Justice Reed and what he said was, "Why can't the little bastard keep his big mouth shut and let us get on with it?"' [8]

Since the presiding judge, if anyone, can control the pace and direction of the oral argument, it is perhaps not surprising that most of the counsel whom I interviewed perceived the senior Law Lords (who preside with the greatest frequency) as having a dominating influence on their colleagues. Such a view appears to be shared by the authors of *Final Appeal*.[9] But Lord Radcliffe has rejected the suggestion, asserting instead that,

> The one who presides has no special weight in the forming of the decision, except in the negative sense that if he patently tries to sway the presentment of the argument, he may provoke a movement of resistance in his colleagues.[10]

It is likely that Lord Radcliffe had Lord Atkin in mind for he told me that Lord Atkin,

> ... was intolerable as a presiding Law Lord because he had no wish that the case should be fully and fairly explored. He'd formed a view and he was going to use whatever odds he possessed ... to try to see that that succeeded. It very often produced a counter-effect, of course, in the people who were sitting with him.

Apart from the president's opportunities to guide the oral interchange, the current Law Lords whom I interviewed generally shared the perception of Lord Radcliffe. As Lord Reid said,

> Oh, he's no more power, but on the other hand I take the view

that I can give a lead very often where perhaps the others couldn't, and if I think that ... mind you I am not always right, but if I think that my colleagues are likely to be going along a certain line, well I can try and crystallise it a bit. But it may turn out I was wrong and I haven't represented the common view. Yes, I think the presiding man can give a lead, but that's all.

His successor as presiding Law Lord, Lord Wilberforce, was of like mind. 'All the Lords can take part in the oral [interchange]', he observed, ' ... but the presiding Lord can suggest possible directions for its development.'[11]

THE LAW LORDS' POWERS OF INTERVENTION

Irrespective of the paramountcy (or otherwise) of the presiding Law Lord, or the relative frequency or infrequency of his interventions, the question remains: 'For what purposes have the Law Lords (and the presiding judge in particular) exercised their restrictive, interrogative and persuasive powers in recent times?' The interviews provided several clues.

[The oral interchange] can be used for a variety of reasons. It may be to clear up some difficulty in your own mind - or maybe you're not sure that you've grasped counsel's argument properly. Or you want to see if he's got a presupposition he's not revealing. Again a new aspect of the problem may strike you and you want to know if he's going to cover it. (Lord MacDermott)

Firstly, to clear up difficulties in my own mind. Secondly, if I was thinking of taking a particular line myself I would want to put it to him even if I didn't think his answer would be likely to help very much but simply so that it couldn't be said that he hadn't had an opportunity of dealing with it. Thirdly, on very rare occasions, to stop a rather futile argument. (Lord Devlin)

In fact, my observations of the court, an analysis of the interviews and a scrutiny of the Law Reports suggested that interventions by the Law Lords have five main motives. These were, to curtail the argument, to test counsel's propositions, to sound out counsel's views on particular points, to obtain clarification of counsel's argument and to persuade fellow Law Lords.[12] Of course one intervention can serve more than one purpose.

CURTAILMENT

Examples of the Lords curtailing the argument of counsel are legion. As we have already seen, the Law Lords will normally restrain advocates from raising new points in the House. Counsel who sidles up to a point not argued below saying 'It is a point that grows on one' will be told by the presiding Law Lord, as the respondent in *Mardorf Peach* v. *Attica Sea Corpration* was, 'Well it will have to grow on us in some other case.'[13]

In other situations the curtailment is couched as a statement, *e.g.* 'Their Lordships do not require to hear argument on ... ' or 'Their Lordships need not trouble you on ... .' Such interventions are the result of discussions by the Law Lords in the informal conferences which they hold throughout the duration of an appeal. Having decided whether further, or indeed any, argument is required on a particular point the Law Lords (through the presiding Law Lord) will normally, though not invariably, communicate this (in open court) to the relevant counsel when he is next addressing them. Such interventions are not made at the commencement of an appeal and they are almost always restricted to situations where one or other, or both, of the parties have already argued the point. The inadequacy of the synopses of the oral interaction in the Lords (published in the official Law Reports - the Appeal Cases), makes it difficult to gauge how often such interventions are made. 'Judicial directives' of this nature are recorded in over 20 per cent of the cases reported in the Appeal Cases for the past twenty-five years, but my observations of the court would suggest that this figure is a considerable underestimate.

Typically such interventions occur at the start, or during the course of argument by the respondent's counsel. Blom-Cooper and Drewry record that the respondent was not even called on to address the Law Lords in 9 cases out of 393 English appeals heard during the period 1952-68.[14] More commonly the respondent will be told that argument is not required on a particular point which has been raised by the appellant. Thus in the course of the

respondent's argument in *Knuller* v. *DPP* the following interaction
ensued,

Lord Reid: Mr Buzzard, their Lordships need not trouble you
further on whether this House should overrule the
decision in *Shaw* [1962] A.C. 220. Mr Hazan
[appellant's counsel], are you still maintaining
that the present case is distinguishable from *Shaw*?

Hazan QC: In the circumstances I would find it difficult to
maintain that proposition.

Lord Reid   Mr Buzzard, their Lordships need not trouble you
further on count 1.[15]

Again in *Hedley Byrne* v. *Heller*[16] Lord Reid makes it clear in his
speech that the respondents were prevented by the Law Lords
from arguing that they were not negligent in their actions, despite
the eagerness of the respondents to take up the point.

It is comparatively rare (in reported cases) for the appellant to
be told that he does not require to reply on any point to the
respondent,[17] although it is commonplace for the House to
indicate that a reply is not required on certain (named) points.[18]
Occasionally, however, such an interruption does not forebode
success on the point for the appellant.[19] For this reason 'statement'
type curtailments should be exercised with caution, for I have
never known counsel to refuse openly to accede to such
'directives'. Any counsel who was told that no argument was
required on a relevant point only to discover later that he had lost
the case on that point would have legitimate grounds for
grievance.

Finally, curtailment may take the form of a request or
suggestion from the Law Lords. As we have already seen,[20] such
requests are not regarded as mandatory by counsel. Thus in *Cassell*
v. *Broome*[21] the appellants' counsel, Roger Parker QC, felt able to
lead the court into a detailed scrutiny of all the defamatory
passages complained of in the litigation, and thus to make a plea in
mitigation in relation to them, even though he received hints from
the Bench that such a course would be inappropriate since there
had been no appeal against the award of compensatory damages.
Later in the same appeal, the respondent's counsel, David Hirst
QC, was faced with the problem of whether or not to challenge
Lord Devlin's exegesis of the law on exemplary damages in *Rookes*

v. *Barnard*, as he had done successfully in the Court of Appeal. As he explained to me later,

> Well, it's the problem of the advocate ... if you've got two points which you think you can win on, do you run the second one even though you think you've won the first? I thought I would win on the first but I had always intended to challenge the narrow interpretation of the second category of damages in *Rookes* v. *Barnard* and I received judicial encouragement [in the Court of Appeal][22] in this direction.

However Lord Hailsham and his brethren (with the exception of Viscount Dilhorne) felt that the respondent could win without adopting such tactics. When Hirst began his argument on *Rookes* v. *Barnard* on the tenth day of the hearing in *Cassell* v. *Broome*, Lord Hailsham suggested that he should desist, adding, 'We can't stop you but the purpose of our hints is to prevent you prolonging the case, *and to save your client's money.*' The following day Viscount Dilhorne asked Hirst to discuss the cases which were superseded by *Rookes* v. *Barnard* and Hirst used this as a way into challenging *Rookes* v. *Barnard*. Hirst's refusal to accept Lord Hailsham's hint cost his side dear, for in the hearing on expenses, *Cassell* v. *Broome* (No. 2),[23] the Law Lords penalised the respondents for the attack on *Rookes* v. *Barnard* (which had prolonged the appeal) by ruling that they would only receive half their expenses in the Court of Appeal and the House of Lords from the appellants. This was a ruling which in the circumstances of the case looked akin to the Law Lords 'eating their cake and having it'.

TESTING

Interventions designed to test the scope and soundness of counsel's argument are the hallmark of the oral interaction both in the Lords and in the United States Supreme Court. Lord Reid felt this keenly,

> Of course you have got to be reasonable, but broadly speaking I would think that the job of the man on the Bench is always to be rather against the man who is on his feet. In other words you are trying to test him out you see, and to find any weak points in his argument.

Lord Hailsham was of like mind. He used the interchange for 'testing the validity of questionable propositions of chains of reasoning'. There were similar comments from those on the other side of the Bar. As one lawyer put it, 'The interaction is the key to the Law Lords' decisions. They are testing things out to see how the jigsaw falls into place. It's a process of discovery and exploration.'

Lord Reid, when he presided in the Lords (as he did from 1962-74), had no equal in this aspect of an appeal. Law Lord and counsel alike were agreed on this. Some considered it his greatest contribution to the Lords and lamented that for the most part his efforts in this area were not recorded. A glimpse of Lord Reid's technique can be seen in the celebrated contempt of court case, *Attorney-General* v. *Times Newspapers*, where the illustrative analogy of the 'Venetian Times' and Shylock, which influenced some of the Law Lords, derived not from counsel's inspiration but from an interruption made by Lord Reid during the submissions of the Attorney-General.

> 'There must be some limitation to this', Lord Reid said. 'Do you taint the source of justice by pointing out to a litigant that he has moral obligations as well as legal ones? Would it have been contempt for someone to have said to Shylock: "You have a sound case in law but your name will reek with your fellow men if you pursue your claim to your pound of flesh",'[24]

A stronger flavour of this master craftsman at work emerged from the interviews. Judge Everett QC recalled,

> You could see him saying to himself, 'Now I'll ask [counsel] so and so, then if he says this, then I shall ask him that, then he'll have to answer in that way, then I'll ask him this and then I shall have him.' It's all testing, testing, testing out, exploring right the way through. 'Would you submit so and so; Well now, what would be the consequences of that; Would you like to develop that line and see where it leads to?'

Lord Pearce gave an equally vivid account of Reid's *modus operandi*.

> Scott Reid when he talks, always gets the argument one stage

further .... He says, 'Well, does what you are arguing really amount to this?', then he puts something clearly and fairly and then counsel is doubtful for a moment, and Scott says, 'Well, I think you have got to put it as high as that, haven't you, in order to make your point that so-and-so and so-and-so?', and then counsel think again, and then he says, perhaps, 'No, I don't think I have got to put it quite like that'. Then Scott Reid says, 'I think you have to, don't you, because if you admit so-and-so', and then perhaps it is agreed either .... It is more often that Scott's right, but often counsel can get out of that one. Scott is not demolishing him, you understand, at all. He just wants to see where all this is leading, and then we have got to another stage in the argument. It is now agreed that if this is the right way of looking at the case, then one has got really to accept proposition A, or to amend it, or to accept proposition B. Well then, you are one forward, you see, then you go on. Well, none of that can ever be got into any brief, because if you start re-writing a brief in the alternative, with about 100 different alternatives, you get nowhere. It doesn't convince.[25]

Testing such as this is not always welcomed by counsel. It is not necessarily even an indicator of how the interrogator is thinking, since he may be adopting the role of the devil's advocate. As one counsel observed with a certain resignation, 'It's like getting hold of a wild horse, you deal with it as it comes ... you try and cope with it. It's a situation you know you are going to meet.' Others, like Mr Justice Ackner were more positive,

As an advocate you've a role to play, a line to take and having worked out the best way of presenting your line, your function is to hang onto it rather like a bull terrier and make sure it's not whipped out of your grasp. The interventions [of the Law Lords] are the way of testing your proposition and if you reckon your proposition is sound the more it's tested the more its strength becomes apparent. It's highly stimulating.

Sometimes, the Law Lords' testing can be very trying for counsel,[26] as D. N. Pritt's autobiography showed. Sometimes their devil's advocacy becomes merely devilment. Lord Justice Russell's experiences in *Gilmour* v. *Coats* were a good illustration of this. When the case came before the Lords, he had to argue that trust funds bequeathed to a Carmelite priory (whose primary work was intercessory prayer), were charitable and therefore tax exempt. To prove this, he required to show that the work of the priory was for the public benefit. While trying to argue that the benefit of intercessory prayer to the public could be assumed without proof, Russell was asked by Lord Normand, 'Is it part of your contention, Mr Russell, that prayer is always answered?' Russell looked at the clock (which showed five minutes to four o'clock), then at Normand, and then again at the clock and replied, 'Perhaps your Lordship would allow me to answer that tomorrow.'[27]

Yet as Lord Radcliffe told me,

> It is very wrong to use interruptions in order to indulge the range and intelligence of your own mind. I mean, this is a terrible weakness which grows upon Law Lords. I think normally one would use the interruption only for the purpose of trying to explain to the counsel some difficulty in your own mind that was going to weigh with you, which he had not met.

SOUNDING

This form of intervention, designed to sound out counsel's views on particular points, is the Law Lords' counter to the restrictive powers of counsel. If the Law Lords give counsel an opportunity to deal with points which counsel has not raised but which the Law Lords consider to be important, it is less easy to accuse them of breaking the rules of the adversary game. But, as we saw earlier, counsel may decline to take the point and thus place the Law Lords in a difficult position.

Sometimes counsel will be asked for his comments on a case or cases which a Law Lord has discovered in his own researches. Lord Hodson did this in *Johnson* v. *Callow*[28] and as a result the appellant abandoned the appeal on the issue of contributory negligence. In *Ridge* v. *Baldwin*[29] at the end of the respondent's submissions Lord Morris produced four cases which favoured the respondent. However the appellant's counsel, Desmond Ackner QC was able to provide six cases[30] to counter those produced by Lord Morris. As his opponent recorded in his autobiography,

[Desmond Ackner] seemed to produce new cases like a

conjuror, and when Lord Reid said quietly that some of those cases (which he produced during his Reply) seemed to have more bearing on the point than some others to which their Lordships had had to listen, I began to lose hope. Lord Devlin, as was his wont, asked one or two deceptively simple questions which were traps to be avoided with care.[31]

More often counsel will simply be told that the Law Lords would like to hear argument on a point which is bothering them. Thus, in *West* v. *Shephard*,[32] Lord Reid asked the respondent's counsel to address the House on whether it was bound by its own previous decisions. Similarly, in *DPP* v. *Nock* Lord Diplock indicated that the Law Lords wished to hear argument on whether their *dicta* in *Haughton* v. *Smith* were *obiter,* and if so whether the House could reconsider them.[33] In very exceptional circumstances, as for instance in *Rookes* v. *Barnard*,[34] the Law Lords may even exercise their power to order a reconvened hearing of a case for argument on points not dealt with at the original hearing.[35]

CLARIFICATION

Perhaps the most common form of judicial intervention is the request for clarification. 'Why did x occur?', 'What do you mean by ...?', 'I'm worried about ... ' and so on. By and large, counsel welcome these interventions. They show where the Law Lords' doubts lie. Thus Justice Jackson believed that counsel should welcome any question from the Bench for, he said,

It is clear proof that the inquiring Justice is not asleep. If the question is relevant, it denotes he is grappling with your contention, even though he has not grasped it. It gives you opportunity to inflate his ego by letting him think he has discovered an idea for himself.[36]

Moreover, clarifying questions can have a significant effect on the course of the oral argument and indeed on the outcome of the case. The fear of 'double counting' by a jury in its assessment of exemplary damages as a result of Lord Devlin's *dicta* in *Rookes* v. *Barnard*, which weighed heavily with several of the Law Lords in *Cassell* v. *Broome*, derived from a remark of Lord Hailsham. On the fourth day of the oral argument in the Lords he said,

My problem in this case ... is in deciding how the jury made the split assessments [of compensation and of exemplary damages]. It's a metaphysical task which is an incitement to double counting.[37]

In *Rogers* v. *Home Office* the oral argument in the Lords took a different course based on public interest rather than Crown privilege (which had been the field of debate in the Divisional Court) because at a very early stage Lord Reid said to the Attorney-General, 'I do not quite understand. Surely the Gaming Board has a separate privilege which has nothing to do with the Crown?' Counsel for the Gaming Board was not satisfied with the Attorney-General's success in claiming Crown privilege for the Board's documents in the Divisional Court. He applied at the same hearing for an order for the Board in its own right, but was refused. Following Lord Reid's intervention in the Lords, the case proceeded and was decided on the basis that the Board did indeed have an individual right to invoke the public interest in protection of its documents.

Again, in *Anisminic* v. *The Foreign Compensation Commission* the appellants' counsel were so pessimistic of success (having lost in the lower courts) that they informed the Judicial Office that they estimated that the hearing would last two only days at the most.[38] Following key interventions by Lord Reid, the appeal took on a different complexion, the hearing lasted for twelve days and the appellants won the case.[39]

PERSUASION

The fifth and final variety of judicial interjection is one of the most interesting since it involves a reversal of roles. Its purpose is to persuade the other Law Lords. When it occurs, the Law Lord's remarks though ostensibly directed at counsel are in reality addressed to his colleagues. As one QC explained,

When a member of the House feels strongly about something, but feels that the point is not being put clearly and persuasively in argument as it could be, he has a go at reinforcing it, to try and get the point over to his colleagues. If you had to apply a percentage to remarks that are made to clear up difficulties in a Law Lord's own mind, in comparison with those made in order to get points across to counsel or to other members of the tribunal, or merely for the satisfaction of the speaker, his way of putting the point, I would say that the great majority falls into the latter classes.

One example of a persuasive judicial intervention occurred in *Knuller* v. *DPP* where a Law Lord who felt that counsel for the appellant was not going far enough with his argument on the second count, persuaded counsel to alter his line of attack to say that conspiracy to outrage public decency was an offence unknown to the common law.[40]

Such judicial adoptions of the advocate's role can ease the burden of counsel for if the latter is prepared to run the argument that he is being offered by the Law Lord he will be able to count on the assistance of that Law Lord should he encounter resistance from other members of the Appellate Committee. As we saw in the last chapter, some of the bolder or more ambitious counsel will even try to win one Law Lord round to their cause, precisely in the hope that he will 'take on the bowling' of his colleagues against the counsel's position.[41] Indeed, in *Gollins* v. *Gollins* and *Williams* v. *Williams*, the presence on the bench of two Law Lords who were known to hold diametrically opposed views on the main issues in the cases, was utilised by the opposing counsel to such effect that the contesting Law Lords occasionally appeared to be bearing the brunt of the argument.

Debates similar to these between Law Lords in the oral argument were not uncommon in hard cases during the period of my research.[42] Some Law Lords seemed to regard them with considerable favour. Lord Radcliffe, for instance, once wrote,

> ... if properly conducted, the legal debate is uniquely effective in enabling a committee of judges to arrive at a matured committee decision. The presence and, under control, the participation of counsel serve as a valuable catalyst. They enable members of the court to advance conflicting views for consideration without direct confrontation with each other or too early commitment to one point of view; and the mere maintenance of the debate is a great help to making progress towards an ultimate conclusion.[43]

This passage seems to me to exaggerate the contribution made by the Law Lords to the oral interaction. However, when taken in conjuction with the examples of judicial intervention discussed in this chapter, it should be clear that the Law Lords have considerable powers with which to influence the length and direction of the oral argument.

REPORTS OF THE INTERACTION

It should by now be apparent that the dialectic between Bench and Bar can have a vital part to play in the decision which is ultimately reached by the House in a particular appeal. Yet no record is kept of the oral interaction in the Lords. The arguments are not tape recorded, as they are in the US Supreme Court and the European Court of Justice, nor could a transcript of the oral argument in an appeal be produced.[44] Even the edited versions of counsel's arguments which appear in the Appeal Cases are derived largely from consultations with counsel after the appeal is over rather than from the law reporter's notes.

This somewhat astonishing state of affairs in the supreme tribunal in the United Kingdom seems to stem from the fact that the hearings before the Appellate Committees are in constitutional theory still parliamentary proceedings and therefore the subject of parliamentary privilege. Under House of Lords Standing Order No. 15,[45] the printing or publishing of anything relating to the proceedings of the Lords is subject to the privilege of the House. It might be argued, therefore, that the publication of several of the oral interchanges reported earlier in this chapter is in breach of the parliamentary privilege asserted in this Standing Order.

But whatever the reason why no adequate records have been kept of the oral interchange, their absence is a serious handicap to any study of judicial decision-making in the House of Lords. Even the reports we have can be seriously misleading - particularly in their omission of the vast majority of interventions by Law Lords.[46] Indeed, of all the instances of Bar-Bench interactions mentioned in this chapter and the last, only two appear in the attenuated versions of counsel's arguments which are published in the Appeal Cases.[47] Inevitably, this means that significant aspects of the decision-making process in the Lords are lost to posterity. Judicial interjections which change the course of appeals go unreported. Interchanges which provide a guide to the Law Lords' 'situation-sense'[48] in appeals go unrecorded. Signs of judicial awareness of political pressure (a rare event in the Lords) go unnoticed.[49] Equally the persuasive influence of counsel's submissions, the pictures they paint, the baited analogies they proffer, the avenues they close in their arguments - all these are left neglected. Worst of all, the lack of proper transcripts helps perpetuate the notion amongst academic scholars that the real work of the Law Lord, and the only important aspect of appeals going to the House of Lords, are the speeches produced at the end of the day. This concentration on the end product, to the exclusion of the process by which it was arrived at, is intellectually dangerous and academically unsound.

CONCLUSION

The aim of this chapter has been to demonstrate that the restrictive and persuasive powers of counsel must be balanced against their counterparts in the hands of the Law Lords. Not only do the Law Lords possess restrictive, interrogative and persuasive powers, they also act as a reference group for counsel sanctioning them negatively and positively for their arguments in appeals.[50] This suggests that the passages from Wetter and Llewellyn which I quoted earlier[51] are misleading. The interchange between Bench and Bar is not one way. It should be seen as a dialectic to which each side contributes. Counsel are not always the authors of their own submissions: frequently they borrow a line of argument from the judgements in the courts below,[52] and this may in turn be appropriated by a Law Lord in his speech. Again, a Law Lord's intervention may commend itself to counsel who incorporates it in his submissions, which may then be taken up by the other Law Lords.

Each side is engaged in a series of 'negotiations' over the role performance of the other and each encounters role conflicts during the interaction. In sum, we may conclude that the oral interchange between Law Lords and counsel can play a significant part in the disposition of appeals coming to the Lords, and that hitherto the importance of this two-way interchange has been unjustifiably overlooked. In the next chapter I shall turn to deal with another form of interaction which affects the decision-making process in the House but which, in Britain at least, has also been neglected. It is judicial interaction.

5 Law Lord Interaction and the Process of Judgement

> You have the enormous advantage of being able to talk things over with them. I don't say agreeing with them or disagreeing with them; but one is much more likely to be right after one's talked it over informally and quietly, not in a forensic way, than one is if one just acts on one's own impressions.
>
> Lord Kilbrandon

BEHIND THE APPELLATE CURTAIN

Contemporary judicial interaction, like the inner working of the British Cabinet, is an activity which it is difficult to write about in an informed way. Hence its neglect by British scholars. Those who are on the inside - judges and officials alike - accept, for a variety of reasons, that their deliberations must remain secret.[1] Only thus can the candid exchange of ideas, the free flow of discussion, which are essential to the efficient operation of the court, be encouraged. Only thus can 'insider dealing', the profiting from leaks of confidential information, be prevented. Only thus can the prestige and the authority of the court be maintained. So run the arguments. Those who are on the outside - counsel, academics and other interested spectators - whether they accept these arguments or not, encounter almost insuperable problems of access. In the past twenty years the diaries and personal papers of several US Supreme Court Justices have become available to researchers, and in 1979 *The Brethren*,[2] a major breach in the wall of secrecy, was published. But British judges have been more reticent - no Richard Crossman or Barbara Castle has emerged from their ranks, as yet. It follows that we now have considerably more information as to the internal proceedings of the Supreme

Court, both in general and in particular cases, than those of the House of Lords. But many problems remain. The writings of any one judge are selective and only partially reliable. Thus, a comparison of the competing accounts left by Supreme Court Justices reveals numerous gaps and not a few contradictions.

Denied first-hand access to judicial interaction, dependent on discrepant and ambiguous second-hand accounts, scholars in their third-hand efforts reconstruct reality in disparate ways.[3] Until the problem of access is resolved, the best that can be done is to put the reader on his guard and whenever possible to examine the compatibility of the judges' writings, actions and interview responses. This I have tried to do.

THE LAW LORDS AND THE COURT OF APPEAL

There are many aspects to judicial interaction. A Law Lord interacts with judges from inferior courts, as well as his colleagues; with judges in the past and in the future as well as those in the present.

Direct interaction between the Law Lords and members of the Court of Appeal, as we saw earlier,[4] is inhibited by geographical and other factors. Nevertheless, in the early 1970s five Lords Justices and five Lords of Appeal were Benchers of the same Inn - the Middle Temple - and this meant that occasions arose not infrequently for them to discuss, if they so wished, appeals from Court of Appeal decisions which were going to the Lords. So far as I could ascertain, most Lords Justices regarded it as improper to talk about such cases until after the House had produced its decision. But one judge I spoke to admitted to having discussed with the Law Lords several cases while they were before the House, which he had dealt with in the Court of Appeal.

Indirect interaction during appeals before the Lords, on the other hand, was welcomed by Law Lord and Lord Justice alike. The Law Lords have on numerous occasions stressed the importance which they attach to having the benefit of the opinions of the judges in the Court of Appeal on particular points which arise in appeals.[5] Thus the principal misgiving voiced by the Law Lords when the procedure enabling cases to 'leap-frog' from the High Court to the Lords was introduced, was that they would be deprived of the judgements of the Court of Appeal in such cases.[6]

It is almost as though the Law Lords regard the judgements in the Court of Appeal as arguments by sophisticated advocates which are additional to the arguments put forward by counsel, rather as in previous centuries the House of Lords would take the advice of the professional judges.[7] And, as with counsel, the Lords will take more account of some judges' views than others.[8]

Members of the Court of Appeal, in their turn, often write their judgements with the House of Lords in mind. Lord Justice Diplock openly admitted in his judgement in *Hardwick Game Farm* v. *Suffolk Agricultural Association* that, 'Its function, if any, is to provide ammunition for the parties in the House of Lords.'[9] Another Lord Justice observed to me that he took more care and precision in expressing his reasons where an appeal was likely to go to the Lords, and that in such cases it might sometimes be desirable to express *obiter* views, where, if the Court of Appeal's decision was to remain unappealed, *obiter* views would be inappropriate. Lord Denning told me that he drafted his dissent in *Conway* v. *Rimmer*[10] with the House in mind. It was also, apparently,[11] intended to help Conway to obtain legal aid for the appeal to the Lords. On occasion, moreover, the wide statements of principle enunciated by Lord Denning in his judgements seem to be designed to force the House of Lords into a broader legal discussion in disposing of an appeal than the Law Lords might otherwise have felt was incumbent upon them.[12]

The House in recent years has not been loathe to respond to such challenges and as we saw in Chapter 3 has several times felt it necessary to rebuke the lower court openly and forcefully.[13] In the nature of things the Law Lords are usually left with the last word in their dialogue with the Court of Appeal, but even this advantage has been tempered by Lord Denning's comments in *The Discipline of Law* on reversals of his decisions by the House of Lords. He was even more explicit in one complex commercial case in 1978 where he is reported[14] to have said,

[In two previous cases] the trade set the court an examination paper with many questions to answer. The Court of Appeal did their best, but recently their papers were marked by the House of Lords in [a decision in 1978][15]. They only gave the Court of Appeal about 50 per cent.

The House of Lords were fortunate in that there was no one to examine them or mark their papers. If there was, his Lordship did not suppose that the House of Lords would get any higher marks than the Court of Appeal.

APPEAL COMMITTEES AND APPELLATE COMMITTEES

Apart from discussion with members of the Court of Appeal or publicity in the media - both relatively rare events - the first a Law Lord is likely to hear of a potential appeal is when he sits on an Appeal Committee. The House of Lords has much less control over the cases that it hears than the US Supreme Court.[16] Eighty per cent of its civil caseload and 60 per cent of its criminal caseload during the period of my study came to the House as of right or by leave of a lower court. Only in the remaining cases had an Appeal Committee of the House consisting of three, or on rare occasions five, Law Lords granted leave to appeal. Appeal Committees are scheduled to sit about fifteen to twenty times a year but the dates assigned to them remain provisional, and should a full appeal hearing continue longer than anticipated the Appeal Committee may be squeezed out.[17] Equally, if a full appeal collapses unexpectedly it may be possible to arrange a sitting of the Appeal Committee at short notice. Selection of the Law Lords to sit on these committees is done by the Principal Clerk to the Judicial Office. Given the circumstances in which the sittings are finally arranged, the Principal Clerk's choice is often effectively reduced to three of the Law Lords who sat on the previous appeal or who are about to sit on the next appeal.[18] He tends not to ask the senior Law Lords to sit and no efforts are made to tailor the panel to the petition under consideration by, for example, picking a Chancery Law Lord to sit on a Chancery petition for leave. Selection for Appellate Committees, a mystery in the eyes of counsel and Law Lord alike, is handled rather differently. No attempt is made to ensure that the Law Lords who sat on the Appeal Committee and granted leave to appeal, are asked to sit on the Appellate Committee which hears the full appeal. Sometimes none of the three sit, sometimes all of them do. Selection, although theoretically in the hands of the Lord Chancellor, is actually delegated to his Permanent Secretary who consults the Lord Chancellor in cases of difficulty. Lord Hailsham described the guidelines which operated in his first period as Lord Chancellor, in the following way,

> Obviously cases which have party political implications should normally be adjudicated by non-political judges.[19] Also the composition of the panel must take account of the nature of the problems to be adjudicated upon, an expert in each of the relevant fields being made available where possible. A Scottish Law Lord should usually sit in all Scottish cases. These special considerations are, however, exceptional. The normal practice is to select the most convenient panel available.

In practice the Permanent Secretary often has remarkably little room for manoeuvre. At the end of each legal term he meets with the Principal Clerk of the Judicial Office and the Judicial Clerk to the Privy Council. Together they compile a provisional list setting out the order for hearings of appeals in the following term in the House and in the Privy Council and the two clerks brief the Permanent Secretary as to the talents needed in the various appeals. If there is a Chancery appeal in the Lords and a commercial case before the Privy Council then other things being equal the Chancery Lords will sit in the Lords. Equally, Chancery Law Lords tend not to sit on criminal appeals.[20] When a Scots appeal comes to the Lords strong efforts are made to ensure that one, if not both, Scottish Law Lords will sit.[21] But of course other things never are equal. If the senior Law Lord is Scottish he may be wanted to head a strong team in the Privy Council or to preside in an English appeal before a second Appellate Committee. A balance has to be struck to ensure that junior Law Lords are not relegated to the Privy Council for more than 50 per cent of the year.[22] Judges who have sat in an appeal in the Court of Appeal and since become Lords of Appeal, have to be excluded when that appeal comes before the Lords.[23] On top of this, because of the difficulty in synchronising the hearings in the Appellate Committee and the Judicial Committee of the Privy Council there is a tendency to keep the same or almost the same panel of Law Lords together for several appeals on end.

As if the logistical problems of organising suitable panels for the House and the Privy Council several weeks or months in advance were not enough, the Lord Chancellor's Office has to cope with subsequent developments - often at the last minute. A case may drastically overrun its estimate,[24] a judge can fall ill, or decline to sit because of an interest in a case,[25] he may want to attend a conference in a foreign country or be asked to serve as Chairman of a Royal Commission or a Public Inquiry. As far as I could gather, when such incidents occur the Permanent Secretary's Secretary will try to exchange the relevant Law Lord with one on the other panel or will call on a retired Law Lord to sit (taking whoever is available). On rare occasions, the Lord Chancellor himself may step into the breach. Such complications go a long way to ensuring that any present-day Lord Chancellor would find it exceedingly difficult to 'pack the court' in cases of a particular type, even if he were minded to do so. They are also the explanation of the occasional 'freak' panel of Law Lords which is thrown up, for example, one with five common Law Lords of Appeal or one which contains no Scottish Law Lord in a Scots appeal.

The Law Lords receive their invitations to sit on the various committees scheduled for a particular week, three weeks in advance, but unless they specifically ask to have them earlier, they will receive the printed Cases only a few days in advance. Although informal discussion could take place at this stage between panel members invited to sit on a particular appeal or (where leave to appeal was granted by the House) between panel members and members of the Appeal Committee, my researches did not suggest that this was a frequent occurence.

INTERACTION IN THE LORDS

Once the hearing of an appeal commences, however, the interchange between the Law Lords begins in earnest. As we saw in the last chapter, many of their interventions during the oral arguments are actually aimed at their colleagues. Outside the Committee Room constant discussions take place between the Law Lords.[26] They commence at the lunch recess. As the judges file from the room, as they wait for the lift, as they descend in the lift and drift towards their rooms, they are conversing together about the morning session. The Law Lords generally lunch together, though in separate groups,[27] and the discussion may continue. If not, the exchanges begin anew as the Law Lords gather prior to returning to the Committee Room. Then at four o'clock, when the day's hearing has ended, the Law Lords meet informally for 15 minutes or so in a corridor[28] off the Chamber of the House of Lords, where several of them have their rooms, in order to discuss the day's developments. Normally,[29] that is the end of the discussion until the following morning when the Law Lords assemble in the House of Lords Library. Depending on when they each arrive, further exchanges may ensue for ten minutes or so until it is time for the hearing to be resumed.

Most Law Lords find this process of continuous consultation (which occurs both in the House of Lords and the Privy Council[30]) extremely valuable. As Lord Salmon explained,

Well, I think discussion is always good and the more you hear of the other man's view the more it helps you to form your own. I suppose it is a matter of temperament ... It doesn't mean that because you are listening to the other man, you necessarily agree with him, but it is very important to know why he is thinking what he is thinking.

Lord Cross added,

You are discussing the case the whole time with your colleagues and ... it is infinitely helpful. From what they have been saying, you may suddenly see a thing in a new light.

Lord Pearson was in agreement.

It is an important feature of our system, I would say, that you get to know what your colleagues are thinking. If you find yourselves all of the same mind, well that is very nice, but if you are differing, you have to argue, though not at great length. These preliminary discussions at four o'clock every day in the corridor or as you are walking into or out of the Committee Room ...[are] important because that is when the minds are not yet made up ... to a greater or lesser degree we are still in suspense.

The debates differ from the dialectic between the Law Lords and counsel. Lord Pearce felt this for he said,

It is a terribly different tempo from the argument in court by counsel. You are arguing shorthand with somebody who has been primed with all the stuff ... It is a very compressed argument. 'But if you say that, then it leads to [such and such] consequences ... ' or somebody says 'No, because in that case, ... '. In that way the issues get pretty well boiled down.

When there are strong differences of opinion between the Law Lords the arguments which began in the corridor may be continued in the presiding Law Lord's room or in the Conference Room. Yet at this formative stage some Law Lords will only have tentative views and it is not uncommon for one or more to change his mind. Lord Reid told me that he had commonly changed his mind during the argument of a case,

You may change your mind off your own bat, or you may change your mind because the respondent has put forward his case in a much better way than you realised was likely, or you may change your mind because of what your colleagues say. I would think that if you can't change your mind then you are a pretty bad judge.

Naturally some of the Law Lords who are more sure of their positions in a particular case will try at this stage to win round their colleagues who are undecided. One of them adverted to this explicitly.

You break off say at four o'clock, then starts the argument. Three people arguing, then up drifts a fourth, and you really thrash the thing out. Then somebody raises a point which you think you can demolish. I mean, another Law Lord, two other Law Lords, you want to convince them that the other point is right. You look at a Law Report when you come in, in the morning beforehand, and casually remark as you gather in the library for a quarter of an hour, that it seems to you that the case of so-and-so really has got the right principle much more. Then the argument starts again. Then [the presiding Law Lord] says, 'Well, we had better get along', then you go into the lift and then you listen to counsel.

THE FIRST CONFERENCE

With the completion of counsel's submissions the hearing comes to an end. An usher calls out 'Clear the Bar' and counsel, solicitors, parties and spectators are swept hurriedly from the room. If it is close to a recess the Law Lords' deliberations will take place in the Conference Room[31] after the adjournment. Usually, however, the Law Lords (now alone apart from the clerk from the Judicial Office[32]) commence the conference in the Committee Room as soon as the Bar is cleared. Having ascertained that his brethren are prepared to express provisional opinions on the case (they almost invariably are), the presiding Law Lord turns to the most junior Law Lord and asks him for his views.[33] Thereafter, each Law Lord, in inverse order of seniority, gives an outline of his impressions and his conclusions. As in the Privy Council[34] and the US Supreme Court,[35] the conference at this stage is more akin to a series of monologues rather than a discussion, for it is rare for the speakers to be interrupted. Most of the Law Lords I spoke to said that it was unusual for their colleagues to spring a surprise at this stage since their provisional views had normally emerged during the discussions between the Law Lords which had been taking place throughout the appeal. Yet some Law Lords play their cards very close to their chests and will not disclose their opinion until the very last minute, while others (although this is rare) may be so undecided that they are reluctant to state even a tentative opinion until they have heard their colleagues' views. Similarly, in the US Supreme Court a Justice may postpone his contribution to the conference until his colleagues have expressed their views.[36]

If, when all the Law Lords have spoken, they are not unanimous, the presiding Law Lord will enquire whether any of his brethren wishes to alter his opinion in any way. As in the Privy Council and the US Supreme Court, a general discussion may then ensue. Thereafter, the judges in the Supreme Court, though not those in the House or in the Privy Council, formally vote on the appeal[37] (in inverse order of seniority).[38] However, where the Law Lords are all agreed for substantially the same reasons, the presiding Law Lord may say, 'Well, look here, there is no point in having five speeches in this case. Who's going to do this?' Taking account of their respective workloads, expertise and interest in the case, the Law Lords may then decide who is to write the major opinion or who is to deal with a particular aspect of the case. This informal arrangement does not prevent any of the other Law Lords writing if they so wish. The Law Lords will also, in an effort to avoid unnecessary duplication, frequently agree that one of their number will deal with the facts of the case in his speech. Although the presiding judge may take the lead in suggesting such arrangements, in the normal course of events these opinion assignments are not made by the presiding judge but are the product of collective agreement. Nevertheless, in very exceptional cases, e.g. *DPP* v. *Smith* or *Heaton's Transport Ltd* v. *TGWU*, a presiding judge may determine that for policy reasons only one opinion of the court should be produced and that it should appear under his name.* In the Privy Council the presiding judge, even if he is in a minority of one, assigns who is to write the opinion of the court.[39] In practice, presiding judges who are in a minority suggest either that the judge who is in the middle of the majority bloc should write the opinion, or simply leave it to the majority bloc to decide which of them will write. In the US Supreme Court on the other hand, the presiding judge (usually the Chief Justice) assigns who is to write the opinion of the court only if he is in the majority. (If he is not, then the senior Justice in the minority assigns the opinion.) This creates a potential for tactical voting by a Chief Justice who can see that the view which he favours is not going to prevail, in that he may vote with the majority in order to control the opinion assignment and thus attempt to minimise the damage inflicted by the decision of the Court on the view which he actually holds.[40]

Yet in many, perhaps the majority of cases in the Lords, it is not cut and dried who is going to write.[41] Where there is substantial divergence of opinion or even if the Law Lords are agreed but it is plain that they are agreed for widely different reasons, it is accepted that the number of speeches cannot be cut, at least at this stage, and the conference comes to an end. In all, the conferences normally last only half an hour or so, though some may be over in ten minutes, while others, where the case is complex or difficult or one in which several different opinions have emerged, may go on

---

*Even then he requires the acquiescence of his colleagues. In *DPP* v. *Smith*, Lord Kilmuir LC insisted that there should be only one judgement. Although it appears under his name, one of the Law Lords involved informed me that it was in fact drafted by the Lord Chief Justice, Lord Parker. In the US Supreme Court there are also cases where the Court strives to attain a united front, *e.g.* *Brown* v. *Board of Education*, *Swann* v. *Charlotte-Micklenburg Board of Education* and *US* v. *Nixon*.

for up to two hours. In only a few, exceptional cases have the conferences exceeded this, e.g. *Ross-Smith* v. *Ross-Smith* (half a day) or *Heaton's Transport Ltd* v. *TGWU* (a whole day). In the Supreme Court, however, the amount of conference time devoted to particular cases can be much greater. In part this is because the Justices have not had the advantage of lengthy oral argument from counsel, interspersed with exchanges with their colleagues. The general discussion which ensues after each has given his preliminary views is their first opportunity for collective consultation on a case. Under Warren Burger's regime, Justices may speak as frequently and as long as they wish,[42] though this may not advance the cause they are pleading. Certainly Justices in the past who were thought by some to speak too much in conference, *e.g.* Pitney,[43] Frankfurter and Harlan,[44] did not endear themselves to their colleagues on this account. On the other hand, the length of discussion in the past has also been drastically curtailed on occasion by a Chief Justice, such as Hughes, who appeared to prefer efficiency to democracy.

THE DRAFTING STAGE

Once the first conference is over, the curious process of drafting opinions begins. In the Lords this takes six weeks on average;[45] in the Supreme Court it may last many months. In the Supreme Court the assigned opinion is normally the first to be circulated (dissents and concurrences come later), but in the Lords and the Privy Council the opinions can emerge in any order. Where there are several speeches, some are produced within a week or so of the conference or the opinion assignment, and then circulated amongst the other judges. The bulk of the remaining speeches are circulated in the next two or three weeks, with one or two speeches taking rather longer. In part, differences in speed of production are attributable to natural differences between the judges. There have always been some Law Lords[46] and Justices[47] to whom writing appears to come more easily and naturally than to others[48] (and others again who will sometimes labour over a multiplicity of drafts before being in any way satisfied).[49] Lord Cross hinted at such differences in our interview,

It is a matter of individual preference. Some people always

want to say something. If I feel that I am in complete agreement
with some other people who will probably enjoy writing more
than I do, I would tend to sit back and wait until I get their
opinion.

Very occasionally, judges who do not normally experience
difficulties in composition encounter cases where the opinion will
not write. In an extreme situation the judge may even end up
writing an opinion the other way, since he is unable to produce
one which he finds intellectually acceptable, which supports his
original view. But such cases are rare.

On the other hand, differences in speed of production can also
be the result of deliberate decisions. In the Lords and the Privy
Council a judge will sometimes produce and circulate his opinion
particularly quickly in the hope of persuading some of his brethren
to change their minds.[50] More commonly a Law Lord will decide
to delay writing. He will usually do so for one of three reasons.
First, the desire to complete opinions for cases heard earlier in the
term, either in the House or the Privy Council. Second, because,
as Lord Cross suggested, the Law Lord may be intending simply
to concur with another colleague's judgement unless it contains
something unexpected with which he cannot agree. Third, where
he is in doubt or the court is heavily divided, a Law Lord may
wish to see what his colleagues produce before writing his own
speech. Five of the fifteen Law Lords whom I interviewed said
they had done this from time to time.[51] Lord Cross said,

> I think in a case where there are five Law Lords, and two of
> them are strong one way and two the other and you really find it
> difficult, then obviously you would say to both sides, 'Well,
> look here, I am open to conviction, I will wait and see what you
> have to say.'

A few Law Lords went further. One confessed that he 'often liked
to see the others' drafts' before writing and Lord Radcliffe added,

> I would have thought one constantly waited when there was a
> division or the question arose whether you should add anything
> to what was going to be the view. Yes, [probably] more often
> than not I waited to see what one or more other opinions were.

But six other Law Lords, Lords Reid, Guest, Denning, Pearce, Hailsham and Gardiner, indicated that they had never waited in this way before writing an opinion - although they did not necessarily think that there would be any impropriety in so waiting. Lord Reid's response was typically forthright,

> I don't think I would do that, no. It is said that before my time there were members of the House of Lords who used to do that, but I don't think one does that nowadays. You write out your stuff if you think you want to write, and if you find that the other man against you has said something that you didn't expect, well then you either cancel what you have said or you alter it, but no, I don't think it is a good way to wait and see how the cat jumps.

MULTIPLE JUDGEMENTS AND THE PURSUIT OF UNITY

Lord Reid's answer raises a further question. What sorts of consideration lead a Law Lord to write anything at all, instead of formally concurring[52] with a colleague's speech? It transpired that there are no hard and fast rules on the matter. Lord Reid told me,

> If you feel that something ought to be said and somebody else is going to give the leading judgement, well then you say it. I think, so as not to complicate the thing too much one concurs if you are in substantial agreement with what the other man says and may add something if you want to. But it's all done extremely ... it's a matter of judgement as you go along, there is nothing like a rule.

Lord Pearson confirmed that it was very much a matter of personal choice,

> If I feel I have got something to say, I write it, or if I feel I have got nothing to add to what everyone else has said, I tend to concur. Personally, I think unless it has been pretty definitely arranged that only one of us should write - that is done sometimes - I would think it otherwise better that two or three should write. But I have no very settled practice in that way: it

depends largely on what you think of the case. I mean, it is a bad thing to write unless you can write carefully ... therefore I would not write unless I had time to take a bit of trouble.

While it did emerge that a Law Lord would be more likely to write if the House was divided, or if it was overruling a unanimous lower court decision, most of the Law Lords whom I interviewed were agreed that unnecessary multiplication of opinions was to be avoided. Accordingly, once all the Law Lords who intend to write have written, it is sometimes possible for the number of opinions to be reduced. But the decision as to which speeches should be cut or pruned is not a collective one. Occasionally, two who have circulated speeches which are substantially on the same lines may agree between themselves that one will withdraw and merely concur with the other, but usually the decision is a voluntary sacrifice by an individual Law Lord.[53] All the Law Lords I spoke to were agreed that there was no expectation that more junior Law Lords ought to defer to their seniors by withdrawing their opinions. There was only one exception, a very junior Law Lord who seemed to feel the natural diffidence that any new member of a 'club' experiences. In fact, since speeches are reported in order of seniority, it is only natural that those coming fourth and fifth should feel more pressure than their seniors to curtail their speeches. Yet it should be realised that the order in which speeches are reported in most cases bears little relation to the order in which they are produced. Some Law Lords like to wait for others to produce their opinions, as we have seen; indeed, some past Law Lords were said to be notorious for waiting till the end and creaming off the best of the others' opinions. Recent critiques[54] of multiple opinions in the Lords, for example Professor Cross's caustic references to 'the second or third speech in the House of Lords which concurs in the result reached by its precursors after the same review of all the authorities with as little reference to principle ...'[55] seem to overlook the fact that the first speech on the record is not necessarily the first to be produced. What do the critics expect of a Law Lord, particularly a junior Law Lord, who gets his opinion out first which deals with the whole case, and circulates it to his colleagues? Later, other speeches are produced saying much the same thing. Is he then expected to withdraw his opinion? He surely cannot be expected to do this very often simply because he is number five on the list. He is entitled to the fruits of his labours and to express his views in his own way. This is all the more true since the opinion of a Law Lord is in constitutional theory a speech delivered in a debate in the Upper Chamber of Parliament, and the 'encouragement' of repeated withdrawals interferes with the peer's freedom of speech.

As we shall see later, the Law Lords when I interviewed them were divided on the issue of multiple opinions. While a large majority favoured having several speeches in common law hard cases there was considerable support for a norm of single speeches in criminal appeals particularly those based on a point of statutory construction. Even as staunch a believer in having more than one opinion as Lord Reid approved of the single judgement of the court given in *Heaton's Transport Ltd* v. *TGWU*.

> You see you have got to take public opinion and public policy into account and that was for consumption by non-lawyers and it might have been confusing. I wasn't in it but I think they were quite right in that case to have one judgement, but there are comparatively few cases in which considerations of that sort would lead you to one judgement and of course they took far more trouble in correlating their own views. We couldn't possibly spare the time to be as thorough as they were in discussing the thing afterwards .... We can't start a sort of committee meeting over a joint judgement, there simply isn't time. Now they tell me in some of these foreign courts they spend weeks discussing their joint judgement. We couldn't do it, we would never get through our work.

The Law Lords of course are quite familiar with the technique of producing a single judgement of the court, because of their experience in the Privy Council. But for this very reason some have reservations about introducing the single judgement with greater frequency in the Lords.[56] Lord Radcliffe considered it one of the strengths of the Privy Council that,

> The people who were accustomed to being in the Council got rather good at rendering one judgement that reflected the opinions of the others. There was a sort of tradition that you didn't take a strong line unless it was one which could be shared by the others.

Other Law Lords were less enthusiastic. Lord Pearce was one of them.

> We all know that in the Privy Council it gave quite a bit of weakness over the centuries to a Privy Council judgement that sentences were put in for the man who thought the appeal was doubtful as to whether it should succeed, and felt that it was more likely it should fail, as against the man who wrote it, who was certain it should succeed, and so he would put in the sentences .... You are getting a compromise judgement in a sense.

Composite judgements of this sort are much rarer in the Lords, though here are some famous, not to say notorious, examples, including - in addition to Lord Wilberforce's judgement of the court in *Heaton's* - Viscount Simon's solo performance in *Duncan* v. *Cammell, Laird & Co.*[57] and Lord Devlin's 'codification' of the law of exemplary damages in *Rookes* v. *Barnard*. As the latter told me,

> Lord Reid had quite strong views about it but because it was purely an English point of law he didn't wish to write on it. I think he said to me, ... well you put something down and I'll see if I agree with it, and I did and the others made a number of suggestions so that it became rather a judgement of the court in that sense. I modified it a good bit to fit in with other people's views.

The other criticism of some Privy Council judgements is diametrically opposed to the first. That is, what purports to be a judgement of the court is in fact that of one man. As Lord Denning recalled,

> You had a case, then six weeks later some chap comes up with his judgement. Well by that time you've forgotten all about it and you can't be bothered about the details and you don't take all that interest, or at least at all events I didn't by that time. I think if you leave it to one, you leave it to him and you don't go through that judgement critically in the ordinary way. That's human nature, you've got other things to do.

Yet, despite the misgivings of some Law Lords over single

judgements, there was in the early 1970s a general willingness (which seems to be on the increase in recent years) on the part of most Law Lords to sacrifice a measure of freedom of speech in the interests of a common front, in a certain minority of appeals.[58] To what extent, if any, did this somewhat tentative support for unity in the court manifest itself in relation to the right to dissent?

In an attempt to answer this question I asked the Law Lords what factors led them to publish dissenting opinions and whether there was any feeling in the Lords that dissents should be discouraged. Commentators have frequently discussed the functions served by published dissents. They provide comfort to judges in the lower courts who are being reversed and to losing litigants, they indicate to the layman that unanimity is no easier to obtain in difficult areas of law than, for example, in the higher reaches of science or theology, they highlight the areas of law which are developing and uncertain, and they indicate possible limits to the legal doctrines espoused in the majority of opinions. Yet the dissenting judge may, and often will, have intended something quite different in producing the dissent. The issue of timing is important. Circulation of a dissent within the court is not the same as making it public. At the first stage, the dissenter has not given up hope of influencing his colleagues and his dissent is part of the ongoing interaction between members of the court. For example, Lord Radcliffe told me,

> If I couldn't persuade my colleagues in the course of the hearing and the discussion afterwards, I tended to leave it alone and see whether, if I really worked hard at my opinion and circulated it before the decision was handed down, I might perhaps knock somebody off his perch.

Even if the dissenter fails to win more support for his position, his dissent may lead to changes in the majority opinion(s). Thus, John Harlan who dissented in 63 per cent of the votes taken on the Warren Court from 1963 to 1967 was well pleased if his heavily researched dissents were plagiarised in a revised majority opinion since the dialogue had worked to produce a better Court opinion. He was much more frustrated when the majority writer declined to enter into a dialogue since he saw no need to respond to the dissent - this Harlan considered to be bad judicial craftsmanship.[59] Whether successful or not some judges withdraw their dissents at this stage, considering that they can serve no further useful purpose.

The decision to make a dissent public may involve different considerations. Often it is an attempt to shift the arena of combat.[60] Having lost in the court, the judge can appeal to history, 'to the brooding spirit of the law, to the intelligence of a future day'.[61] It is in this situation that Law Lords can be said to be interacting with future judges, including their successors. In the words of one Law Lord,

> I think one of the most important justifications of dissent is in consequence of the 1966 Declaration [permitting the House to overrule a previous decision of its own]. One hopes that a dissent might influence a court which has to reconsider the matter.

Sometimes the alternative arena[62] is a law reform body, such as the Law Commission, or even the legislature. Several Law Lords mentioned the possibility of reform as a reason for publishing a dissent.[63]

Again, the dissent may be designed to circumscribe the effect of the majority opinion(s). Lord Radcliffe considered this to be the principal merit of a dissent,

> This is the value, I think, of the dissent process, that it does enable you to try to limit what you regard as an unsatisfactory line by some reasoned and carefully worked out contribution of your own.

Lord Pearson made a similar comment,

> I think it is regarded as useful to dissent, first of all it gives satisfaction to the dissenter, that he is not thought to believe in something which he does not believe in, and secondly, when the next case arises and it is a little bit further along the line or a bit short of the line, the dissent may be valuable. There is a difference between a unanimous decision in the House of Lords and a 3:2 conclusion. You look at the dissenting opinions for that reason.

At other times a judge dissents because he just cannot help

himself. Thus in the Privy Council before 1966 when dissents could not be published or recorded at length in the judgement book,[64] some were written none the less, not only in an attempt to influence the majority but also because they had a cathartic value for the writer. As one Law Lord informed me,

> All of us feel there is no point in dissenting just because you disagree. One often does and there is no object in recording a dissent. It is sometimes necessary to dissent in order to show one of the parties that their case has been sympathetically listened to. In other cases, it is necessary to dissent in order to encourage some review of the law. In other cases you just can't help it.

Some commentators have argued (Professor Cross amongst them[65]), that too frequent resort to the right to dissent 'creates gnawing uncertainty in the law',[66] and have suggested that judges should exercise a measure of self-restraint in publishing them. There was some support for this view from about half my sample of Law Lords.[67]

> I think there should be unanimity if possible, and it has been said that there is too much dissent. I am inclined to think that maybe there is. (Lord Salmon)

> I don't think in an important matter of law I would dissent unless I were pretty sure. (Lord Kilbrandon)

> If there was a split and the other four were all strongly of one opinion I would probably acquiesce or give a dubitante opinion. (Lord MacDermott)

> If you are a bit wobbly and the other four are going one way, well then the sensible thing to do is simply to say, 'Well I am not quite sure about this, but anyway I won't dissent.' There is no good in dissenting unless you think you are right. (Lord Reid)

Even Lord Denning said, 'I don't think any of us would want to dissent unless we felt strongly about it ... I don't dissent unless I feel sufficiently strongly in a sense.'

It seems, however, that this is an area of conflicting role

THE PROCESS OF JUDGEMENT

perceptions, where the pressure for unanimity or unity, for collegiality and community, has to be balanced against the right to judicial individualism and judicial independence. As Lord Guest explained,

> I think there are two conflicting pressures. I think there's the one you mentioned, that dissent tends to diminish the authority of the decision, on the other hand I feel strongly that if one has anything to contribute one should express it, because you see one never knows whether in the future it may be that the dissenting judgement may become of importance.

It seems also that this is an area of changing expectations, for Viscount Radcliffe told me,

> When I first went to the Lords in 1949 there was a bit of an olde worlde feeling, you know, that we all ought to hang together and you oughtn't to expose the differences in the House of Lords because it weakened its authority.... Dissent was regarded as a more serious thing then.... Personally, I thought this was all nonsense, but it was there.

However, he added that by the time he retired in 1964 that view no longer prevailed. He could not remember anyone advancing it at that stage. If Lord Radcliffe was correct, then the pressure for unity in the court had declined, in this period, from being a relevant or even pivotal expectation to being a peripheral one in the role of a Law Lord. At any event, by the early 1970s the bulk of the Law Lords like Lord Guest clearly considered that in most circumstances the right to individual expression was more central to their role than any pressure to present a united front to the public.[68] Lord Reid was characteristically robust in his response to the question whether there was any feeling in the Lords that dissents should be discouraged. 'Oh, I think that's a piece of nonsense. I don't see why anybody who really does dissent shouldn't say so.' Lords Gardiner, Hailsham, Devlin, Denning and Radcliffe agreed. So too did Lord Cross,

> Is there any feeling against dissents? Oh, not in the least. On the whole they are all great individualists.... I do not think people think it is a sign of strength for all to agree. I think the

attitude is much more, we are all individuals and we all take our own line. The fact that we disagree with one another doesn't matter tuppence.

Lord Pearson,

No, I don't think so. One prefers to have a unanimous conclusion. It is nice to be all thinking the same, but there is no pressure on people not to dissent. Of course, if it is a 3:2 division, you can see that there might be rather strenuous arguments with somebody who might be persuadable, but on the whole I think, no.

and Lord Pearce,

I doubt that. They are fairly determined people by the time they get to the House of Lords. They are not going to be pushed off their view because four other people think it is wrong. Naturally, you regret to see your colleagues are so misguided, and you use your best arguments to stop them going down the wrong way.... If it dilutes the authority, so be it.

In certain European courts on the other hand, dissents are not encouraged, indeed in a few of them it is still not possible to publish dissents.[69] The dissent rates in the US Federal Courts of Appeals vary by circuit but are all markedly less than in the Supreme Court in recent times. On some circuits there is an unwritten rule that one does not dissent unless the issue is one about which the judge has exceptionally strong feelings.[70] Canon 19 of the Canons of Judicial Ethics promulgated by the American Bar Association is in a similar vein.

It is of high importance that judges constituting a court of last resort should use effort and self-restraint to promote solidarity of conclusion and the consequent influence of judicial decision. A judge should not yield to pride of opinion or value more highly his individual reputation than that of the court to which he should be loyal. Except in cases of conscientious difference of opinion on fundamental principle, dissenting opinions should be discouraged in courts of last resort.

Nevertheless in the Supreme Court itself, the rate of published dissents has fluctuated throughout its history. When Taft and Hughes were Chief Justices (1921-41), there were relatively few dissenting opinions. Thus, between 1930 and 1937 the ratio of dissenting opinions to decisions of the court was 1 to 9 (0.11). In 1938 the number of dissents began to rise (the ratio was 0.25), in 1948 it was 93:124 (0.75) and it remained at around this figure for ten years before reaching a peak in 1960 of 111:118 (0.94). Thereafter, the rate fell to 0.71 (between 1961 and 1968) but, with the appointment of Warren Burger as Chief Justice in 1969 and further Nixon nominees in the early 1970s, the rate rose once more and for the first time the number of dissenting opinions exceeded the number of opinions of the court.[71]

Commentators attribute these fluctuations in the frequency of published dissents not just to changes in the ideological balance in the Court[72] but also, as in the House of Lords, to changes in the judges' roles. Danelski has argued that in the Taft and Hughes Courts it was an accepted norm that a Justice should not dissent unless it was absolutely necessary.[73] Both Taft and Hughes supported this norm. Taft never really approved of dissents except as a last resort, regarding them as a breach of institutional loyalty and an attack on certainty in the law.[74] Hughes, like Taft, readily adopted the role of mediator or 'social leader',[75] endeavouring to reduce tensions and to reconcile differences amongst his brethren. His purpose, it has been said, was 'to secure as great a degree of unanimity as possible without compromising the integrity of the majority opinion'.[76] Stone, who as an Associate Justice had smarted under the 'restricted dissent' tradition, when he succeeded Hughes as Chief Justice in 1941 made it clear to his colleagues by deed and word that his perception of the role of the Chief Justice did not include suppressing dissent in any way. 'He did, of course, seek out all grounds for an honest reconciliation or accommodation of views within the Court', wrote one of his law clerks,[77] 'but he did not believe it proper to go further.' In fact, Danelski's account of his activities in conference casts doubts on whether he went even this far.[78] It seems he offered very little in the way of leadership to his colleagues, who very quickly acquired a taste for the new freedom for individual expression and the consequent change in their role. Subsequent Justices have never relinquished this freedom, yet as late as 1954 Justice Jackson could write,

Each dissenting opinion is a confession of failure to convince the writer's colleagues, and the true test of a judge is his influence in leading, not opposing, his court.[79]

Earl Warren, it is true, offered his colleagues a very effective form of leadership - though its essence was not always easy to define.[80] What evidence we have suggests that he frequently played the role of social leader in his Court[81] and that where he considered that circumstances warranted it, for example in *Brown* v. *Board of Education* he would work long and hard to obtain a unanimous opinion of the Court.[82] But his perception of his role as Chief Justice does not seem to have extended, in normal circumstances, to trying to reduce dissents.[83] Under Burger the Justices have, if anything, been even less inhibited in their use of dissent. Like the Law Lords, they clearly do not seem to think that there is any expectation that dissents should be discouraged.

In the light of the American studies, I asked the Law Lords whether they thought that the presiding Law Lord ought to adopt the role of a mediator who tries to reconcile differences in the court. The great majority of the Law Lords, including Lord Reid (then the senior Law Lord) had no doubts. The presiding man had no such role. As Lord Guest put it, 'No. It is no part of the presiding Law Lord to try and reconcile differences of opinion unless some question of public policy is involved.' Yet it is worth noting that there was a minority who gave some qualified support to the proposition.

Yes, but this is the responsibility of each of us. (Lord Wilberforce)

I think there's something in this as a description of the general corporate will of members of the Court, who will go as far as they can to give effect to it. But I don't know that it is a function of the presiding judge to try to enforce it. (Lord Kilbrandon)

Well, I think it is not the function of the presiding judge any more than the function of any other of the judges. I mean, any other of the Law Lords. I think we should all be striving to see if we can agree, but you cannot agree unless you are persuaded that the view propounded is correct in law. (Lord Salmon)

In the consultation which precedes the delivery of judgement the presiding judge should always consider whether further consultation will produce agreement. But he should never seek to blunt the edge of genuine differences which emerge after adequate consultation. (Lord Hailsham)

In fact as Lord Hailsham's remarks suggest, it is possible for the presiding judge to convene a second conference in the Lords if he feels that it would be of assistance in reducing the disparities between the circulated opinions. This happens as one Law Lord told me 'not very often, but not seldom'. Thus between March 1971 and March 1972 there was only one such conference. It took place when Lord Donovan reconvened the Committee which had heard *Albert* v. *MIB* and *MIB* v. *Meanen*, in a vain endeavour to reduce the number of separate judgements. In the following year there were two or three reconvened conferences. One of the most celebrated second conferences in recent times occurred in *Rookes* v. *Barnard* when the majority switched after a second conference and a re-hearing was requested. Some Law Lords told me that a case could be made for holding a conference more frequently after the circulation of opinions, particularly in cases like *Indyka* v. *Indyka* or *Boys* v. *Chaplin* where there were a multiplicity of divergent opinions. But even they conceded that there were practical drawbacks to such a suggestion. Apart from the sheer logistical difficulties in getting the same five Law Lords together, as one Law Lord put it, '[I]t would take up time and energy, and I think what one wants to avoid is any sort of undue pressure on people to change their minds.'

Other Law Lords opposed the suggestion, particularly Lords Reid and Guest,

Well, I don't think that's a very good plan. You see, by the time you will reach that stage it will be three or four weeks after the hearing and your recollection has got a little bit dull. If you started doing that it would mean a tremendous lot more work, and we really wouldn't have time to do it properly and, unless you are going to do it properly you had better not do it at all. That's my view anyway. Well, now take for example that Rhodesian UDI case in the Privy Council.[84] We had a good deal of conference about that and I changed what I said in some respects, but we couldn't do that as a general rule. There again

you ... really had to try and show a united face because of
political reasons. (Lord Reid)

I think that's an ideal solution, but I'm afraid it wouldn't work
in practice, because as you probably know, when one case is
finished you start on another one. And if you had a logjam of
discussions facing you of cases which have been heard perhaps a
month ago, I think it would be very difficult to keep up. It's
difficult enough to keep up in the House of Lords, writing your
judgements in the evening, at the same time as hearing
argument in other cases. I have known cases where the House
has had a further meeting to discuss points, and I think that has
been useful. But there is a limit to the discussions which can go
on, and if people have formed views they're unlikely to change
them. On the whole I think the system which we have works
really tolerably well. (Lord Guest)

In the Court of Appeal conferences after the preparation of
reserved judgements are exceedingly rare, but, as in the US
Supreme Court, there have been significant differences in role
perception between presiding judges. Thus Lord Justice Slesser
wrote of Scrutton LJ,

I do not think that, as Chairman of the Court, he thought it any
part of his duty to make others concur. In this respect he was in
great contrast to Lord Hanworth, who, in the other [division of
the] Court, would take endless pains to get agreement if he
could. In Scrutton's view, each should state his own conclusions. If we concurred, so far so good, if we did not, the
majority would settle the matter.[85]

Lord Denning's views and practice are almost identical to
Scrutton's in this area.[86]

We may conclude then from this excursus on multiple
judgements, dissents and the pursuit of unity, that the prevailing
ethos on these matters in the House of Lords is that of *laissez-faire*.
By and large, it is up to the individual Law Lord whether he writes
or not, and whether he dissents or not. Except in a small minority
of appeals the support for unity in the court is only tentative, there
is little resistance to dissents on the ground that they are
detrimental to the authority of the court and attempts to reconcile

differences in the court are the exception rather than the rule. These findings have two significant implications, first, for bargaining in the court and, secondly, for the character of judicial decision-making in the Lords.

Bargaining amongst the Justices of the US Supreme Court is an everyday occurrence, as repeated studies have shown us.[87] The 'necessity'[88] of a court opinion supported by five Justices, the value placed on a court opinion with unanimous or near unanimous support in cases of great constitutional significance, the divisive effect of concurring opinions and the view (held by many Justices, past and present) that dissents undermine the precedent value of a decision, all combine to produce a situation which is highly conducive to negotiations and bargains. Each Justice has effective bargaining counters in his vote, his ability to write a separate opinion (concurring or dissenting) and even his ability to keep silent. Time and again (but particularly where the Court is heavily divided), the majority opinion writer is forced into an accommodation with his colleagues, inserting or deleting sentences under the threat of a separate concurrence or even a dissent (possibly losing him his majority).[89] Thus, as in the Privy Council, the opinion of the Court may begin to resemble one written by a committee with all the attendant vices of such mode of production, for example, internal inconsistencies, disjointedness, compromise and confusion. In the House of Lords few if any of the factors which lead to bargaining in the Supreme Court or the International Court of Justice[90] are present. No opinion of the court is required and this together with the prevailing *laissez-faire* ethos on concurrences and dissents ensures that in normal circumstances 'threats' to write or to dissent, or 'offers' of silence carry little weight in the Lords. Accordingly, I would conclude that bargaining is much less common in the Lords than in the Supreme Court.

DECISION-MAKING IN THE LORDS: FIVE INDIVIDUALS OR A GROUP?

Does the collegiate nature of appellate courts mean that appellate judicial decision-making is a collective process? Some jurists and political scientists, particularly in North America, have tended to assume that it does and in consequence have turned for

enlightenment to 'small group analysis'[91] and other approaches
derived from social psychology. In the case of the House of Lords
this assumption cannot so easily be made. On paper, decisions of
the House could conform to three patterns, solos, quintets or
concertos. Solo decisions might occur in one of two ways. First,
where only one judge writes and his colleagues merely concur
without contributing anything of value to the decision. Secondly,
where five opinions are produced but each is a solo effort, *i.e.*
written without taking into account the arguments and opinions of
the other judges.[92] In either situation each judge who writes is
performing as if he were sitting on his own. Judicial decision-
making of this sort could not meaningfully be described as group
decision-making. Quintets are the antithesis of solos and the acme
of group decision-making. Fully collaborative performances with
continuous discussions, arguments and exchanges throughout the
hearing and the conferences, quintets would normally produce a
single joint judgement of the court. Concertos fall half way on the
continuum between solos and quintets. As such, they would
contain both group and individual elements with exchanges
between them.

    To which of these models do actual decisions of the Lords
conform? My researches suggested that the House was a delicate
balance of collegiality and individualism. Interaction between the
Law Lords takes place at various stages in an appeal, as we have
seen. Sometimes it takes the form best described as five individuals
in action,[93] sometimes it is genuinely collaborative,[94] mostly it is
somewhere in between the two.[95] Thus in any given case, and
often at different stages of it, the House may conform to any one of
the three models.

    Solo opinions of the first type occur in about 9 per cent of civil
appeals coming to the Lords.[96] Some interaction will have occurred between the Law Lords during and after the hearing, it is
true, but thereafter significant contributions to the single speech
by the writer's colleagues are relatively infrequent, either because
they are too busy or because the subject-matter of the appeal is
highly specialised. The second type of solo decision, with five
independent speeches and practically no interaction between the
Law Lords, is relatively rare. All five Law Lords deliver a speech
in 35 per cent of appeals[97] but in most of them there will have been
constructive exchanges both during and after the hearing. Where
such exchanges have been lacking (or sometimes even where they

have occurred) and five disparate opinions emerge, the House is likely to come under fire from the critics of multiple opinions.[98] Group decisions from which a single judgement emerges after long consultations between Law Lords are equally rare,[99] although more common in criminal cases.[100] The bulk of appeals, however, involve both group and individual elements. The importance of the *laissez-faire* ethos on concurrences and dissents in this connection is that it encourages more individual and less group oriented decision-making in the House.

GROUP MEMBERSHIP AND THE ROLE OF THE DECISION-MAKER

In keeping with the finding that only a small minority of appeals are quintets as opposed to concertos, my interviews suggested that only some of the Law Lords avail themselves of such opportunities as exist in the House to try to influence their colleagues. Some Law Lords recognise that, in order to influence the development of the law in cases coming before them, they must acquire the art of persuading their colleagues to adopt their point of view. Those who are successful at this need not figure with any prominence in the law reports - indeed, they may well employ the tactic of offering to withdraw their opinion in return for an amendment which they desire in a colleague's speech. Other Law Lords, who may appear with greater frequency in the law reports, are either uninterested in trying or unwilling to try to persuade their colleagues except by the power of the printed word. Such differences are in part due to differences in perception of that part of a Law Lord's role which relates to decision-making. Individualists who attach only peripheral importance to the attribute of group membership in deciding an appeal (at least outside the Committee Room), perhaps because they view group decision-making as inimical to judicial independence, consider it illegitimate or pointless to try to win their colleagues round. As far as I could trace, only a small group of Law Lords in the past twenty-five years were of this persuasion. Lord Guest was one of them. I asked him if he thought it legitimate to try to persuade his colleagues to adopt a particular view. He replied,

No. I do not consider that one judge has any right to influence another judge's decision ... I usually made up my mind at the end of a case and drafted out very roughly the opinion that I was going to express, and it's very rarely that I changed that opinion by listening to the views of my colleagues. I have done so, of course, on several occasions, but I'm not sure that it's a good thing to be influenced too much by one's colleagues in what I consider to be the wrong direction.

Lord Hailsham considered it perfectly legitimate to try to persuade his colleagues but added that he seldom did it. Lord Denning replied in similar terms indicating that as a rule he didn't find that his colleagues changed their minds much in discussion after the end of the hearing.[101]

The bulk of the Law Lords in the past twenty-five years or so seem to have taken the view that group membership was at least a relevant attribute in their decision-making role. They have been prepared to argue at length with their colleagues, but usually only in a group context, for example in the corridor, the Conference Room or the Library. Law Lords in my sample who were of this persuasion included Lords Cross, Gardiner, Kilbrandon, MacDermott, Pearce, Pearson, Radcliffe, Reid and Salmon. There were, however, differences between them. Some appeared to restrict their discussions very much to a group context. Thus Lord Reid while observing that, 'We might often have a talk ... if we're two or three on the one side, we might often have a talk amongst ourselves, that's not uncommon', was sceptical about the value of trying to win round dissenters.

Well, of course you can't hope to convince your colleagues. Remember most of the cases that come up to us are cases of difficulty, and it is not sensible to suppose that five people are always going to agree, you know perfectly well they are not.

Lord Radcliffe would argue for his point of view in the course of the hearing and the conference afterwards but rarely tried to influence his colleagues in discussion thereafter. It was not that he considered such behaviour to be illegitimate, it was simply that he preferred to rely on his circulated speech. Other Law Lords were prepared to try to persuade their colleagues individually as well as in a group. Lord Devlin replied, 'If I thought it an important point and if a man was doubtful I might have a go at persuading him.' Lords Cross, Gardiner and MacDermott were in agreement, though Lord Cross added that his efforts were more usually directed at those with whom he was concurring and that he saw little point in trying to win round a dissenting colleague.

Lastly, there was a third group of Law Lords who perceived the attribute of group membership as pivotal to their role as decision-makers. They were well aware that only three Law Lords are required to constitute a majority and would push for their point of view from an early stage. They were prepared to lobby any colleague in his room (and elsewhere) in the hope of winning him round. As far as I could ascertain, at least three of the nineteen Law Lords in my samples fell into this category. One of them explained how in a difficult case he would frequently, 'go into a colleague's room, particularly a sympathetic one, one you hope to enlist for your point of view, to try to share ideas with them'. Another, however, observed that there were limits which there was no point in trying to exceed.

> If I can influence or control the majority, it is not worthwhile arguing [the dissenters] round. It merely tires them and tires me. I think it was Disraeli who said, 'A majority is the best repartee'.

It also emerged from my interviews that certain celebrated Law Lords of the past had been in this camp, notably Lord Atkin and Viscount Simonds. The latter in particular disliked being in a minority and would use his best endeavours to win round anyone whom he considered to be persuadable. As one Law Lord told me,

> Gavin minded very much if anybody whose opinion he respected didn't agree with his. He felt it personally.... He wasn't the only Law Lord who did that, but he did feel it very much.

ANGLO-AMERICAN COMPARISONS

In the US Supreme Court there have been Justices, for example Douglas,[102] who, apart from when they were assigned to write the opinion of the Court, seem to have preferred to operate in isolation from their colleagues. Nevertheless, the greater prevalence of bargaining and group discussions in important cases in the Supreme Court as compared with the Lords, not to mention the 'necessity' of a Court opinion, have ensured that the great bulk of recent Associate Justices have viewed group membership as a 'pivotal' or at least a 'relevant' attribute in their role. Yet curiously there are probably as many private discussions between individual Law Lords concerning an appeal as take place between individual Supreme Court Justices. This is largely due to two institutional factors.

First, the Justices have their own chambers with several law clerks, secretaries and a messenger. Each functions as a small, independent law firm. The Justice relies on his law clerks for discussion on a case and collaborates with them while drafting his opinion.[103] Thus he has less need to confer with his colleagues on difficult points than his transatlantic counterpart. Justice Powell has even gone so far as to assert that,

> The [Supreme] Court ... is perhaps one of the last citadels of jealously preserved individualism .... The informal interchange between chambers is minimal, with most exchanges of views being by correspondence or memoranda. Indeed, a justice may go through an entire term without being once in the chambers of all of the other eight members of the Court.[104]

Access to the diaries of Burton and Frankfurter, the private papers of other Justices and to a lesser extent, *The Brethren*, suggests that Powell's assertion that the majority of intra-court exchanges outside the conference room are written rather than oral is probably accurate.[105] On the other hand, they also show that there have been Justices in recent times such as Frankfurter, Black and Brennan who believed strongly in lobbying their colleagues in private.[106]

Secondly, while the Justices frequently write comments on, or memoranda in response to, a colleague's circulated opinion, in the House of Lords[107] this is practically never done. Either the Law Lord will comment orally to his colleague on the opinion or he will simply adjust his speech to take account of the points made in the circulated opinion.

> At the stage where the opinions are circulated one's colleagues are very polite. If there is an obvious omission you draw

attention to it, but you would seldom re-argue the merits. (A Law Lord)

Generally you'd leave it alone unless it was a case where you'd agreed that only one judgement would be delivered or if you were going to follow a particular man you might go to him and say, 'Look I'm really almost in entire agreement with you so I just propose to say, "I agree" but I'm a bit stuck about this [phrase] ...' You might do that. (Lord Devlin)

You would more frequently [comment] when the judgement was agreeing with yours, but if it was dissenting from you altogether, there would not be much point in doing it .... But in cases where the judgement is concurring with yours, you might say, 'Well, do you think we want to put it quite as you put it?' But then you would probably go and do that orally. You go and see the man. You would not circulate a formal statement saying I cannot agree with paragraph 4b in terms. You go round to the man and say, 'Oh, that was a wonderful piece of work you did', whether you thought it was or not, 'But don't you think perhaps this sentence might be modified, doesn't it go too far?' (Lord Cross)

You would not, I think, *write* comments. You would make them orally in the Library. It is most important to emphasise the informality of this: but it is not the less effective for that. This must be an extreme difference from a court in which there are recognisable political or ideological differences between groups of judges. (Lord Kilbrandon)

Nor does the presiding judge have any particular role in this area. Lord Guest commented,

It's not his duty to vet the speeches of the other judges, they're their own responsibility. Very, very seldom does the presiding judge make any comment to a member of the House upon his written judgement, unless there's something which he plainly wants to ask about or which he thinks is plainly wrong.

Lord Reid (who presided from 1962-75) concurred,

I very, very seldom criticise anybody else's opinion when we get them in draft. They are always circulated and we readjust our own in the light of what anybody else says, but I very seldom have suggested to anybody that it would be better to leave something out, and if I do it's more from the point of view that it wouldn't be tactful, than anything else.

THE VIRTUOSO PERFORMER

Of course virtuosity as a performer in a quintet or a concerto requires more than merely being willing to participate. Danelski's work[108] in applying 'small group analysis' to the Supreme Court suggests that not only are there social leaders[109] on the Court but also 'task leaders'. The latter 'exercise effective leadership concerning decisional outcomes', leadership which is affected by 'personality, esteem within the Court, intelligence, technical competence, and persuasive ability'.[110] Task leadership in the Lords is a characteristic most likely to be found amongst those who percieve group membership as pivotal to their decision-making role, *i.e.* the lobbyists, and the most effective lobbyists, at that. Here personalities and personal relationships inevitably play a part. Where a judge is doubtful he is more likely to be influenced by the way those whom he respects, or whose 'way of thinking' he often shares, or even those to whom he is attracted (*i.e.* his reference individuals) respond to the problem. He may even be moved by flattery[111] - or at least more so than by the comments of those with whom he is frequently at odds. Close friendships have existed between certain Law Lords and between certain Justices particularly those with a similar cast of mind, *e.g.* Simonds and Radcliffe, Burton and Frankfurter,[112] Burton and Harlan,[113] Frankfurter and Harlan[114] and Warren and Black.[115] There have also been long-standing antagonisms in the two Courts, *e.g.* Frankfurter and Douglas,[116] and Black and Jackson.[117] It cannot, however, be assumed that just because judges snipe at each other in their speeches, *e.g.* Lord Simonds' or Lord Russell's attacks on Lord Denning's judgements,[118] or harangue each other in the heat of conference as Black and Frankfurter did, that the opponents are personal antagonists. Despite Frankfurter's acid comments on Black in his diaries, it seems clear that a strong bond of friendship existed between them.[119] Nevertheless, judges who, like Black and

Frankfurter, fight 'hard, long and loud in the conference room and out'[120] for their views run the risk of alienating their colleagues. Jackson publicly accused Black of using bullying tactics in conference,[121] and Frankfurter's pontifical 'lectures' to his brethren led some of them to regard him as a 'puffed up professor'.[122] Even in the House of Lords, which has many fewer cases involving issues of fundamental principle or constitutional significance, the Law Lords can have fierce arguments. As Lord Radcliffe put it,

> It's good for a Law Lord, since he's essentially a member of a group, to be peaceable and temperate in his approach to the law, however passionately he may be involved in a particular case, and people do occasionally get tremendously worked up about their cases.

Similarly, a lobbyist who is too persistent or too entrenched in conference or too long-winded in his opinions is likely to alienate his colleagues. Lord Atkin frequently lobbied his colleagues. His daughter later recalled,

> He continued to use his powers of persuasion when he was sitting as a Lord of Appeal and would come home and say that he thought he had won his brothers over to his side or 'so and so is still not convinced but I think he may be tomorrow'.[123]

But it irked his colleagues that he was not open to persuasion in return. Lord Dunedin described him as 'obstinate if he has taken a view and quite unpersuadable',[124] and Lord Simon, whose overtures in *Liversidge* v. *Anderson* had been rejected by Atkin,[125] recorded in Atkin's obituary,

> I think he relied less than many members of [the House of Lords and Court of Appeal] do on the conference and discussion which takes place after the arguments are over. He was, therefore, a strong judge ...[126]

Again, Lord Radcliffe as we saw earlier,[127] considered that Atkin's obstinacy as a presiding Law Lord sometimes produced a counter-effect in his colleagues.[128]

The acid test for the group-oriented Law Lord is whether he can persuade one or more of his colleagues to share his point of view, particularly where this will result in a switch in votes or even a reversal of the existing majority position. Such successes do occur but are remarkably hard to document. The final judgement cannot be taken at face value. A unanimous decision may eventuate from a court divided at the first conference. Equally there have been 3:2 decisions where none of the participants have ever felt any doubt. From the interviews it emerged that most changes of mind take place during the hearing, but that they also occur between the first conference and the final judgement - though not with the frequency with which they occur in the Supreme Court at this stage.[129] As one Law Lord put it, 'It is unusual, though, of course, by no means unheard of ... for people to change their mind after ... the end of the oral hearing.' Another Law Lord admitted that he had changed his mind on several occasions after the first conference and that sometimes the majority even changed, but added that 'on the whole people are reluctant to change their positions after the first conference'; while a third Law Lord said that in the cases he had sat in between 1971 and 1973 there had only been two instances of a Law Lord 'coming right round' and switching his vote after the first conference. Viscount Radcliffe indicated that he very rarely changed his position after the hearing and neither Lord Denning nor Lord Devlin could recall ever changing at this stage, in the Lords.

Occasionally, Law Lords will make it clear in their speeches that they have had a change of heart since the first conference. Sometimes the change is merely attributed to 'further reflection' e.g. Lord Russell in *Anns* v. *London Borough of Merton,*[130] Lord Diplock in *Suffolk County Council* v. *Mason*[131] and Lord Russell in *Waugh* v. *British Railways Board.*[132] More often it is attributed to 'further reflection' and reading other Law Lords' speeches, *e.g.* Lord Normand in *National Anti-Vivisection Society* v. *IRC*[133] (after reading Lord Simonds' speech), Lord Hodson in *Gardiner* v. *Motherwell Machinery and Scrap Co.*[134] (persuaded by Lord Reid's speech), Lord Simon in *Federal Steam Navigation Co. Ltd* v. *Dept of Trade and Industry*[135] (convinced by the speeches of Lords Salmon and Wilberforce), Lord Kilbrandon in *Walker* v. *Leeds CC*[136] (after considering Lord Wilberforce's speech), Lord Hailsham in *The Siskina*[137] (persuaded by Lord Diplock's reasoning), Lord Russell in *MacShannon* v. *Rockware Glass Ltd*[138] (dissuaded by his colleagues' views), Lord Edmund-Davies in *Dias Compania Naviera SA* v. *Louis Dreyfus Corporation*[139] (satisfied by Lord Diplock's speech) and Lord Fraser in *Tyrer* v. *Smart*[140] (convinced by Lord Diplock's speech). In addition there are the cases where one or more Law Lord switches his opinion but this is not apparent from the law reports. One celebrated case in which this occurred was *Rookes* v. *Barnard* where after the initial hearing Lord Devlin was in a minority of one (or possibly two) favouring the appellant. After a second conference Lord Reid reconvened the Appellate Committee, further argument was heard and a unanimous decision upholding the appeal finally emerged. Lord Pearce was one of those who switched. His speech indicates the difficulty he experienced in the case and that he was persuaded by the speeches of Lords Reid and Devlin. It does not reveal that in fact he had initially written it in favour of the respondent but found it 'so feeble and wrong' that he then rewrote it the other way. Lord Evershed's speech seems to indicate that he was the last to switch.[141]

In none of the foregoing cases were the changes of mind attributed to persuasive discussions with fellow Law Lords. We may be sure that such discussions took place,[142] perhaps in a majority of the cases, but to go further and to assert that the vote changes were the outcome of effective lobbying by group-oriented Law Lords would be mere speculation. What can be said from a study of these and other recent cases where the House has been heavily divided is that Law Lords who perceive group membership to be pivotal to their role as decision-makers usually end up on the majority side. To what extent this simply reflects a pragmatic tendency to 'cut one's losses' rather than be forced into a dissent is impossible to say.

CONCLUSION

This chapter has focused on judicial interaction and its significance for decision-making, both in the formative period before the end of the oral argument in the House and in the later stages when the speeches are being drafted and circulated. We have seen that the relative influence exercised on the decision-making process by each Law Lord varies, in part as a result of their role perceptions and in part from their differing abilities to exercise task leadership. Two further factors affect a Law Lord's relative influence. First, where the Law Lord in question is the presiding Law Lord he has a certain edge over his colleagues, even though he lacks the power to assign an opinion of the court. The edge derives from the lead he can provide for his brethren at the hearing stage, from the fact that it is slightly easier for him to exercise task and social leadership than for his colleagues, and from his power to convene a second conference of the Law Lords. Lord Reid, when presiding Law Lord, seems to have believed more in leadership by example[143] than task or social leadership. Viscount Simonds, on the other hand, did endeavour to exercise task leadership, as is clearly suggested by some of his colleagues' *dicta* in *National Anti-Vivisection Society* v. *IRC*.[144] He was certainly prepared to reconvene the Law Lords if he considered it worthwhile. One Law Lord observed,

> You [had] a strong man like Lord Simonds who so hated being in a minority that he would have two or three meetings trying to get everybody round to his point of view ... he'd work desperately hard to try and get the others with him.

Yet it is difficult to say how effective his task leadership was. On the face of it, he was not outstandingly successful in cases where the court split 3:2,[145] but his efforts may well have persuaded his colleagues to modify their speeches even when he was in a minority. He probably did not try to exercise social leadership. As one Law Lord commented, 'I didn't look upon [his approach] as mediating and getting an agreed point of view so much as getting his own point of view over.'

The second factor affecting a Law Lord's relative influence is the operation of 'opinion deference'.[146] With the possible exception of one junior Law Lord, the Law Lords I interviewed were agreed that there was no expectation that more junior Law Lords should defer to their more senior colleagues. On the other hand, they were almost unanimous in agreeing that there was a tendency to give extra weight in particular appeals, *e.g.* Scots, Patent, Chancery, Commercial, *etc.* cases, to the opinions of Law Lords with specialised experience in these fields by those Law Lords who had not. One or two Law Lords also added that they would be slow to come to a conclusion which was diametrically opposed to that of certain of their colleagues whose intellectual prowess they respected, *e.g.* Lord Radcliffe or Lord Reid.[147]

These findings on the relative influence of Law Lords have two significant implications. In the first place, it means that the traditional measure of a stature or success in a Law Lord, *i.e.* the long term standing of his reported judgements[148] is inadequate. A Law Lord who exercises task and social leadership may appear very little in the law reports, though profoundly influencing the outcome of the cases in which he sat. As Lord Cross put it,

> [It all depends] what you mean by 'successful'. One man may be regarded as a tower of strength by his colleagues but thought little of by academics, while another may be a great man to academics but a mere nuisance in the eyes of his colleagues.

The second, and perhaps more important, implication is that the values and role perceptions of Law Lords who exercise task leadership are likely to play a disproportionate part in the outcome of hard cases coming to the Lords.[149] It is to the Law Lords' role performances in such cases during the period 1957-73 that the next two chapters are devoted.

6 The Role of a Law Lord: Conflict and Change

> It is no doubt unsafe to generalise about judicial process. For after all it is a generalisation about the work of individual men. In no field of special knowledge does one man pursue its technique or exercise its art precisely in the same way as another .... There is no place where the inequalities and variations of men can be seen more clearly than when the men are up on a Bench.
>
> Sir Owen Dixon, 'Concerning Judicial Method'[1]

INTRODUCTION

Decision-making in the Lords involves group and community processes quite apart from those adverted to in the last chapter. This is because, as we saw earlier,[2] a Law Lord is influenced not just by his own conception of his role but also by his fellow Law Lords and their predecessors, and to a lesser extent by other groups in the wider legal and non-legal community. 'Pivotal' to his role when deciding an appeal is the expectation, held within and without the legal community, that he should justify his decision by reasoned argument. Furthermore, within the legal community itself there are more or less shared understandings as to what constitutes a valid and acceptable argument for a Law Lord to employ, and as to what standards he may relevantly appeal when justifying his decision.[3] Such understandings are in no small way the product of a common socialisation pattern, a traditional training with a received body of knowledge and learning.[4] Indeed it has been argued that such traditional practices and ideas, nurtured by a legal caste, are the very essence of the common law.[5]

Where the case to be decided is a 'hard' one, on the other hand, Ronald Dworkin and other scholars have argued that a judge should transcend not only his own notions of fairness but also those of the legal community by looking to those prevailing in the wider non-legal community, to the 'plane of expectations' - the sense of justice of societal groups.[6] Yet, as we shall see in this chapter, in many cases coming to the Lords contradictory expectations which are held in this wider community create a situation of conflict for the Law Lords. As we shall also see, the differing responses of the Law Lords to this conflict during the period 1957-73 were in accordance with the typical responses to role conflict which have been identified in previous research. Concomitantly, I shall demonstrate that there have been significant changes in the Law Lord's role during this period.

JUSTICE v. CERTAINTY

My premiss is that there is a tension between the drive for stability and certainty in the common law, which requires that disputes be adjudicated in accordance with previously announced norms and the drive for adjudication on the basis of individuated justice, which in certain cases will require that previously announced norms be radically altered or departed from. The former drive is concerned with fulfilling that aspect of justice which asserts that like cases should be treated in like manner and thus also with meeting the reasonable desire of businessmen and others to know in advance the rules which will be applied to their conduct. The latter is concerned with ensuring that certainty does not become the certainty of injustice, by challenging the application of a norm that is considered unjust or no longer suitable to the conditions of the time of the instant case. R.W.M. Dias has pointed out[7] that this dialectic involves different aspects of (or perhaps different views about) justice, but in accordance with established usage I shall refer to the conflict as being between justice and certainty.

As Lord Devlin once observed,

> The object of a rule is to ensure that similar cases are similarly decided; if they were not, then there would not be justice at all ... [yet] any rule, however well phrased, may occasionally interfere with judgement on the merits. Justice for all carries

with it the possibility of something less than justice in the individual case.[8]

The judicial obligation to do justice according to law indicates the tightrope that judges sometimes must walk between justice and certainty.* The aphorism 'Hard cases make bad law' reflects the consequences of the judges falling from that tightrope. It is perhaps not surprising that it has been said that the competing goals pose a severe problem for law-givers,

> That of proving to mankind that the law is fixed and settled, whose authority is beyond question, while at the same time enabling it to make constant readjustments and occasional radical changes under the pressure of infinite and variable desires.[9]

This analysis, of course, exaggerates the dichotomy between the competing poles. The common law contains many elements which ameliorate the tension, ranging from the evolution of broad principles (as opposed to narrow rules) and variable standards, *e.g.* reasonableness, to 'categories of illusory reference',[10] leeways of precedent[11] and legal fictions. Nevertheless the competing goals of justice and certainty arise in many hard cases for they are reflected in the conflicting normative expectations held by the parties and their advisers. The Law Lords have long been aware of this conflict in their role as the following quotations show:

> The Layman ... would like the law to be at once certain, speedy and inexpensive in its operation, and yet also to produce decisions which fit in with his notions of fair play and justice ... [T]he central question of practical jurisprudence ... is, how far can we reconcile certainty in the law with the achievement of justice in each particular case?[12]

> People want two inconsistent things; that the law shall be certain, and that it shall be just and shall move with the times.[13] (Lord Reid)

---

*Learned Hand seeking to provoke Mr Justice Holmes once said to him 'Well sir, goodbye. Do Justice!' Holmes turned quite sharply and ... replied 'That is not my job. My job is to play the game according to the rules.' (Account derived from M. Mayer, *The Lawyers* (New York: Harper & Row, 1966) p. 520.)

[W]hatever a judge does, he will surely have his critics. If, in an effort to do justice, he appears to make new law, there will be cries that he is overweening and that he has rendered uncertain what had long been regarded as established legal principles. On the other hand, if he sticks to the old legal rules, an equally vocal body will charge him with being a reactionary, a slave to precedent, and of failing to mould the law to changing social needs. He cannot win and, if he is wise, he will not worry, even though at times he may ruefully reflect that those who should know better seem to have little appreciation of the difficulties of his vocation.[14] (Lord Edmund-Davies)

There are two very desirable things about a system of justice; one is that it should be certain, because nothing is worse when people go to a solicitor, and he says, 'I cannot tell you what the answer is. It entirely depends which judge we get.' On the other hand, it is desirable that the law should be flexible so as to meet changing social and economic conditions, and these two very desirable things are in permanent conflict.[15] (Lord Gardiner)

Well, you do get into that great trouble if you want something certain and you want something just, and if you lay down any certain rule, it is liable to produce injustice. But that is inherent in society.[16] (Lord Pearson)

In the interviews the Law Lords were asked whether they perceived conflicts between such ideals as justice and certainty or stability and flexibility as playing a large part in the appeals that came to the Lords. Without exception all eleven active Law Lords interviewed (and the four retired Law Lords) answered the question in the affirmative. As one of them replied,

That's just the debate. You say to yourself when you're considering the case, if we deal with it in this way we shall be accused of undue formalism. If we decide another way we shall be charged with being sociologists.

Lord Radcliffe, it is true, perceived the clash to take place less frequently than some of his colleagues. Yet he gave greater recognition to the conflicting demands in his extra-judicial writing.[17] In addition, three of the Law Lords whom I did not interview, Lords Diplock,[18] Morris[19] and Upjohn[20] have recorded in print their recognition of the conflicting demands.

The Law Lords' actions matched their words. Their collective Statement[21] on Precedent in 1966 expressly cites the conflict as its *raison d'être*,

> Their Lordships regard the use of precedent as an indispensable foundation upon which to decide what is the law and its application to individual cases. It provides at least some degree of certainty upon which individuals can rely in the conduct of their affairs, as well as a basis for orderly development of legal rules.
>
> Their Lordships nevertheless recognise that too rigid adherence to precedent may lead to injustice in a particular case and also unduly restrict the proper development of the law.

Not surprisingly, in cases where the new freedom has been discussed the conflict between justice and certainty has featured strongly in the speeches of the Law Lords, *e.g.* Lord Morris in *Conway* v. *Rimmer*,[22] Lords Reid, Dilhorne and Diplock in *Jones* v. *Secretary of State for Social Services*,[23] Lord Pearson in *British Railways Board* v. *Herrington*,[24] Lords Wilberforce and Simon in *Miliangos* v. *George Frank (Textiles) Ltd* [25] and Lord Diplock in *Davis* v. *Johnson*.[26] It also featured in other cases. Thus in *Gollins* v. *Gollins*[27] Lord Reid observed,

> Judges, bound by the existing state of the law, have shown much ingenuity where justice demands a remedy ... [In] spite of the difficulties created by artificial tests there are very few reported cases where they have not been circumvented when justice required that.

Again, in *Boys* v. *Chaplin*[28] Lord Wilberforce, having restated the basic rule of English law with regard to foreign torts, concluded,

> It remains for me to consider (and this is the crux of the present case) whether some qualification to this rule is required in certain individual cases. There are two conflicting pressures: the first in favour of certainty and simplicity in the law, the second in favour of flexibility in the interest of individual justice.

CLARIFYING THE CONFLICT

Since the Law Lords consider that conflicts involving justice and certainty emerge in many hard cases, the question arises as to what measures, if any, the Law Lords take to 'resolve' the conflict. To answer this question it is first necessary to recognise that the expectations we have been considering are only two of a larger group of connected expectations which are potentially in conflict with each other. This group includes the following expectations for a Law Lord in deciding a hard case:[29]

1. That he ought to reach a conclusion in his speech which produces a decision between the parties to the appeal on at least one of the issues raised by the parties, and which does not go beyond the issues raised in the case (the 'decide the case' expectation).[30]
2. That his decision ought to be justified by reasoned argument and framed[31] as a judgement between the competing claims of right made by the opposing parties. Thus he may not overtly adopt the role of the mediator and endeavour to reach a compromise between the parties which involves each side giving up a part of their claim (the 'provide justification' expectation).[32]
3. That in his efforts to do justice according to law he ought not to usurp the role of Parliament (the 'don't legislate' expectation).
4. That his decision ought to be consistent with the existing rules and principles of the law as laid down in precedents and statutes, either as being a direct application of such rules and principles or as being an application of rules and principles derivable by close analogy from the established rules and principles. In other words, that the community's need for certainty and stability in the law be taken into account (the 'be consistent' expectation).
5. But also, the decision given ought to be based on a rule or principle which, taking account of contemporary social conditions, achieves a fair and just result as between the parties (the 'be fair' expectation).

The potential for conflict between these expectations is further exacerbated by the fact that 'hard' cases fall into at least four broad and overlapping categories. These are:

(a) Cases where there is a binding or strongly persuasive precedent whose *ratio* is clear and in point but which the court is being asked to overrule or distinguish. In such cases the 'be consistent' and the 'be fair' or the 'don't legislate' and the 'be fair' expectations may conflict.

(b) Cases where there are alternative strands of ostensibly relevant precedents or competing principles confronting the court.[33] Here a conflict between the 'provide justification' and the 'be consistent' expectations can arise.

(c) Cases for which there is a closely analogous precedent whose *ratio* is unclear, or which fall within the penumbra of uncertainty of an ostensibly relevant rule.[34] In such cases the 'don't legislate', the 'be consistent' and the 'be fair' expectations may conflict.

(d) Cases where there are no strongly persuasive (as opposed to merely permissive) legal rules or precedents in point in the existing law.[35] In these situations the question whether to extend an existing rule by analogy or to create a new rule or to apply an existing legal principle may involve a clash between the 'don't legislate' and the 'be fair' expectations or between the 'decide the case', the 'provide justification' and the 'don't legislate' expectations.

In the discussion of the judicial role which follows, I shall concentrate primarily on cases which fall within the first category of hard case, although some reference will be made to examples drawn from the other categories. The concentration can be justified on two grounds. First, that such cases are easier to recognise and classify uncontroversially than those in the other three categories. Secondly, and more importantly, it is in these cases that the potential conflict between the 'don't legislate', the 'be consistent' and the 'be fair' expectations is most clearly marked. Should the hypothesis, that a conflict between these expectations frequently exists and significantly influences the behaviour of the Law Lords in such cases, not be confirmed, then it is unlikely to be confirmed in any other category of hard case.

RESPONSES TO THE CONFLICT

Research by role analysts has shown that individuals confronted by role conflict react positively, adaptively and by withdrawal.[36]

These typical responses can be grouped as follows:

I *Positive responses*
(a) *Innovation:* Where the individual (or a group of individuals) endeavours to achieve a redefinition of the role whereby the conflict is reduced or institutionalised.
(b) *Convening one's role-set* or significant reference groups:* In the case of the Law Lords this would include a meeting with their primary reference group (themselves) to discuss conflicts in their role. As I shall argue later, this occurred prior to the announcement of the 1966 Practice Statement on Precedent in the House of Lords.

II *Adaptive responses*
(a) *Ranking the competing expectations:* As we saw in the earlier chapters the Law Lords frequently utilise this technique for handling conflicting expectations. The ranking of the expectations may be done according to the individual's perception of their legitimacy, their weight, or the consequences of complying with one rather than the other(s).

Thus a Law Lord who declares that his task is to apply the law as it is and not as it ought to be implies that the 'be fair' expectation is a less legitimate expectation for a lay person to hold of a Law Lord than the 'be consistent' expectation.

In Chapter 2 I argued that even those who have attained the status of a Law Lord may be influenced in their choice between competing sets of expectations by the desire to avoid antagonising their colleagues.[37] Even if this were not the case, it is, as we shall see, commonplace for a Law Lord to take account of the social or legal consequences of his decisions. It is also common for a Law Lord to rank competing expectations according to his perception of their weight or functional importance for the proper performance of his role. Thus he might accord 'pivotal' status to one or more expectations and 'relevant' or 'peripheral' status to the remainder. For example, Lord Atkin was of the opinion that, 'Finality is a good thing, but justice is a better.'[38] Lord Wright was of like mind, 'I should', he said, 'be sorry if the quest for certitude were to be substituted for the quest for justice.'[39] Justice Brandeis on the other hand once declared,

---

*A role-set is the group of individuals with whom a person typically interacts when performing his role.

It is usually more important that a rule of law be settled than that it should be settled right. Even where the error in declaring the rule is a matter of serious concern, it is ordinarily better to seek correction by legislation.[40]

Interestingly, when the 'don't legislate', the 'be consistent' and the 'be fair' expectations are ranked against each other, the end products turn out to be categories with which judicial scholars have some familiarity. Such typologies as Llewellyn's 'Formal Style' and 'Grand Style',[41] Pollock's 'Judicial Caution' and 'Judicial Valour',[42] Lord Denning's 'bold spirits' and 'timorous souls',[43] Lord Hailsham's 'reformer' and 'traditionalist',[44] Lord Reid's 'legal reformers', 'black-letter lawyers' and 'common sense men'[45] and Glick and Vines' 'Law Maker', 'Law Interpreter' and 'Pragmatist'[46] can be represented, I would argue, as the product of different rankings or balances between the three expectations according to the suggested criteria.

(b) *Evasion:* This technique though also found in other forms[47] is most frequently found amongst the Law Lords in the form of 'dissimulation'* - masking the existence of the conflict in their words, though not in their deeds. Thus, in hard cases, this mechanism often involves the claim that there is no conflict between the 'don't legislate', the 'be consistent' and the 'be fair' expectations. The Law Lords imply that compliance with each of the expectations involves no breach of the others, when in truth they actually violate one or more consequent on a ranking according to the criteria above mentioned or according to the comparative ease with which the expectations' violation can be concealed.

This technique has a long history in the law for it is exemplified in the device of the legal fiction. As a recent extensive survey of the history and function of legal fictions concluded,

Judicial fictions have played an extremely significant and beneficial role in the development of the law. By concealing their lawmaking activities behind the facade of fictions, judges were able to ameliorate, adapt and extend legal rules in order to render just and good decisions.[48]

---

*It must be emphasised that this is a technical term. It is used purely descriptively and is not intended to convey a value judgement.

III *Withdrawal*

(a) *Psychological:* Where an individual's self concept and his perception of his role conflict, a form of psychological withdrawal is often the outcome, namely, 'role-distancing'.[49] This activity consists in the individual letting it be seen that he, as a human being, dislikes the course of conduct which his role obliges him to follow and that although he is prepared to continue to act in accordance with this role, he is not fully committed to it. When Law Lords are deciding hard cases this response occurs with some frequency. Every genuine case of 'judicial regret',[50] where a Law Lord is moved by the merits of an appeal (*i.e.* the 'be fair' expectation) but feels bound by precedent to decide the other way (*i.e.* to favour the 'be consistent' expectation) involves 'role-distancing'. In the words of Cardozo,

> Judges march at times to pitiless conclusions under the prod of a remorseless logic which is supposed to leave them no alternative. They deplore the sacrificial rite. They perform it, none the less, with averted gaze, convinced as they plunge the knife that they obey the bidding of their office. The victim is offered up to the gods of jurisprudence on the alter of regularity.[51]

and Piero Calamandrei in 'The Crisis in the Reasoned Opinion' wrote,

> [T]he judge is a human being ... even if he stifles the voice of his conscience, when he is obligated to apply a law in which he does not believe, it is only natural that he will apply it mechanically, as an official duty, with a cold bureaucratic pedantry; he cannot be expected to vivify or to recreate a law that is extraneous or actually hostile to his philosophy.[52]

Yet as Coleridge J once remarked,

> Perhaps the most efficacious mode of procuring good laws, certainly the only one allowable to a Court of Justice, is to act fully up to the spirit and language of bad ones, and to let their inconvenience be fully felt by giving them full effect.[53]

This observation suggests that the motivation of a judge in

pronouncing a 'judicial regret' may not always be the passive acquiescence which is typically associated with such statements.[54] 'Role-distancing' usually operates in conjunction with the *Adaptive* response of ranking, a fact which illustrates that the various responses need not operate independently of each other. Nor need an individual be consistent in his responses every time he encounters a similar form of role conflict.

(b) *Physical:* With the exception of Lord Denning's departure from the Lords to be Master of the Rolls,[55] there is no evidence that I am aware of to suggest that any recent Law Lord has experienced such problems in handling role conflicts in hard cases as to lead him to resign or retire.

THE LAW LORDS IN 1957

When applied to the Law Lords' actions and their perceptions of their role during the period of my research (1957-73), this taxonomy produces interesting results. I propose to divide the period into three parts (1957-62, 1962-66, 1966-73) and shall begin with 1957-62, during which time Lord Simonds was the senior Law Lord (and therefore usually the presiding Law Lord). In April 1957, following the promotion of Denning LJ to the Lords, the body of active Law Lords consisted of Viscount Kilmuir LC, Viscount Simonds, and Lords Morton, Reid, Radcliffe, Tucker, Cohen, Keith, Somervell and Denning. Other Law Lords who were likely to be invited to sit included, Earl Jowitt, Lord Goddard, Lord Oaksey, Lord MacDermott and Lord Evershed. With the exceptions of Lords Reid, Radcliffe, Denning and MacDermott, a reasonable consensus existed amongst the Law Lords as to their role in hard cases. This consensus, dubbed 'Substantive Formalism' by Robert Stevens[56] might be summarised as,

(a) Favouring precedent to general principle.[57]
(b) Refining rather than rationalising the law.[58]
(c) Applying the law as it is, not as it ought to be.[59]

Perhaps the clearest articulation of such a role was that made, before my first period, at an Australian law conference by Viscount Jowitt LC in September 1951. During a discussion of the case of *Candler* v. *Crane, Christmas & Co.* he said,

It is quite possible that the law has produced a result which does not accord with the requirements of today. If so, put it right by legislation ... [P]lease do not get yourself into the frame of mind of entrusting to the judges the working out of a whole new set of principles which does accord with the requirements of modern conditions. Leave that to the legislature, and leave us to confine ourselves to trying to find out what the law is. If this does come to the House of Lords, if we examine it and discover that there is a case which is precisely in point, then whether we like the decision or whether we do not, whether we think it accords with modern requirements and conditions or whether we think it does not, we shall follow loyally the decision which has already been come to. In that way and that way only can we introduce some certainty into the law.[60]

In fact, the Law Lord who expounded this conception of the judicial role most frequently and forcefully in decisions of the House immediately prior to 1957 was also the most active task leader in the court,[61] Viscount Simonds. It was his dominance of the court while senior Law Lord which had, I believe, much to do with the continued strength of this concept of the Law Lord's role (which had emerged in the early 1940s) until the early 1960s.

Lord Simonds' restrictive attitude to precedent can clearly be seen in *Jacobs* v. *LCC*[62] where, in considering a previous decision of the House he said,

... it would, I think, be to deny the importance, I would say the paramount importance of certainty in the law to give less than coercive effect to the unequivocal statement of the law made after argument by three members of this House ...

Similarly, in *Chapman* v. *Chapman* he remarked,

It is ... possible that we are not wiser than our ancestors. It is for the Legislature ... to determine whether there should be a change in the law and what that change should be.[63]

And in a well-known series of pronouncements directed at what he considered to be deviance on Lord Denning's part, Lord Simonds reinforced the majority view of the judicial role.[64]

Lord Cohen, too, had indicated his preference for precedent

and certainty when he wrote that

> Uncertainty in the law is a supreme disadvantage and if we
> abandon the principle of *'stare decisis'* we open the door wide to
> uncertainty ... I think there is much to be said for a rule which
> prevents the Judiciary from usurping the function of the
> legislature and tends to certainty in the law.[65]

Similarly Lord Goddard, in the leading opinion in *Best* v. *Samuel
Fox*[66] rejected a wife's claim for damages for loss of consortium
with the following words,

> If the wife is to have a cause of action it must be found in
> principle or authority ... never during the many centuries that
> have passed since the reports of the decisions of the English
> courts first began has recovery of damages for such injury been
> recorded.[67]

In fact in a series of cases[68] in the years prior to 1957 the Law
Lords, in accordance with the role perceptions which I have
outlined, declined to develop the law* beyond the existing
precedents or to take anything other than a passive stance when
faced with legal authority. Their response to the potential conflict
between the 'don't legislate', the 'be consistent' and the 'be fair'
expectations in hard cases, was to rank the first two much more
highly than the last. The ranking remained the same whether
based on (a) the perceived consequences of breaches of the
respective expectations, (b) their weight,† or (c) their legitimacy.
By this means the bulk of the Law Lords defined out of existence

---

*When I use descriptive words such as 'creative', 'conservative', 'activist',
'passive' and the like, I am not making value judgements. It is no part of my
argument that judge-made law is always good law or that judicial activism is
better than judicial restraint. My use of 'creative' or 'activist', *etc.* is (unless
otherwise stated) simply intended to be descriptive and directional.[69]

†The strength of the commitment of most of the Law Lords to the 'be
consistent' expectation and precedent in particular, at this time, is graphically
illustrated in an anecdote recounted by J.D. Wilson.[70] He records that he once
asked Lord Normand, a Scottish Lord of Appeal in the early 1950s, what he did
in the House of Lords. 'Do? Oh we try to knock a little sense into them.' And he
gave an instance of a recent case in which the English Law Lords were seeking
for a precedent which led them right back to the reign of Edward III. 'Like a
pack of dogs,' he said, 'smelling up an almost interminable avenue!'

the potential role conflict in hard cases. So far as I could trace, 'role-distancing' was uncommon during this period[71] and only Lord Reid[72] evidenced the response of *Innovation*. However there was some evidence of *Evasion*. Thus in the two cases in which the Law Lords were prepared to develop the law in the face of precedent,[73] there is little or no overt discussion of the limits of judicial law-making, policy considerations, social or legal consequences or keeping the law in touch with changing social conditions.[74]

Two factors which seem to suggest that at least four Law Lords (Lords Reid, Radcliffe, Denning and MacDermott) did not subscribe to the prevailing orthodoxy in interpreting the judicial role in 1957, were their preference for principles rather than precedents and their willingness on occasion to take account of the need to keep the common law in step with changing social conditions.[75]

THE LAW LORDS IN 1962

If such was the balance of judicial opinion (and thus in large measure the judicial role)[76] in 1957, what was the position in April 1962 when Viscount Simonds retired? At first sight very little appears to have changed. The intervening years had seen a series of dicta from Viscount Simonds reinforcing the dominant role perception of 1957 and earlier years. In *Plato Films Ltd* v. *Speidel*, he observed,

> In effect ... the plea of the appellants was that the law was not what it ought to be. That is a plea to which this House is not inclined to listen when it is sitting as a supreme appellate tribunal.[77]

And in 1961 he delivered his most celebrated dictum on the judicial role, in *Scruttons Ltd* v. *Midland Silicones*.

> ... to me heterodoxy, or, as some might say, heresy, is not the more attractive because it is dignified by the name of reform. Nor will I easily be led by an undiscerning zeal for some abstract kind of justice to ignore our first duty, which is established for us by Act of Parliament or the binding authority

of precedent. The law is developed by the application of old principles to new circumstances. Therein lies its genius. Its reform by the abrogation of those principles is the task not of the courts of law but of Parliament.[78]

Lord Cohen, too, reaffirmed his respect for precedent in January 1961 in his speech in the seven judge case of *Ross Smith* v. *Ross Smith*. Although he considered that the decision of *Simonin* v. *Mallac* made in 1860 was wrong, Lord Cohen declined to overrule it because it had stood for over 100 years and had been followed or applied in a large number of cases not only in England but in the Commonwealth. Yet he recognised that to overrule the case would neither upset anyone's expectations nor have any side effects. Lord Morris similarly believed the decision to be wrong but was reluctant to overrule it because of its great antiquity.[79]

This passive approach to developing the common law was stressed in extra-judicial writings by two Law Lords, Lord Evershed[80] and Lord Devlin. The latter in a treatise on judicial law-making which largely reflected the articulated version of the prevailing orthodoxy, concluded,

Judges have tended more and more to leave new instances to Parliament as well as new principles ... I doubt if judges will now of their own motion contribute much more to the development of the law.[81]

And in 1961 one leading academic, Rupert Cross, recorded with evident regret that '[It] is more difficult to get rid of an awkward decision in England than almost anywhere else in the world.'[82] Like Professor Goodhart[83] he considered that the English doctrine of precedent was more rigid then than it ever had been in the past. As he concluded, 'The truth is that the judges' power of making law is very limited.'

Yet, in 1963 C.K. Allen wrote,

There seems to be less reluctance than formerly in superior courts either to overrule previous, and sometimes old, precedents, or else to sterilize them by the semi-fictions of 'distinguishing' them on tenuous grounds of fact or law by recourse to the doctrine of incuria. With the help of a certain degree of 'judicial valour', new opportunities seem to be opening up of escaping from the bondage which carries 'consistency' or 'loyalty' to unprofitable extremes ... [84]

Allen's remarks suggest that the Law Lords no longer felt able to rely on arguments based on certainty and 'not usurping the function of Parliament', as a complete defence to the criticism of those who expected the courts to produce 'justice as fairness' or decisions in line with changing social conditions. From being a peripheral expectation, the 'be fair' expectation had become a relevant one. Two factors certainly contributed to this change in attitude. First, there had been alterations in the personnel of the House. Lords Morton, Somervell, Cohen, Keith and Tucker had retired, to be replaced by Lords Jenkins, Morris, Hodson, Guest and Devlin. On the basis of my interviews with Lords Guest and Devlin and from the comparative performances of the two groups it seems that the latter group of Law Lords tended to give more weight to the 'be fair' expectation than their predecessors.

Secondly, and more importantly, during this period Lords Denning and Reid began to make their mark in the House. Both of them recognised that hard cases sometimes involve a clash between the 'be consistent' and 'be fair' expectations. Both of them sought to respond to the conflict by *Innovation*. Their aim was to bring about an alteration in the rules concerning precedent in the House of Lords. Lord Denning had long since declared his desire for a 'new equity' in order to mitigate the hardship caused by a rigid adherence to precedent.[85] His views on this matter were in many ways the direct antithesis of the judicial orthodoxy prevailing in 1957. He did not believe in the rigid dichotomy between the law as it is and as it ought to be. He ascribed a far higher status than the majority of his colleagues to the 'be fair' as opposed to the 'be consistent' expectation. For him, doing justice in the individual case was central to the judicial role.[86] In interview, he said,

I take firmly the view that judges oughtn't just to be saying I am only going to apply the law. I think that the law ought to be developed, the judge ought to do justice in the particular case, not leave it to Parliament years afterwards, who don't do anything about justice in the particular case. It means that the poor individual has got to go away without justice.

Turning to his performance in decided cases between 1957 and 1962, we can see how Lord Denning approached the conflict in practice. In *London Transport Executive* v. *Betts*[87] he dissented from the majority who were following a precedent of the House, saying,

It seems to me that when a particular precedent - even of your Lordships' House - comes into conflict with a fundamental principle, also of your Lordships' House, then the fundamental principle must prevail.

His dissents in *Ostime* v. *Australian Mutual Provident Society*[88] and in *Close* v. *Steel Co. of Wales*[89] ran along similar lines.

At one time Lord Denning regarded the rule that the House of Lords was bound by its own precedents as too firmly entrenched to be removed judicially.[90] His dissents show that he had departed from this position and that he was prepared either to outflank that rule, or to mount a frontal attack upon it.

There can be little doubt that Lord Denning during his time in the Lords was consciously trying to redress the imbalance which he perceived to exist between the 'be consistent' and the 'be fair' expectations in the perceptions of the judicial role held by most of his colleagues. He sought through *Innovation* to mitigate the rigid operation of *stare decisis* in the House. A self-styled iconoclast, assailing cherished beliefs or venerated institutions,[91] he endeavoured to influence others to accept his concept of the judicial role.[92] Yet he had doubts as to the success of his efforts and in a recent interview he conceded that he might have achieved more if he had been more circumspect.

Irrespective of the success of Lord Denning and Lord Reid at this time in undermining the rigid operation of the theory of precedent in the House, their activities made it no longer possible for the majority of their colleagues to treat the 'be fair' expectation as merely 'peripheral' and thus to minimise any conflict which might arise between it and the 'don't legislate' and the 'be consistent' expectations. Its emergence as a 'relevant' expectation in the dominant conception of the judicial role by 1962 can be traced through the judicial role performances between 1957 and 1962.

In *National Bank of Greece* v. *Metliss* even Viscount Simonds was to be found declaring,

But my Lords, in the end and in the absence of authority binding this House, the question simply is: What does justice demand in such a case as this?[93]

Although the majority had felt unable to evade precedents of the House of Lords in *London Transport Executive* v. *Betts*, *Ostime* v. *Australian Mutual Provident Society* and *Close* v. *Steel Co. of Wales Ltd*, they did not experience the same problem in *Public Trustees* v. *IRC*, *Thomson* v. *Moyse*, *Unit Construction Co.* v. *Bullock*, *Cavanagh* v. *Ulster Weaving Co.*, *Pyx Granite Co.* v. *Minister of Housing and Local Government*, and *Scruttons Ltd* v. *Midland Silicones Ltd*. Only in *Ross Smith* v. *Ross Smith* did the Law Lords once again reveal the extent of the dissension in their ranks over the competing claims of the 'be consistent' and the 'be fair' expectations. While overall this case owes more to the prevailing role perception of 1957 than to that of later years, even then four of the Law Lords would have been prepared to overrule the 1860 precedent, despite its antiquity, but only three (it was a seven judge case) considered that the precedent had been wrongly decided. Yet in most of the cases which I have just listed the Law Lords adopted a creative approach to the *ratio* or dicta in a precedent of the House itself. The technique which the Law Lords deployed in these cases was 'Dissimulation', for in them they appeared to maintain the compatibility of the 'be consistent' and the 'be fair' expectations, whereas in reality they were violating the former expectation in favour of the latter.*

On the other hand, as in the period just prior to 1957, I found little trace of 'role-distancing' as a judicial response to the conflict. Two exceptions were Lord Reid in *Adamastos* v. *Anglo-Saxon Petrol Co.* and several of the Law Lords in *IRC* v. *Hinchy*. Again there was no attempt to convene the role-set to deal with the role conflict, so far as I could trace.

---

*I have deliberately not elaborated my discussion of these cases, and of the Law Lords' use of 'Dissimulation' in them, because to have done so would have involved the repetition of the cogent arguments set out by G. Dworkin in '*Stare Decisis* in the House of Lords', 25 *MLR* (1962) 163 (esp. pp. 165 and 170). I would propose instead to adopt his descriptions of the Law Lords' performances in these cases as part of my argument. I would only add that the *Scruttons* case is a further example of the danger of evaluating precedent orientation as passive or non-activist.[94]

THE 'FACADE' APPROACH

The period 1957-62 was significant for the study of the judicial role in hard cases for another reason. This was the publication of Lord Radcliffe's Rosenthal Lectures, given in 1960, under the title of *The Law and its Compass*.[95] In these lectures Lord Radcliffe discussed the creative role of the judge more openly than possibly any English judge (with the exception of Lord Denning) who had put his views into print prior to that date. In so doing I believe he provided the explanation of the increasing use of 'Dissimulation' by the Law Lords in the early 1960s.

So long as the prevailing orthodoxy of 1957 retained its sway the Law Lords could assign such a low status to the 'be fair' as opposed to the 'don't legislate' and 'be consistent' expectations as virtually to deny the possibility of a conflict between them. This had the effect of minimising the Law Lords' role as law-makers* and thus no issue of legitimacy arose. Once the Law Lords had come to perceive the 'be fair' expectation as a 'relevant' part of their role in hard cases, however, the potential role conflict could no longer be ignored. Faced with *Innovation* from Lords Denning and Reid, it was harder for the other Law Lords to continue consistently to rank the 'be fair' expectation below the other two. This in turn meant that the 'don't legislate' expectation could no longer be interpreted as an absolute prohibition on judicial creativity. But opening up the issue of judicial law-making meant that the question of its legitimacy would also arise. Lord Radcliffe's solution was simple. Whilst recognising 'the judge's law-making capacity, a capacity which only the judges themselves, and that for excellent reasons, are likely to dispute ...' he suggested that the judges should deny it in public. He added,

> If judges prefer the formula - for that is what it is - that they merely declare the law and do not make it, they do no more than show themselves wise men in practice. Their analysis may be weak, but their perception of the nature of the law is sound. Men's respect for it will be the greater, the more imperceptible

*I am aware of the semantic problems attached to the use of this word. (See Twining, 87 *LQR* (1971) 398 at p.400.) It is used in this and the following chapter simply to denote that Law Lords in deciding points of law in hard cases have, and most perceive themselves as having, a certain room for choice between the various alternative solutions (see Chapter 8 below).

its development.[96]

Lord Radcliffe later elaborated his views on this point and for reasons of convenience I shall quote them now. In 1967 in an address to Harvard University Law Faculty he said,

> [We] have to make some assessment of the Judge as a maker of the law in his own right .... His duties and his failures in this capacity constitute very much a contemporary theme although I doubt whether its elaboration is not likely to prove more of a curse than a blessing. It is so easy to start, and it seems so hard to know where to stop. Would anyone now deny that judicial decisions are a creative, not merely an expository, contribution to the law? There are no means by which they can be otherwise, so rare is the occasion upon which a decision does not involve choice between two admissible alternatives .... [Yet we] cannot run the risk of finding the archetypal image of the judge confused in men's minds with the very different image of the legislator .... Personally, I think that judges will serve the public interest better if they keep quiet about their legislative function.[97]

From these quotations it will be seen that Lord Radcliffe recognised the potentiality for conflict between the 'don't legislate', the 'be consistent' and the 'be fair' expectations. To give effect openly to the 'be fair' expectation at the expense of the other two, he implied, could raise acutely the problem of the legitimacy of judicial law-making. A judge who is seen to be developing the law runs the risk of undermining his (and his brethren's) authority[98] by revealing that on occasions he acts as a legislator without democratic authority.[99] On the other hand Lord Radcliffe found it equally unacceptable to adopt the orthodoxy of 1957 which in most cases involved the rejection of the 'be fair' expectation in favour of the other two. His solution to the conflict was 'Dissimulation'. The judge should appear to uphold all three expectations and yet in reality violate whichever of the three he considers necessary in any given case. In accordance with this view Lord Radcliffe told me that he regarded the 1966 Practice Statement on Precedent as 'a very foolish statement to make, because his own view was that this wasn't needed'. He continued,

I never did understand how a declaration of a century ago was any more sacrosanct than any other House of Lords' judgement. It was just standing on its own tail, really.

In the same interview he remarked, 'If a judge of reasonable strength of mind thought a particular precedent was wrong, he must be a great fool if he couldn't get around it.'*

But the facade approach did not (and does not) solve the problem of the legitimacy of judicial law-making. It defined it out of existence by judicial fiat and swept the issue under the carpet. It also had considerable disadvantages for the profession, for it created uncertainty. By refusing to discuss judicial law-making it left the limits of judicial law-making in practice, and the content of the 'don't legislate' expectation in particular, largely undefined. C.K. Allen in *Law in the Making* illustrated the consequences of this when he asked,

[Is] it possible to extract any general principles which tell us, with some measure of probability, when a superior court will rid the law of what are generally agreed to be errors or blemishes? It seems impossible to predicate anything very definite .... The plain truth is that in this important matter our judicial technique does not seem to have developed any consistent principle; *quot judices tot sententiae*.[100]

On the one hand this flexibility enabled the Law Lords to refuse to develop the law in the years before 1957 by hiding behind the 'don't legislate' expectation, yet on the other hand it permitted the same judges to indulge in judicial law-making of the calibre of *Shaw* v. *DPP*. The absence of a specific content for the 'don't legislate' expectation in the late 1950s and early 1960s not only undermined the 'reckonability'[101] of decisions by the profession. It also meant that there was less restraint on a judge implementing his value preferences in a decision,† as some of the Law Lords in

---

Cf. his comment in 'The Judges', a Thames Television interview in 1971. 'I'm bound to say I think that a man who is ... lively minded ... who is not overreverential towards the great men of the past of his profession, can generally find a way of dealing according to his conscience with problems that come before him, even though in theory they may be dogged by precedents of the past.'

†It will be recalled that 'Dissimulation' may involve ranking expectations according to the ease with which their violation can be concealed. It is easier to conceal the violation of an amorphous standard than a more specific one.

Shaw v. *DPP* appeared to do. This weakness in the Law Lords' role, which allowed their personal sympathies to creep in, is perhaps what led Robert Seidman to conclude as late as 1969 that, ' ... there are no commonly accepted norms defining the judge's role in deciding the hard cases'.[102]

THE LAW LORDS IN 1966

The second period of my study, from the date of Viscount Simonds' retirement in 1962 to the announcement of the 1966 Practice Statement on Precedent on 26 July 1966, was one of considerable judicial law-making. I do not think it can be denied that the more activist approach to precedent which appeared (albeit under the guise of 'Dissimulation') in 1957-62 was maintained if not increased in the four succeeding years. The list of hard cases contains such celebrated cases as *Hedley Byrne & Co.* v. *Heller*, *Ridge* v. *Baldwin*, *Gollins* v. *Gollins*, *Burmah Oil Co.* v. *Lord Advocate*, *ICI* v. *Shatwell*, *Rookes* v. *Barnard*, *Stratford* v. *Lindley*, *National Provincial Bank* v. *Ainsworth*, *Carl-Zeiss Stiftung* v. *Rayner & Keeler*, *Suisse Atlantique* v. *Rotterdamsche* and *Myers* v. *DPP*. But even in these cases the Law Lords by and large did not discuss their activitism openly.[103] References to judicial law-making were rare,[104] overt references to policy considerations were infrequent[105] and 'Dissimulation' was still resorted to as the principal response to the role conflict inherent in hard cases. But even in the four years the position was changing. The ease with which the Law Lords departed from a principle of 100 years standing in *Button* v. *DPP* was in marked contrast to the agonies of *Ross Smith*. In *Hedley Byrne* v. *Heller* and *National Provincial Bank* v. *Ainsworth* the House of Lords faced up to and overruled precedents of the Court of Appeal which some lawyers had considered well established. The tenor of the period was, I would suggest, one of adapting the law to changing social conditions.[106] No longer was the emphasis on the separation between the law as it is and as it ought to be, as heavily defined as in 1957,[107] and more stress was being placed on legal principles as opposed to legal rules.[108]

The suggestion that a more activist approach to precedent was being taken than in the years immediately prior to 1957 is not a rationalisation following the appearance of the 1966 Practice Statement. Rather, I would argue that the Statement was the

culmination of a period of increasing willingness by the Law Lords
to take a freer attitude to precedent. This assertion has support
from a variety of sources. C.K. Allen in *Law in the Making* wrote,
in 1963,

> There is, ... at the present time, a marked disposition to
> mitigate, by various devices, the severity of precedent when it
> tends merely to perpetuate error, and the whole system seems to
> be passing through a critical phase in its long history.[109]

Professor Lloyd writing in 1965 said,

> ... there are signs that the present House of Lords is adopting a
> rather freer attitude towards its earlier decisions than was
> previously manifested.[110]

Similar views were expressed in the same year by Robert
Stevens[111] and Allen[112] again. Even Professor Cross whose summary of the state of the doctrine of precedent in England I quoted
earlier, a mere five years later was able to write,

> [T]here has been a considerable relaxation in the rigour with
> which the rule of *stare decisis* is applied in this country ... indeed
> ... the process of relaxation has, it is submitted, gone far
> enough to call for a radical restatement of the English doctrine
> of precedent.[113]

The views of the Law Lords whom I interviewed largely
supported the thesis that the Practice Statement was the
culmination of a period of increasing willingness by the Law Lords
to take a freer attitude to precedent. These views, of course, were
perceptions by the Law Lords of a change in their role. Lord Reid
considered that prior to the Statement, 'Most of us were prepared
to get round a decision that we couldn't stomach. We'd reached
the stage that we could find a way round any such decision.'[114]
Another commented,

> I don't think the Practice Statement was meant to produce any
> revolutionary change. I don't think in this House it has made
> much difference because one has always treated precedent with
> a certain amount of liberty here, and I haven't yet noticed that

it has changed our spirit.

Lords Denning, Devlin, Guest and MacDermott all shared the view that the Practice Statement saved the House from attempting to distinguish the indistinguishable.* Lord Pearson also provides an insight ino the prevailing attitude to precedent in the House of Lords when he joined it in 1965, in the following observation,

> ... on coming to the House of Lords, one has to adapt one's attitude and outlook quite considerably. You bear in mind that not only has one been in the Court of Appeal, but also at first instance, and at the Bar, and one did, in the earlier stages, develop a very strong regard for precedent. And one did seek to find authority in favour of one's propositions and was more keen to find authority, perhaps than to work out the principle. And I dare say one should have worked out the principle more, but when one comes here, one finds one is very much engaged in working out the principle without too much regard to what has been previously decided in all the lower courts.

Finally Lord Upjohn - no supporter of an activist approach to precedent (on his own admission)[115] - said in 1968,

> I may be wrong - I hope so - but I think there has been a tendency perhaps over the last ten years to draw fine distinctions between earlier cases, in order to do what is called justice in the particular case; I may be old fashioned but I deplore that attitude.

These quotations from the Law Lords and from the academic commentators are important. They demonstrate that between 1957 and 1966 the role of a Law Lord in the first category of hard case was changing from a passive attitude to precedent to a more activist one. It was not just that the role performances had changed; the role perceptions had also changed. Moreover, as we

---

*However, Lords Guest and MacDermott considered that the Statement had been a 'very violent change' and 'a significant change', respectively. I think these assessments are more akin to Lord Pearson's description of the Statement as 'a UDI'. They reflect a change from the facade approach, *i.e.* a change in candour which was significant, rather than a violent change in outlook towards precedent.

shall see, they had changed in the direction favoured by certain of
their reference individuals and by academic commentators (acting
in their limited capacity as a reference group). The change
involved a different attitude to the role conflict between the 'don't
legislate', the 'be consistent' and the 'be fair' expectations (when it
arose), to that enshrined in the prevailing orthodoxy of 1957 and
the years immediately prior to that. This included the elevation of
the 'be fair' expectation to 'relevant' status and a willingness on
occasion to violate the 'don't legislate' and the 'be consistent'
expectations under the guise of 'Dissimulation'. What the 1966
Practice Statement represented was a further development in
which the conflict was publicly stated to exist, coupled with a
recognition that on occasion it would be legitimate for the Law
Lords to rank the 'be fair' above the 'be consistent' expectation.

Stevens, in *Law and Politics*,[116] is clearly correct to argue that the
changing social and political climate of the 1960s contributed to
this change in attitude to precedent (and thus to a change in the
role of the Law Lord in a hard case), but foremost amongst the
other contributory factors to which I have already adverted, was
Innovation on the part of Lord Reid. It was his activities, more than
any other Law Lord's, I would argue, which brought about the
change and also the 1966 Practice Statement.

LORD REID: INNOVATION AND PRECEDENT — THE MAKING OF A PRACTICE STATEMENT

We saw earlier that Lord Reid was acutely aware of the layman's
expectation that the law be both certain and just. He set out his
response to the conflict in 'The Judge as Law Maker', where he
said,

> People want two inconsistent things; that the law shall be
> certain, and that it shall be just and shall move with the times. It
> is our business to keep both objectives in view. Rigid adherence
> to precedent will not do. And paying lip service to precedent
> while admitting fine distinctions gives us the worst of both
> worlds. On the other hand too much flexibility leads to
> intolerable uncertainty .... Of course we must have a general
> doctrine of precedent - otherwise we can have no certainty. But

we must find a middle way which prevents precedent being our master.[117]

Lord Reid, therefore, favoured a balancing solution. Understandably, he was not satisfied with the solution adopted by the prevailing orthodoxy in the House of Lords in the early 1950s, of giving very little weight to the 'be fair' as opposed to the 'be consistent' expectation. He set out to redress this imbalance in a series of dicta. The first was in *Nash* v. *Tamplin*, where he said,

> My Lords, it is very unsatisfactory to have to grope for a decision in this way, but the need to do so arises from the fact that this House has debarred itself from ever reconsidering any of its own decisions. It matters not how difficult it is to find the *ratio decidendi* of a previous case, that *ratio* must be found.[118]

He referred again to the House's self-imposed shackles in *IRC* v. *Baddeley*[119] and in the Second reading of the Occupiers' Liability Bill he stated,

> the justification for the present rule is that it is supposed to lead to certainty in the law - a most desirable thing, if one can achieve it. But a good deal could be said to the effect that it has exactly the contrary effect.[120]

Again in *London Transport Executive* v. *Betts*,[121] Lord Reid expressly stated that he would favour a modification of the 'strict practice' of the House being bound by its own decisions. And in *Scruttons* v. *Midland Silicones*[122] came his well-known remarks about the 'three classes of case where ... we are entitled to question or limit' a House of Lords' precedent.

Lord Reid's next attack occurred in *West and Son* v. *Shephard* when he invited Mark Littman QC to review the authorities on the rule, even though the point was not essential to the case. His last published statement on the issue prior to the Statement, appeared in the *Chancery Lane* v. *IRC* case where he said,

> This House still regards itself as bound by the rule that it must not reverse or depart from a previous decision of the House. But it would in my view be pedantic and unreasonable to apply that rule to the present case ... [123]

Lord Reid then declined to follow the precedent in question even though it was indistinguishable on the facts, because he said the reasoning in that case had been based on a mistaken view of the facts.

On the basis of these statements, it would seem that Lord Reid was actively seeking to negotiate a change in the definition of his role as a Law Lord in hard cases.* Although he was prepared on occasion to attempt to erode the doctrine of precedent in the Lords, as in *Scruttons* or the *Chancery Lane* case, this was always a tactic which he regarded as 'the less bad of the only alternatives'[124] open to him. His desire was that the doctrine should be openly modified in order that a proper balance between justice and certainty could be struck. Such a modification he believed would actually reduce uncertainty at the same time as reducing the potential for conflict between the 'be consistent' and the 'be fair' expectations. Lord Reid's argument was that the old view that any departure from rigid adherence to precedent would weaken existing certainty in the law, was erroneous. He continued,

> It is notorious that where an existing decision is disapproved but cannot be overruled, courts tend to distinguish it on inadequate grounds .... But this is bound to lead to uncertainty for no one can say in advance whether in a particular case the court will or will not feel bound to follow the old unsatisfactory decision. On balance it seems to me that overruling such a decision will promote and not impair the certainty of the law.[125]

We may conclude, therefore, that Lord Reid's response to the conflicting expectations was *Innovation* (endeavouring to effect a change in one's role in such a way that role conflict will be reduced or institutionalised).† Lord Reid's views certainly influenced his colleagues, the more so since he fulfilled Lord Diplock's stipulation that,[126]

---

*Lord Reid's repeated statements on the rule of *stare decisis* in the Lords were not accidental. Repetition was, as we shall see, a tactic which he adopted on several issues in which he wished to influence his brethren.

†I did not ask Lord Reid explicitly whether he had been seeking to bring about a relaxation in the doctrine of precedent in the House of Lords. But when I asked him (in 1972) whether he thought that the House had taken a freer line as regards precedent in the last fifteen years, he replied 'Yes. I think there's been quite a significant relaxation in our approach to precedent. I'm less conservative than Lord Simonds was.'

He who sets out to alter the habits of mind of judges must be possessed of stamina and patience and, if he hopes to see some positive results, blessed with longevity ...

The impetus for change depends upon the personal persuasion of someone who is accepted as a member of the community.

Another person who influenced some of the Law Lords, who also objected to the rigid doctrine of precedent in the Lords, was Professor Goodhart.[127] In this he was joined by most of the contemporary jurisprudence textbook writers.[128] Inasmuch as this group or members of it acted directly or indirectly as a reference group or reference individuals to the Law Lords on this issue, then their opinions were a further contributing factor to the introduction of the Practice Statement.*

What may be said with hindsight was that the innovatory activities of Lords Reid and Denning, taken together with the academic consensus as represented by these writers, had contributed to an atmosphere receptive to the change. It required but a catalyst.

The catalyst came from an unexpected source - the Scottish Law Commission.[129] Its first programme contained a proposal for legislation declaring for the avoidance of doubt that the rigid doctrine of precedent in the House of Lords did not apply in Scottish Appeals. The English Law Commission were then sorry[130] that they had not included a similar item in relation to English Appeals in their first programme. A plan of campaign was agreed on between the Law Commissions which involved the Scottish Commission in drafting a Bill, which they duly did. After consideration of the constitutional problems, the Chairman of the Scottish Law Commission (Lord Kilbrandon), decided to consult the Lord Advocate and the Lord Chancellor. A letter on the matter reached the Lord Chancellor on or about 17 March 1966. At or about the same time the English Law Commission approached the Lord Chancellor with their proposals. Lord Gardiner was sympathetic and decided to ask the Law Lords what they thought. He accordingly spoke to Lord Reid. Sir Denis Dobson (the Lord Chancellor's Permanent Secretary) then invited

---

*Lord Reid told me that the Law Lords, when they decided to issue the 1966 Practice Statement, were aware that various academic writers did not like the rigid doctrine.

the Law Lords (incuding the retired ones) to a formal meeting in the House. (Such formal meetings of all the Law Lords do take place at rare intervals - another one was held when it was decided that dissents in the Privy Council should be published.)[131]

Before the meeting various judges drew up memoranda on the issue[132] and the Law Lords read the Scottish Commission's proposals.[133] The meeting was attended by the existing Lords of Appeal (Lords Reid, Morris, Hodson, Guest, Pearce, Upjohn, Donovan, Wilberforce and Pearson) and certain of the other Law Lords including Lords Denning, Devlin and Parker, Viscount Radcliffe, Viscount Simonds and Lord Tucker.[134] The meeting decided that the strict doctrine should go. As Lord Gardiner recalled,

> They came along to my room eventually and they said, 'Well we have been thinking about this, and we do not think in these days that the House of Lords ought to be bound by judicial precedent: but we would use this power sparingly and not where contracts have been made on the state of the previous law, particularly as far as property and investment are concerned. But we think that we ought not to be strictly bound as we now are, and we could change this by saying so.' Well, far be it from me to say the Law Lords do not know the law, but I was a little surprised that they all said 'It is not a rule of law: it is a rule of practice, and we can alter our practice, and we would quite approve if you would get up and make a statement on our behalf that in the future ...'

and he added later,

> ... my recollection is, they all came to my room and we discussed it, and who actually drafted the Statement out, I forget. I do not think I altered it at all. I dare say Lord Reid did.

I asked Lord Reid whether he had drawn up the actual Statement and he replied 'No. I had a hand in it, but I didn't compose the whole thing.'

Lord Morris later asserted that the change had the full concurrence of all the Lords of Appeal in Ordinary;[135] in fact some of the Law Lords at least, had reservations. Lord Reid commented,

Well, one or two were dubious about the change, but no one was prepared to dig his heels in. If one or two had dug in then it couldn't have been done. If only one had done so then he might have been persuaded to keep quiet. It couldn't have been got through in my early days as a Law Lord.*

On the basis of this account several observations can be made. First, that Lord Gardiner, despite his desire for the reform,[136] took relatively little active part in bringing it about. He did not act until approached by the Law Commissions and he left the decisions as to whether a change should be made, and if so, how,[137] to the Law Lords.† Lord Reid as senior Law Lord seems to have played a more active part than most of his colleagues[138] - a finding which supports the thesis that Lord Reid's favoured response to the problem of precedent was *Innovation*.

Secondly, the mode adopted for bringing about the change, viz. by a Practice Statement, was premised on the Law Lords' assertion that the rule of precedent in the House of Lords was one of practice. In this they seem to have taken advantage of the fact that in constitutional theory appeals to the Lords are petitions to the whole Upper Chamber of Parliament. Since Parliament cannot bind its successors the Law Lords saw no reason why a rule

---

*Lord Guest confirmed that there was a minority of Law Lords against it and Viscount Radcliffe indicated that he had been sceptical about it. Lord Reid's final sentence raises the issue of whether there had been discussions amongst the Law Lords in the past on the question. Lord Denning insisted that there had been such earlier discussions when Viscount Simonds was the senior Law Lord and that 'Lord Simonds wouldn't have it at all'. See also *The Discipline of Law*, p. 296. Lord Pearce confirmed that Viscount Simonds had been very much against the change even as late as 1962. Of the others who attended the meeting several, including Lords Reid, Guest, Pearce and Pearson all told me that they favoured the change. Lords Upjohn (see his address 'Twenty Years On' p. 657) and Devlin (see his article 'Judges and Lawmakers' 39 *MLR* (1976) 1 at p. 13) have expressed the same view in print. Of the active Law Lords only Lord Cross considered that it had been a mistake.
†Lord Gardiner certainly played an important passive role, for without his acquiescence it is unlikely that the change could ever have been made. Despite his comments in *Law Reform NOW* Lord Gardiner adopted the same passive stance on whether a third tier of appeal was necessary. He remarked,

> I have never had any strong views as to whether we ought to retain the House of Lords as a judicial body or not. I waited as Lord Chancellor, and encouraged people to say what they thought about it, and nobody ever did, really.

set up by their predecessors could not be altered by themselves.* If precedent at this level is a rule of practice it is hard to see why the same does not apply to the Court of Appeal. I share the doubts of Cross,[139] Glanville-Williams[140] and Dias[141] concerning the 'status of pronoucements by one court concerning the practice to be followed by a court below it in the hierarchy with regard to the previous decisions of that lower court'.[142] The House of Lords, undaunted, has persisted in making such pronouncements in relation to the Court of Appeal, usually ascribing the force of law to the rule that the Court of Appeal is bound by its own decisions.[143] Yet Lord Salmon in a recent Privy Council case[144] asserted with the concurrence of Lords Simon, Fraser, Russell and Scarman that pronouncements by the House of Lords about the rule could only be of persuasive authority.

Cross concludes that the *ratio-obiter* distinction has no bearing on these pronouncements.[145] I agree. Discussions relating to the 1966 Practice Statement and to precedent in the Court of Appeal which are couched purely in terms of law, or practice, or of constitutional convention do not seem to me to be particularly illuminating. On the other hand, if the issues are approached from the standpoint of role analysis, some of the complications disappear. The rules of *stare decisis* are then seen to be 'pivotal' expectations in the role of appellate court judges in hard cases. What happened in 1966 was that as a result of role conflict in one category of hard cases, the

---

*See Lord Reid in 'The Judge as Law Maker', p. 25 and Lord Cohen in 'The Court of Appeal', p. 11. See also Viscount Dilhorne in *Davis* v. *Johnson*, at p. 336F-H.

In 1966 consideration was given to whether as a matter of law this House was bound to follow its earlier decision. After considerable discussion it was agreed that it was not .... This House is not bound by any previous decision ... whether or not the House is sitting to discharge its judicial functions. That is the ground on which those who were parties to the announcement made in 1966 felt, I think, that it could be made without impropriety.

The same argument was used by the Law Lords in the re-hearing on costs in *Cassell* v. *Broome* (No. 2), to justify departing from a procedural precedent which would have prevented the appellants from successfully challenging the Court's initial ruling on costs. Lord Simon of Glaisdale, though in favour of the change, expressed doubts during the oral argument in *Jones* v. *Secretary of State for Social Services* as to the status of Lord Gardiner's statement, but counsel was not prepared to argue the point. Lord Simon's later view was that the Statement was a 'constitutional convention having the force of law', see *Knuller* v. *DPP* at p. 485 and *Miliangos* at p. 472C. I do not think the Law Lords in 1966 would have agreed with this description.

Law Lords (for the reasons already outlined), adopted the unusual *Positive* response to role conflict of convening their most significant reference group,[146] namely, themselves, in order to deal with the conflict. In thus altering one of the pivotal expectations in their own role the Law Lords, by definition, brought about a change in their role in hard cases. Members of the Court of Appeal, however, having a lower status in the legal hierarchy than the Law Lords, possess less relative autonomy in the definition of their own role. The Law Lords certainly perceive themselves to be a reference group for the members of the Court of Appeal, if we are to judge from some of their recent attempts to sanction Lord Denning for deviant behaviour.[147] I would suggest that comments by Law Lords on the Court of Appeal being bound by its own precedents can most easily be understood as the expression and reinforcement of a role expectation for the conduct of members of the Court of Appeal by one of their reference groups. If I am correct, even if Lord Denning succeeds in persuading almost all the members of the court[148] to accept a change in the doctrine of *stare decisis*, this may not be sufficient to effect such a change if the Law Lords do not also agree.

Finally, if my analysis is acceptable, it provides an answer to the problem which has exercised some writers,[149] viz., how can a rule of practice acquire prescriptive authority? For the change in role to succeed it requires that the new role be accepted by the Law Lords' reference groups. Since they are their own primary reference group it would take strong objection by other lesser or symbolic reference groups, *e.g.* Benchers, the legislature or the public, for the change to be effectively challenged.*

---

*The account given of the way the 1966 Practice Statement came about, and the interpretation given of it and of *stare decisis* in the Court of Appeal, are relevant to the juristic controversy concerning the status of H.L.A. Hart's 'rule of recognition', in particular concerning the way in which he attaches that concept to activities of officials (*The Concept of Law,* pp. 107 and 113). It supports Hart against the criticism voiced by Sartorius in 'Hart's Concept of Law' in Summers (ed.), *More Essays in Legal Philosophy* (Oxford: Basil Blackwell, 1971) p.159 that 'the rule of recognition exists only as a complex ... practice seems to be patently false', for it seems quite consistent with Hart's claim that in this area nothing succeeds but success.

7 The Law Lords in 1973 and Beyond

The final period of the original study ran from 1966 to 1973. It was marked not only for the amount of judicial law-making[1] which it contained but also for the candour with which it was undertaken. For the first time the Law Lords as a body began to discuss judicial law-making and policy issues openly in a series of cases,[2] as opposed to the occasional dictum in an isolated case. Concomitantly the enigmatic response of 'Dissimulation' began gradually to fall out of favour, though curiously, as we shall see, in the initial cases where there were attempts to invoke the 1966 Practice Statement (the pronouncement of which had been a body blow to the facade approach) the movement away from 'Dissimulation' was less marked than in other hard cases.

The key discovery to emerge from the Law Lords' interviews and their performance in decided cases in this period, however, was that Lord Reid's *Innovation* and his influence on his colleagues extended beyond his attitude to precedent. He sought also to elucidate the circumstances in which the Practice Statement ought to be invoked, as part of a wider ranging articulation of the limits of judicial law-making in the Lords.

LORD REID: INNOVATION AND PRECEDENT — THE USE OF THE PRACTICE STATEMENT

Lord Reid had no illusions about the potential for creativity in the judicial role.[3] As he once declared,

> There was a time when it was thought almost indecent to suggest that judges make law - they only declare it .... But we do not believe in fairy tales any more.[4]

154

While discussing the *raison d'être* of the House of Lords he told me,

> I think our real function is twofold, (a) to clear up the messes of which there are many and (b) occasionally to be a bit bold and innovate a bit. Take that recent case about the child trespassers ... [*British Railways Board* v. *Herrington*] Well now, we just had to take the bit between our teeth, there was nothing else to be done, and I don't suppose we all said the same thing, but we all came to the same result.

Moreover, he considered that in a democratic society the legitimacy of such judicial law-making was a problem that had to be confronted. Lord Radcliffe's solution of publicly denying one's creativity while privately exercising it - the 'facade' approach - was not acceptable to Lord Reid. 'I don't think we should do that', he said, 'That would be unreal in this day and age. The public wouldn't stand for it'.[5] Thus in a famous address he asserted,

> [We] must accept the fact that for better or worse judges do make law, and tackle the question how do they approach their task and how should they approach it.[6]

On the other hand Lord Denning's bold assertions of the scope for judicial discretion and his appeals to substantive rationality (or even irrationality?) were too untrammelled for Lord Reid's liking. His solution to the problem, which remained an abiding concern of his throughout his career in the Lords, was to set limits to judicial law-making. In short, his response once more was *Innovation* - an appeal to normative guidelines. More than any of his colleagues he spelt out what he considered to be the limits of legitimate judicial law-making in the House, and in our interview he assured me that this had been a deliberate strategy. I asked him whether he was hoping that the other Law Lords would take up these guidelines and he replied,

> I think perhaps I've had a little influence, you know, in that way ... trying to draw the line between the cases when we can innovate and those where it would be wrong to try.

In demarcating thus between Parliament and the Judiciary,

Lord Reid faced up to the task which Lord Radcliffe had failed to tackle, viz., giving greater content to the expectation that the courts should not indulge in 'legislation'. He recognised, moreover, that the more clearly defined and delineated version of the 'don't legislate' expectation which he was advocating, inevitably involved both the expectation that existing principles and precedents should be adhered to (the 'be consistent' expectation) and the expectation that the principles and precedents applied in a case should be in accord with contemporary notions of fairness and justice (the 'be fair' expectation). Indeed, his new version of the 'don't legislate' expectation was based in part on different rankings between the 'be consistent' and the 'be fair' expectations in different areas of law.

Once the 1966 Practice Statement had been made Lord Reid's desire to elucidate the limits of judicial law-making led him to formulating guidelines which stipulated the typical situations in which the freedom asserted in the Statement should be exercised - a task closely akin to delineating the content of the 'don't legislate' expectation. Once again, *Innovation* (for he was really suggesting additions to the Law Lords' role[7]) was his response to the conflict between the 'be consistent' and the 'be fair' expectations which arose whenever there was an attempt to invoke the Statement. In a series of cases between 1966 and 1975 Lord Reid articulated at least seven criteria relating to the use of the new freedom. They were:

1. The freedom granted by the 1966 Practice Statement, ought to be exercised sparingly (the 'use sparingly' criterion).[8]
2. A decision ought not to be overruled if to do so would upset the legitimate expectations of people who have entered into contracts or settlements or otherwise regulated their affairs in reliance on the validity of that decision (the 'legitimate expectations' criterion).[9]
3. A decision concerning questions of construction of statutes or other documents ought not to be overruled except in rare and exceptional cases (the 'construction' criterion).[10]
4. (a) A decision ought not to be overruled if it would be impracticable for the Lords to foresee the consequences of departing from it (the 'unforeseeable consequences' criterion).[11]
(b) A decision ought not to be overruled if to do so would involve a change that ought to be part of a comprehensive reform of the law.

Such changes are best done 'by legislation following on a wide survey of the whole field' (the 'need for comprehensive reform' criterion).[12]

5. In the interest of certainty, a decision ought not to be overruled merely because the Law Lords consider that it was wrongly decided. There must be some additional reasons to justify such a step (the 'precedent merely wrong' criterion).[13]

6. A decision ought to be overruled if it causes such great uncertainty in practice that the parties' advisers are unable to give any clear indication as to what the courts will hold the law to be (the 'rectification of uncertainty' criterion).[14]

7. A decision ought to be overruled if in relation to some broad issue or principle it is not considered just or in keeping with contemporary social conditions or modern conceptions of public policy (the 'unjust or outmoded' criterion).[15]

In setting out these criteria Lord Reid showed that like Lord Wilberforce,[16] his successor as senior Law Lord, he believed that the discretion asserted in the 1966 Practice Statement ought to be exercised according to set principles or guidelines. It is also clear that in his pronouncements on this matter, particularly his seminal excursus on the purpose and parameters of the Practice Statement in the *Jones* case, he was consciously seeking to influence his colleagues.

How successful these efforts were is difficult to gauge. At the very least we can say that his dicta on this topic were cited and have continued to be cited approvingly by his colleagues with a frequency denied to any other Law Lord,[17] or even to the Practice Statement itself. Further, when the perceptions of his colleagues in 1973 are examined, Lord Reid appears to have represented the dominant consensus amongst them. The consensus on the 'use sparingly' criterion was, and continues to be, overwhelming. Five of the Law Lords interviewed (including Lords Cross, Guest, Kilbrandon and Salmon) said that the freedom should be used 'sparingly' or 'very sparingly'. Lords Dilhorne,[18] Diplock,[19] Hailsham,[20] Simon[21] and Upjohn[22] all recorded similar views in print and so too, in more recent times, have Lords Edmund-Davies,[23] Keith[24] and Wilberforce[25] (and by implication,[26] Lords Fraser, Russell and Scarman).

Lord Reid's 'legitimate expectations' criterion (his second), also enjoyed wide support. It is impliedly contained in the terms of the

Practice Statement itself. Lords Guest, Pearson[27] and Kilbrandon expressly mentioned it in the interviews. As Lord Kilbrandon observed,

> The House ... will regard reform as a Parliamentary duty where a doctrine has long ago been laid down and long acted upon, *e.g.* by merchants and lawyers concerned with advising clients.

Elsewhere it has been articulated by Lords Morris,[28] Donovan,[29] Wilberforce,[30] Pearson,[31] Diplock,[32] Dilhorne,[33] Edmund-Davies[34] and Scarman.[35] It was largely on account of the weight which the Law Lords attached to this criterion (it was clearly 'pivotal' to their role[36]) that they began to discuss the technique of prospective overruling,[37] a device which would permit them to change the law for the future without upsetting the legitimate expectations of the public.[38]

Lord Reid's 'construction' criterion (his third) undoubtedly featured in the prevailing consensus amongst the Law Lords in 1973. Lords Cross and Pearson referred to it in the interviews. It was explicitly stated in the *Jones* case[39] by Lords Reid, Morris, Wilberforce, Pearson, Diplock and Simon; in *Taylor* v. *Provan*[40] by Lords Wilberforce, Simon and Salmon; and in *Farrell* v. *Alexander*[41] by Lord Simon. It was applied, by implication, in *O'Brien* v. *Robinson*[42] by Lords Morris and Diplock. The criterion would seem still to be part of a Law Lord's role for it was adverted to with approval in *Vestey* v. *IRC*[43] by Lords Dilhorne and Edmund-Davies and, by implication, by Lord Wilberforce. It was also supported by Lord Diplock in 'Judicial Development of Law in the Commonwealth'.[44]

Lord Reid's fourth criterion came in two forms. Both were closely related to the expectation that the Law Lords ought not to usurp the functions of the legislature. The first (the 'unforeseeable consequences' test), attracted a certain measure of support both before and after 1973. Lord Simon in particular argued vehemently for it in several cases, *e.g. Miliangos* v. *George Frank*,[45] *DPP* v. *Lynch*[46] and *DPP* v. *Shannon*;[47] Lord Kilbrandon endorsed it in *Lynch* as did Lords Dilhorne and Fraser in *Hesperides Hotels* v. *Muftizade*.[48] The second form (the 'need for comprehensive reform' test) was relied on by a majority of Law Lords in *Cassell* v. *Broome*[49] and in recent times has gained considerable currency.[50]

The fifth criterion, that a decision's incorrectness does not, on its own, justify overruling it, might seem to merit the rebuke that, 'some judges are like the old bishop who having begun to eat the asparagus at the wrong end did not choose to alter'.[51] In fact, it is a manifestation of the Law Lords' view that the decision whether or not to exercise the 1966 freedom is 'one of legal policy into which wider considerations enter than mere questions of substantive law'.[52] Support for it can be found in the *Jones*[53] case from Lord Simon; in *Knuller*[54] from Lords Morris and Simon, in *Geelong Harbour Trust* v. *Gibbs Bright*[55] from the whole committee and in *Miliangos*[56] from Lord Simon and Cross. More recently, it was endorsed in *Fitzleet* v. *Cherry* by the whole Appellate Committee, Lords Wilberforce, Dilhorne, Salmon, Edmund-Davies and Keith, and in *R* v. *Cunningham* by Lords Hailsham and Edmund-Davies. There have, however, been some dissenters. Lords Denning and MacDermott when interviewed said that the freedom should be exercised whenever the Law Lords considered that the previous decision was wrong. Lord Diplock appeared to side with the dissenters' position, in *Knuller*,[57] but subsequently accepted the fifth criterion in the *Geelong* case. The minority's position prevails in the US Supreme Court but even there it has been acknowledged that sometimes it is necessary to preserve an 'incorrect' decision,[58] just as in this country the Law Lords have been known on occasion to subscribe to the doctrine of *communis error facit ius*.

Lord Reid's 'rectification of uncertainty' criterion (the sixth) has received rather less support. It was accepted by Lord Diplock and rejected by Lord Simon in *Knuller*,[59] and accepted by both Lord Diplock and Lord Simon in the *Oldendorff*[60] case, endorsed by Lord Elwyn-Jones LC in an adress[61] and upheld by Lord Edmund-Davies in *Fitzleet* v. *Cherry*.[62] On the other hand Lord Reid's final criterion, the 'unjust or outmoded' test, or a close approximation to it has been supported by his colleagues on numerous occasions. In or interview Lord Pearson stated that the Law Lords had overruled *Addie* v. *Dumbreck* in *Herrington's* case because it was,

> simply obsolete, and just would not do for modern conditions. That was a case in which a decision of the House could not stand with prevailing conditions ... [and] ideas of what was just. There may well have been changes in the popular outlook.

A version of the criterion featured in several of the speeches in *Indyka* v. *Indyka*, in Viscount Dilhorne's speech in the *Oldendorff* case,[63] in Lord Diplock's speech in *R.* v. *Hyam*,[64] in those of Lords Wilberforce, Simon and Cross and Edmund-Davies in *Miliangos*[65] and in Lord Kilbrandon's (Lords Dilhorne, Diplock and Edmund-Davies concurring) in *Dick* v. *Burgh of Falkirk*.[66] Again, in 'Twenty Years On'[67] Lord Upjohn suggested that decisions of the House should be overruled if they are 'out of step with modern ideas and situations and no longer represent an acceptable view of the law'. In more recent times a version of the criterion was supported by the appellate committee in *Fitzleet* v. *Cherry* and *DPP* v. *Camplin*, and by Lords Wilberforce, Salmon and Keith in *Hesperides Hotels* v. *Muftizade*.[68] The criterion itself was expressly accepted by Lords Dilhorne, Edmund-Davies and Keith in *Vestey* v. *IRC*.[69]

It is clear, therefore, that whether it is fair to attribute it to his influence or not, Lord Reid's criteria reflected very accurately the dominant consensus amongst his fellow Law Lords both at the time of the interviews (1972-3) and of his retirement (January 1975).[70] So accurately that apart from the criteria already mentioned, only one further criterion not suggested by him (though he probably accepted it) had received much support from his colleagues by the date of his retirement. This eighth criterion was the expectation that a decision in criminal law ought to be overruled only in exceptional circumstances, in view of the especial need for certainty in criminal law.*

Lord Reid's success in providing a lead for his colleagues or in encapsulating their views was all the more noteworthy in that it was not (so far as I could ascertain) the result of formal or informal discussions. Moreover, there has been no shortage of alternative criteria suggested by his colleagues which have failed to achieve widespread support. An attempt by Lord Hailsham to introduce as a criterion for overruling a precedent, that it involved a 'logical

---

*This criterion appears in the wording of the Practice Statement itself and was mentioned in their interviews by Lords MacDermott, Pearson, Salmon and Devlin. It has also been voiced by Lords Morris,[71] Wilberforce,[72] Simon[73] and Edmund-Davies.[74] It was not the basis of Lord Reid's reasoning in *Knuller* v. *DPP*, though curiously his final remarks in *Shaw* v. *DPP*[75] indicate that he considered that there was a particular need for certainty in the criminal law. The criterion has recently been endorsed by the whole Appellate Committee in *R.* v. *Cunningham*.

impossibility' has been rejected more than once by his brethren.[76] The Law Lords have also been divided as to the importance to be attached to the age of the precedent under review. Lord Dilhorne's reluctance to interfere with long-standing precedents (voiced in the *Jones*[77] case) was shared by Lord Kilbrandon (and possibly Lords Diplock and Edmund-Davies) in *Dick* v. *Burgh of Falkirk*.[78] Further, in *The Albazero* Lord Diplock (Lords Dilhorne, Simon and Fraser concurring) concluded that 'the almost complete absence of reliance' by litigants on a House of Lords case for over 120 years did not provide 'a sufficient reason for abolishing it entirely'.[79] On the other hand Lord Simon (with the express concurrence of Lords Wilberforce, Cross and Fraser on the point) held in *Miliangos*[80] that the maxim *Cessante ratione cessat ipsa lex* was a relevant consideration in deciding whether to overrule a previous decision of the House. To add to the confusion, Lord Dilhorne's suggestion[81] that it is easier to depart from a recent case than one that has stood for a long time was rejected by Lord Pearson in his interview, by Lord Diplock in the *Jones*[82] case and by Lord Reid in *Conway* v. *Rimmer*.[83] Yet in *DPP* v. *Nock*[84] Lord Scarman (Lords Diplock, Edmund-Davies, Russell and Keith concurring) gave as a reason for not overruling a decision of the House, the fact that it was 'very recent'. In point of fact none of the arguments relating to the age of the precedent in question seem as yet to have acquired particularly widespread support amongst the Law Lords except to the extent to which they are really a restatement of Lord Reid's second criterion.

The disagreements extended to other criteria. As we shall see,[85] some Law Lords considered arguments based on 'parliamentary inactivity' to be acceptable in this area - others did not; some relied on a 'floodgate' argument to justify inaction - others did not. One Appellate Committee[86] argued that judicial unanimity in a precedent was a reason for it not being overthrown. Yet, another Appellate Committee[87] the year before had held that the converse was not true, *i.e.* that the lack of unanimity in a precedent was not a reason for it being overthrown. Acceptance of a precedent in other common law jurisdictions has been used to justify retaining it;[88] yet the rejection of a precedent in other common law jurisdictions,[89] has not proved a strong argument for overruling it here. Similarly, acceptance of a precedent by textbook writers has been used to justify its retention;[90] yet overwhelming criticism of a precedent by academics and textbook writers[91] has not proved a strong argument for overruling it here.

These disagreements prompt us to consider further questions. What part did and do the criteria play in the Law Lords' decisions in actual cases? What has happened when the criteria have come into conflict with each other? In order to shed light on these matters let us look at the Law Lords' behaviour in cases in which the question of using the new freedom has been raised.

Table 7.1 contains the twenty-nine cases in which the Law Lords were invited to overrule one of their own precedents, together with those in which one or more Law Lords raised the issue without the prompting of counsel, during the period 1966-80. It excludes cases where given different counsel or a differently composed Appellate Committee or even a different approach by counsel or the Appellate Committee, the possibility of exercising the new freedom might have been raised. The size of this invisible figure is hard to gauge, but applying a broad test, namely any case reported in the Appeal Cases (and not contained in Table 7.1), in which a precedent of the House was applied or distinguished, there were about twenty such cases during this period. Of these, even allowing a margin for error, in only half at the most could a serious argument for overruling the precedent have been maintained.

1. The 'use sparingly' criterion has clearly been complied with. Eight or so[92] overrulings in fourteen years can fairly be described as a sparing use of the power. Yet the success rate of more than one in four (28 per cent) is quite appreciable and in eighteen out of the twenty-nine cases at least one Law Lord was prepared to overrule the previous decision of the House.*

2. With the possible exception of *Miliangos* none of the appeals which led to an 'overruling' involved a breach of the 'legitimate expectations' criterion. In *Lynall, Schuler, O'Brien* and *Lim PC* it was expressly cited as a reason for not

---

*Counsel clearly have an influence on these figures. In the early years counsel seemed prepared to run the argument that the House should depart from its previous decision in more or less every case where the precedent was against them. Once the criteria for the use of the Practice Statement began to coalesce counsel became more cautious and in the period 1975-80 there was a marked increase in the number of cases where counsel could reasonably have tried to invoke the Statement but declined to do so.

TABLE 7.1 Cases relating to the 1966 Practice Statement on Precedent in the period 1966–80

Case	How raised	Majority response	Margin[a]
1. *Indyka* v. *Indyka* (1967)	Respondent	Overruled[b]	?
2. *Conway* v. *Rimmer* (1968)	Appellant	Overruled[c]	3:2
3. *Anisminic* v. *FCC* (1968)	Appellant	Distinguished[d]	0:5
4. *Owen* v. *Pook* (1969)	Lord Pearce	Distinguished[e]	1:2
5. *Nat. Bank of Greece* v. *Westminister Bank* (1970)	Lord Hailsham	Distinguished[f]	0:5
6. *FA & AB* v. *Lupton* (1971)	Respondent	Distinguished	2:3
7. *Thomson* v. *Gurneville Secs.* (1971)	Appellant	Distinguished	2:3
8. *Lynall* v. *IRC* (1971)	Appellant	Refused	0:5
9. *The Jones Case* (1971)	Appellants	Refused	3:4
10. *Herrington's Case* (1972)	Respondent	Overruled[g]	3:2
11. *Cassell* v. *Broome* (1972)	Respondent (Case only)	Refused	1:6
12. *R.* v. *Sakhuja* (1972)	Respondent	Distinguished[h]	1:2
13. *Knuller* v. *DPP* (1972)	Appellants	Refused	1:3
14. *Schuler* v. *Wickman* (1973)	Respondent (Case only)	Refused	0:3
15. *O'Brien* v. *Robinson* (1973)	Appellant	Refused	0:5
16. *Oldendorff* v. *Tradax* (1973)	Appellant[i]	Overruled	4:1
17. *Taylor* v. *Provan* (1974)	Appellant	Distinguished/ Refused[j]	0:3
18. *R.* v. *Hyam* (1974)	Appellant	?[k]	2:2
19. *The Miliangos Case* (1975)	Respondent	Overruled	4:1
20. *Dick* v. *Burgh of Falkirk* (1975)	Appellant	Overruled	5:0
21. *The Albazero* (1976)	Appellant	Distinguished	0:4
22. *Anns* v. *Merton Borough Council* (1977)	Lord Salmon[l]	Distinguished	1:4
23. *Fitzleet Estates* v. *Cherry* (1977)	Appellant	Refused	0:5
24. *DPP* v. *Camplin* (1978)	The Law Lords	Overruled[m]	5:0
25. *DPP* v. *Nock* (1978)	Respondent	Refused	0:5
26. *Hesperides Hotels* v. *Muftizade* (1978)	Appellant	Refused	0:5
27. *The Despina R* (1978)	Respondent	Distinguished[n]	1:4
28. *Lim Poh Choo* v. *Area Health Authority* (1979)	Appellant	Refused	0:4
29. *Vestey* v. *IRC* (1979)	Respondent	Overruled	5:0

Notes to table overleaf

NOTES TO TABLE 7.1

a.   This category refers to the division between the Law Lords on the issue
     of overruling the previous case.

b.   Although technically this cannot be an exercise of the new freedom,
     Lords Reid and Pearson told me that they regarded it as such, because
     the Privy Council case they were overruling was too well established to
     be got rid of in any other way. See also Lord Reid, 'The Judge as Law
     Maker', p. 25.

c.   There is considerable disagreement amongst academics as to whether a
     majority of the Law Lords in this case invoked the new freedom. Dias,
     Jurisprudence, 4th edn p. 286; Stone, '1966 and All That!', and
     'Liberation of Appellate Judges', 35 *MLR* (1972) 449; Traynor, *Quo
     Vadis*, p. 15; R. Cross, 'The House of Lords and the Rules of
     Precedent', p. 159; Stevens, *Law and Politics*, p. 543; and Wade 84 *LQR*
     (1968) 171 at p. 183 all conclude that a majority of Law Lords did not
     invoke the Practice Statement in this case. On the other hand Dias (!),
     Jurisprudence, 4th edn p. 170; L. Jaffe, *English and American Judges as
     Lawmakers* (Oxford: Clarendon Press, 1969) p. 25; Blom-Cooper and
     Drewry, *Final Appeal*, p. 70 and MacCormick, *op. cit.*, pp. 134-5
     conclude that a majority did. Lord Reid told me that he considered that
     the freedom had been used by a majority in the case, and Lord Pearson
     said the same. Lord Upjohn has implied it also, see 'Twenty Years On',
     p. 657, and in *D. v. NSPCC* at p. 240H Lord Simon states that the
     freedom was used in *Conway* v. *Rimmer*. Moreover Lord Pearce (over
     whom the commentators are divided) told me that he himself had used
     the freedom in the case. Since most commentators accept that Lords
     Morris and Hodson invoked the Statement it seems fair to conclude that
     this case was the first (at least technically speaking) in which the new
     freedom was exercised.

d.   Only Lord Pearce (at pp. 200-1) states that if he could not distinguish
     the previous case he would reconsider it, but Lords Reid and
     Wilberforce might well have agreed with him.

e.   Of the three judges in the majority only Lord Pearce stated that he was
     overruling *Ricketts* v. *Colquhoun*. Lords Guest and Wilberforce merely
     distinguished it.

f.   Lord Hailsham in the sole judgement distinguished *Foulsham* v. *Pickles*
     but indicated that it might have to be overruled at some stage.

g.   Some scholars have doubted whether the new freedom was exercised in
     this case, *e.g.* Cross, 'The House of Lords and the Rules of Precedent',
     p. 159 and Stevens, *Law and Politics*, p. 619. I have treated it as an
     'overruling' case because: (1) most scholars agree that Lord Morris
     exercised the freedom; (2) a close reading of Lord Reid's speech reveals
     that he did also, and he confirmed this in his interview; (3) Lord
     Pearson, whose speech tends to suggest that he is exercising the
     freedom, also confirmed that he had done so, in his interview.

h.   While Lord Dilhorne was prepared to overrule *Pinner* v. *Everett*, Lords
     Cross and Salmon expressly stated that they were not. In the end four
     Law Lords distinguished it.

i.   The appellant's counsel told me before the case that he did not expect to win it (a view shared by other members of the commercial Bar). He attributed his success to the adverse comments in the lower courts.

j.   All five Law Lords distinguished *Ricketts*'s case but only three expressly refused to overrule it.

k.   Two Law Lords wanted to overrule *DPP* v. *Smith* and two declined to do so. The fifth (Lord Cross) merely distinguished it.

l.   Lord Salmon implied (at p. 766G) that he would have been willing to overrule *East Suffolk Rivers Catchment Board* v. *Kent* but his colleagues preferred to distinguish it.

m.   Although little recognised it is quite clear that in this case the Law Lords on their own initiative and not at counsel's request, overruled so much of *Bedder* v. *DPP* as had survived the Homicide Act 1957. See [1978] A.C. 705 at pp. 718E and 727C.

n.   Only Lord Russell used language which showed that he was 'departing from' the earlier precedent (p. 704F). I find it difficult to know how to characterise Lord Wilberforce's leading judgement; it is possible that he was overruling the precedent but it seems more likely that he was only distinguishing it.

---

overruling the case in question. In at least *Indyka* and *Dick* one reason given by the Law Lords in support of overruling the earlier precedents was that no issue involving this second criterion arose in the cases.

3.   The 'construction' criterion (the third), was only deviated from in *Oldendorff* and *Vestey*. In *Oldendorff* the *raison d'être* for the criterion (that it promotes certainty) was not present and accordingly the 'rectification of uncertainty' criterion (the sixth), was applied. In *Vestey* the conflict between the third and seventh, the 'unjust or outmoded', criteria was severe. At least two Law Lords at the close of the hearing favoured the third criterion but later changed their minds.[93] Although in the end the Law Lords ranked the seventh criterion above the third in this particular case, in other situations the ranking might well be reversed. In *Jones* the third criterion was expressly relied on to justify not overruling the precedent in question, and it was applied by implication in *Lynall*, *Sakhuja*, *O'Brien*, *Taylor* and *Fitzleet*.

4.   Whether Lord Reid's fourth criterion (in either form) was breached in any of the overruling cases is difficult to say. Lord Simon seemed to think the first form of the criterion, the 'unforeseeable consequences', was being infringed in *Miliangos*. On the other hand both forms have frequently

been relied on by the Law Lords in refusing to take action; *e.g. DPP* v. *Myers*, *Morgans* v. *Launchbury*, *Cassell*, *Dick*, *Nock*, *Hesperides* and *Lim PC*.

5. The 'precedent merely wrong' criterion (the fifth), was upheld in all the 'overruling' cases. It was relied on in *Jones*, *Knuller* and *Fitzleet* to justify not overruling the previous cases, and seems to have played a part in similar refusals in *Lynall*, *O'Brien*, *Taylor* and *Hyam*.

6. The 'rectification of uncertainty' criterion (the sixth), has rarely been invoked. It was applied by a majority of those sitting in *Oldendorff* and by the three minority Law Lords in *Jones*.

7. Lord Reid's final criterion, the 'unjust or outmoded' test, in one form or another, has applied in all eight cases where an 'overruling' occurred. Its absence was used as a reason for refusing to overrule a precedent in *Jones*, *O'Brien*, *Fitzleet* and in *DPP* v. *Majewski*.

8. The Law Lords' 'criminal cases' criterion (the eighth), was breached in only one of the 'overruling' cases *Camplin*, and in that case the 'breach' was largely done by Parliament. The criterion was applied in *Sakhuja*, *Knuller*, *Hyam*, *DPP* v. *Majewski* and *R.* v. *Cunningham*.

These results show that in this area, contrary to Professor Griffith's assertions,[94] there was and continues to be a considerable consistency between the Law Lords' views, their statements and their actual behaviour. Clearly the criteria were of different weights. The second, third, fifth, seventh and possibly the eighth were 'pivotal' expectations in the role of a Law Lord in the period 1966-80. The fourth and sixth were at least 'relevant' expectations, but the others, for example the arguments relating to 'parliamentary inactivity', the 'floodgates' of litigation or the age of the precedent, had only 'peripheral' status in this period.

In most cases more than one criterion was applicable. Usually this plurality was used to cumulative effect in the Law Lords' speeches - to strengthen their argument that the House should or should not depart from the precedent in question, *e.g. O'Brien* where the second, third, fourth and sixth criteria all led in the same direction. Occasionally, as in *Fitzleet*, the cumulative effect derived from the presence of one or more criteria pointing to one conclusion and the absence of any criteria pointing to another.

Inevitably there were cases where criteria leading to different conclusions were applicable. Such conflicts were usually 'resolved' by the Law Lords 'ranking' the criteria in accordance with their perceptions of the criteria's weight, legitimacy and the consequences of their application or non-application. As we have seen the first eight criteria were relatively well established so questions of legitimacy only arose in relation to the other suggested criteria. Weight, on the other hand, was often the crucial factor in resolving the conflict. Thus in *Oldendorff* the 'construction' criterion (the third), was outweighed by the 'rectification of uncertainty' criterion (the sixth), and in *Anisminic* the third criterion might have been outweighed by the 'unjust and outmoded' criterion, (the seventh), had the court not been able to evade the precedent concerned. Where, as in *Vestey*, the weights of the conflicting criteria were finely balanced the perceived consequences of not applying the seventh criterion *i.e.* reaching an 'arbitrary, potentially unjust and fundamentally unconstitutional'[95] result, were sufficient to tilt the balance. As MacCormick asserts,[96] consequentialism has a part to play in this area. In any event, despite the relative autonomy of the Law Lords in defining their own role (which ensured that the Law Lords sometimes applied the criteria in different ways), in general, the problems posed by conflicting criteria do not seem hitherto to have prevented the criteria from fulfilling their original purpose, which was to reduce or institutionalise the broader conflict between the 'be consistent' and 'be fair' expectations.

But what impact has the Practice Statement had? Some commentators[97] have concluded, perhaps because of the paucity of clear cases in which the new power has been exercised, that its practical importance has been very limited. This conclusion focuses on the instrumental aspects of the Practice Statement rather than its symbolic dimension. On the other hand several commentators have argued that the importance of the Statement was largely psychological, *i.e.* in the change in attitude to precedent which it encapsulated.[98] In the words of Robert Stevens,

> The importance of the 1966 Practice Statement ... was largely psychological, adding legitimacy to a process that had been going on since the late fifties and was accelerating in the early sixties.[99]

As we saw in Chapter 6 this statement accords closely with the views of the Law Lords themselves.[100] Most of them saw the Statement as a relaxation in their attitude to precedent rather than as a revolutionary change, though they, and I, would argue that the Statement has been used more often than commentators seem to think. What misled the commentators was that like the US Supreme Court which 'rarely overturns decisions in explicit terms, preferring instead to squeeze the life from them'[101] by a narrowing process, the House of Lords, at least in the initial period, seemed to have 'a preference for getting round earlier decisions rather than for pushing them over'.[102] This preference for the evasive* response of 'Dissimulation' to the conflict between the 'be consistent'and the 'be fair' expectations (which arises in most cases where the invoking of the Practice Statement is suggested), can be seen from Table 7.1. To many scholars the first case in which the power was exercised did not come until *Oldendorff*. It was almost as though the Law Lords were taking the view that since they now had the power to overrule their precedents they could get rid of cases they disliked by the apparent use of traditional means even though they would not have felt able to use these means had the Practice Statement not existed.[103]

What was the explanation for this lack of candour? First, the understandable caution of 'new boys' seeking to establish their role in an uncharted terrain. Secondly, the fear, prompted in part by the frequency with which counsel in the early 1970s were prepared to invoke the Statement, that what they considered should be a trickle of cases might develop into a flood. (A fear that the existence and use of the new power might undermine certainty in the law may well explain why so many of the guidelines as to the use of the power related to certainty.) Thirdly, and most significantly, because of the Law Lords' ambivalence towards Lord Radcliffe's 'facade' approach to law-making. As we saw earlier this approach was the predominant response in the period 1962-6 to the conflicts between the 'don't legislate', the 'be consistent' and the 'be fair' expectations which arose in certain hard cases. Although Lord Reid preferred the response of *Innovation* as to the content of the 'don't legislate' expectation to

---

*The Law Lords were not alone in this. The mere fact that in five of the eight occasions when the Statement has been successfully invoked the invitation came from the respondent, is a testimony to the evasive abilities of the Court of Appeal.

the 'facade' approach, not all his brethren were in agreement. While in practice they might share (or come to share) his belief in certain guidelines for the use of the new freedom, guidelines which embodied variable rankings between the 'be consistent' and 'be fair' expectations, such rankings did not have to be overt. In 1972-3, at the time of my interviews, the Law Lords were heavily divided over the 'facade' approach.[104]

Apart from Lord Reid, Lords Gardiner, Kilbrandon, Salmon, Denning and Pearce were opposed (and Lord Edmund-Davies has since indicated[105] his opposition) to the suggestion that the House should keep its activities as to law-making hidden behind a facade of discovering the law and never making it. On the other hand four at least were in Lord Radcliffe's camp, including Lords Guest, Hailsham and Devlin. In Lord Devlin's view,

It is facile to think that it is always better to throw off disguises. The need for disguise hampers activity and so restricts the power. Paddling across the Rubicon by individuals in disguise who will be sent back if they proclaim themselves is very different from the bridging of the river by an army in uniform and with bands playing.[106]

Several others including Lords Pearson, Simon[107] and Cross seemed ambivalent on the issue, as was Lord Justice Russell (as he then was).

Given the Law Lords' understandable caution in relation to the Practice Statement in the early days and the existence of such judicial disunity on the need for candour, it is perhaps not surprising to discover the Law Lords unwittingly complying with Lord Radcliffe's dictum on the proper use of the new power, 'Do it, and don't make a fuss about it.'[108] Even in recent times when, as Table 7.1 suggests, candour is becoming more common in this field, it is likely that to the extent that the majority of an Appellate Committee (which has been invited to overrule a precedent of the House), favours the 'facade' approach, to that extent the chances are reduced that the new freedom will be overtly exercised.

LORD REID: INNOVATION AND JUDICIAL LAW-MAKING

When we turn to consider the broader area of judicial law-making in general in the years 1966-73 and thereafter, it becomes clear that Lord Reid's innovativeness was not restricted to overruling precedents. The Law Lords, he believed, had a role to play in developing the common law to meet changing economic and social conditions.[109] Nevertheless he was equally convinced of the necessity of setting limits to such judicial law-making - limits marking the boundary between what it was legitimate for the courts to do and what ought to be left to Parliament. Here several strands of Lord Reid's judicial philosophy came together. The identification of these limits - which he derived from the public and from Parliament (acting as symbolic reference groups) and from his own notions of common sense, legal principle and public policy[110] - represented for him not just the primary method of legitimating judicial law-making in a democratic society but also the solution to the central question of practical jurisprudence: how far judges could reconcile certainty in the law with the achievement of justice in each particular case.[111] Thus, as before, his response to the conflict between the 'be consistent' and 'be fair' expectations was *Innovation* - suggesting normative guidelines for his own and his colleagues' behaviour. Predictably the guidelines proffered by Lord Reid were closely correlated to those which he was putting forward in relation to the 1966 Practice Statement.

His basic tenet was that the scope for judicial law-making and the balance to be struck between justice and certainty varied with the area of law with which the House was concerned.* 'I think we must treat different branches of law in different ways', he said.[112] In some areas, *e.g.* Property Law,[113] Contract Law[114] and the law governing Settlements[115] and Criminal Law[116] he considered the public's demand for certainty in the law outweighed their demand for justice in individual cases or for the law to adjust to changing social conditions. Thus in 'The Law and the Reasonable Man' he said,

*For a similar argument in relation to judicial activism in Appellate Courts in the United States see M. Schapiro, 'Political Jurisprudence' in R. Wolfinger (ed.), *Readings in American Political Behaviour* (New Jersey: Prentice Hall, 1966) pp.160-1 and R. Leflar, 'Appellate Judicial Innovation', 27 *Oklahoma L.R.* (1974) 321 at p.334.

When we are dealing with property and contract it seems right
that we should accept some degree of possible injustice in order
to achieve a fairly high degree of certainty.[117]

His objection to law-making in these areas was that the
retroactivity of judicial decisions was incompatible with the
stability of the settled law which people rely on as a guide to their
conduct[118] or when entering into contracts or property
settlements.[119]

On the other hand he thought that the judges ought to have
more freedom to develop the law of Tort, since the need for
certainty in that area was, he felt, less than in some others and
accordingly considerations of justice and flexibility could play a
greater part, particularly in cases of Negligence.[120] Similarly he
appears to have favoured the 'be fair' expectation over the 'be
consistent' expectation in the field of Constitutional and Administrative Law.[121] Lord Reid also drew a distinction between,

> cases where we are dealing with 'lawyers' law' and cases where
> we are dealing with matters which directly affect the lives and
> the interests of large sections of the community and which raise
> issues which are the subject of public controversy and on which
> laymen are as well able to decide as are lawyers. On such
> matters it is not for the courts to proceed on their view of public
> policy for that would be to encroach on the province of
> Parliament.[122]

Lord Reid left the limits of the former category (in which the
judges had more freedom of movement) unspecified though it
probably included parts of Tort Law, of Public Law and of
Conflict of Laws.[123] In the latter category he included aspects of
Family Law[124] and Criminal Law.[125] He elaborated his feelings on
this category in 'The Judge as Law Maker' where he said,

> When public opinion is sharply divided on any question -
> whether or not the division is on party lines - no judge ought in
> my view to lean to one side or the other if that can possibly be
> avoided. But sometimes we get a case where that is very difficult
> to avoid. Then I think we must play safe. We must decide the
> case on the preponderance of existing authority. Parliament is

the right place to settle issues which the ordinary man regards as controversial.[126]

Lord Reid's remaining guideline had two aspects to it and was in effect the same as the fourth criterion which he advocated in relation to the use of the 1966 Practice Statement. First, he believed that the Law Lords ought not to develop the law if to do so would involve a change that ought, because of the unsatisfactory state of the area of law in question, to be part of a comprehensive reform. To introduce a minor change in such a situation would entail the risk of further undermining certainty in the law by adding to the distinctions and qualifications already existing in that field. As he stated in *Myers* v. *DPP*,

> If we are to extend the law it must be by the development and application of fundamental principles. We cannot introduce arbitrary conditions or limitations .... The only satisfactory solution [to this problem] is by legislation following on a wide survey of the whole field.[127]

Secondly, he believed that the Law Lords ought not to develop the law if 'it would be impracticable to foresee all the consequences of tampering with it'.[128] Thus he declined to change the law in *Treacy* v. *DPP* because,

> changes of that kind are apt to have side effects which would elude us in any such examination of a problem as we can make in reaching a decision in a particular case.[129]

Similarly in *The Atlantic Star* he observed,

> I cannot foresee all the repercussions of making [such] a fundamental change in English law and I am not at all satisfied that it would be proper for this House to make such a fundamental change.[130]

These and other[131] dicta indicate that Lord Reid took the view that certain complex legal problems exist which are not amenable to solution by judges developing the law in particular cases. Such problems have been labelled 'polycentric' by legal scholars, because they have, many centres of stress and direction of force, only some of which are likely to be the focus of attention when a decision in the area is made .... Because [they] have these many different critical areas and because they are all inter-related a decision's immediate effects are likely to be communicated in many unforeseeable ways and affect many other areas of human concern.[132]

As we have seen, these efforts by Lord Reid to delimit the scope of judicial law-making were deliberate essays in *Innovation*. How successful was he in influencing his colleagues? Certainly he commanded the respect of those of them whom I interviewed. Lord Guest, for example, told me that much of the acclaim 'for the present enlightened policy in the House in relation to making the law' ought to go to Lord Reid who had had 'a lot to do with the House's attitude to the development of the law'. Lord Pearce commented, 'I found myself on the same wavelength as Scott Reid. I am a great admirer of him, because I found generally we had the same approach.' And Lord Devlin in 'The Greatest Judge of Judges'[133] expressed the view (shared apparently by Lords Hailsham[134] and Scarman[135]) that, 'In substance [Lord Reid] is the man who in the last decade has more than any other, shaped the law of Britain.'

Moreover, as with the 1966 Practice Statement, it can be shown that his guidelines in this area encapsulated the views of most of the Law Lords in the early 1970s. Of the nineteen Law Lords who were 'active' between 1967-73, at least twelve (Lords Cross,[136] Devlin,[137] Diplock,[138] Donovan,[139] Gardiner, Guest,[140] MacDermott,[141] Pearce,[142] Pearson,[143] Reid, Salmon[144] and Wilberforce[145]) considered that the Law Lords had an obligation to develop the common law to meet changing social conditions. This marked a considerable shift from the dominant orthodoxy in 1957 which had held that the Law Lords ought to confine themselves to applying existing principles to new situations of fact. Such was the scale of the change that of the remaining Law Lords only four (Lords Dilhorne,[146] Kilbrandon,[147] Simon[148] and Upjohn[149]) could be said, on the basis of their public pronouncements, to prefer the old orthodoxy to the new. Interestingly the sample of the Bar whom I interviewed shared Lord Reid's perceptions on this issue in an even greater proportion than his colleagues, and coupled with the advent of the new orthodoxy, this is likely, as we saw in Chapters 2 and 3 to have had a considerable impact on the discourse between Bar and Bench during cases in this period. Nor would it appear that the dominant orthodoxy has changed greatly since 1973, for at least three (Lords Edmund-Davies,[150] Russell[151] and Scarman[152]) of the six Law Lords appointed between 1973-9 adhere to it.

THE IMPORTANCE OF CERTAINTY AND CONSISTENCY

The wording of the 1966 Practice Statement, my interviews with the Law Lords and their speeches and votes in decided cases made it clear that the bulk of the active Law Lords in 1972-3 shared Lord Reid's belief that the importance of certainty in the law varied with the area under consideration. Its especial importance in relation to contracts and property settlements was explicitly mentioned in the Practice Statement. At least eight of the active Law Lords (Lords Diplock,[153] Guest, Kilbrandon, MacDermott, Reid, Salmon,[154] Simon[155] and Wilberforce[156]) and two of the 'inactive' ones (Lord Denning and Devlin) endorsed this view. Moreover, the Law Lords' decisions in commercial and property cases during the period 1966-73 and thereafter,[157] support this conclusion. As we saw in relation to the 1966 Practice Statement some of the Law Lords during this period also felt that there was a particular need for certainty in the criminal law. This was evidenced not only in the express wording of the Statement but also in statements made by Lords Hailsham, MacDermott, Morris, Pearson, Salmon, Simon, Wilberforce and Devlin and more recently by Lords Hailsham, Edmund-Davies and Elwyn-Jones.[158] It has to be admitted that some decisions of the House in criminal appeals at this time do not appear to attach too much importance to certainty *e.g. Swain* v. *DPP, Knuller* v. *DPP, R.* v. *Kamara, DPP* v. *Withers* and more recently *R.* v. *Lemon.* Three of these, however, related to the law on conspiracy and did not greatly add to the uncertainty which had been produced by their precursor - *Shaw* v. *DPP.* In fact, in these cases some of the Law Lords were trying to rectify the damage done to certainty in the law by *Shaw's* case, for since the day it was decided there has always been a bloc of Law Lords opposed to the decision. *Shaw,* it will be recalled, was made easier by the absence of clear guidelines on judicial law-making when it was decided. As these have begun to emerge so opposition to *Shaw* has, if anything, increased. Thus when Lord Reid retired in 1974 at least eight Law Lords (Lords Diplock,[159] Elwyn-Jones,[160] Gardiner, MacDermott, Salmon, Pearce, Radcliffe and Reid) considered that *Shaw* was wrongly decided.*

THE IMPORTANCE OF FAIRNESS

On the other hand the dominant view in 1973 probably[161] attached less importance to certainty and rather more to justice as fairness in Tort cases. Of the active Law Lords, three (Lords Kilbrandon, MacDermott and Reid) expressed such views in interviews and Lords Diplock,[162] Pearson[163] and Simon[164] have provided supportive dicta elsewhere. Three 'inactive' Law Lords (Lords Denning, Devlin and Pearce) took a similar position when interviewed. Once again the Law Lords' decisions in hard cases were consistent with this perception, *e.g. Hedley Byrne* v. *Heller, Parry* v. *Cleaver, Home Office* v. *Dorset Yacht, The Tojo Maru, British Railways Board* v. *Herrington, Indyka* v. *Indyka*[165] and *Boys* v. *Chaplin.* The two aberrant cases, *Rondel* v. *Worsley* and *Cassell* v. *Broome* served only to show that the Law Lords' tendency to activism in these fields could be overborne - in the one case by the Law Lords' perception of public policy, in the other by their belief that the abolition of exemplary damages was too fundamental a change in the law for the House to undertake. The incremental development of these fields has continued in the Lords in more recent years, *e.g. Cookson* v. *Knowles, Anns* v. *London Borough of Merton, MacShannon* v. *Rockware Glass, Pickett* v. *British Rail,* and *Lambert* v. *Lewis,* although as before there has been the occasional hiccup, *e.g. Moorgate* v. *Twitchings, Lim Poh Choo* v. *Area Health Authority,* and *Gammell* v. *Wilson* .

Curiously, amongst the Law Lords in the 1970s only two, Lords Diplock and Edmund-Davies publicly suggested that Public Law was a suitable area for judicial creativity.[166] Yet it would be difficult to gainsay the former's assertion that under the aegis of Lord Reid the House produced a stream of creative decisions in

---

*Lord Kilbrandon, however, told me (before *Knuller* had been heard), that, I'm absolutely certain that if you stopped the first thousand men and women in the Strand and explained what Mr Shaw had been doing, every one of them would say he didn't get a day too much ... It's only the [academics] who get so excited about this sort of thing, but the man in the street doesn't give a damn, I'm quite sure.

this field.[167] Lord Diplock added, '[I]f I have my way, we have not
finished yet.'[168] Recent decisions of the House on public interest
and the disclosure of documents in litigation, *e.g. D.* v. *NSPCC*,
Waugh v. *BRB*, *SRC* v. *Nassé* and *Burmah Oil* v. *Bank of England*
suggest that his colleagues are in agreement.[169]

LAWYERS' LAW AND AREAS OF PUBLIC CONTROVERSY

Lord Reid's distinction between these areas attracted little overt
support from his colleagues. When taken separately, however,
each of Lord Reid's suggestions had a measure of support with a
considerable overlap between the supporters. Thus Lords Guest,
Reid, Simon[170] and Pearce considered that the Law Lords had a
greater freedom to develop the law in lawyers' law areas than in
others. Likewise Lords Morris,[171] Wilberforce[172] and Edmund-
Davies[173] took the view that they had more room for manoeuvre in
the common law areas which Parliament had traditionally left for
development by the judiciary. On the other hand Law Lords who
argued for judicial restraint in areas of public controversy included
Lords Guest, Reid, Simon,[174] Pearce, Kilbrandon[175] and
Wilberforce[175] and more recently Lords Elwyn-Jones[177] and
Scarman.[178]

Lord Reid's assertion that in certain unsatisfactory areas of the
common law, reform was best done by legislation following on a
wide survey of the whole field rather than by the House
introducing minor changes, which would only compound the
existing confusion, seems to have struck a sympathetic chord with
some of his colleagues. This criterion however should be seen as an
affirmation that major, comprehensive reforms in the law are
beyond the scope of the Law Lords[179] and not as a denial of the
incremental nature of judicial law-making.[180] As Lord Reid
himself expressed it,

> The common law has not been built by judges making general
> pronouncements: it has been built by the rational expansion of
> what already exists in order to do justice in particular cases.[181]

or as Lord Wright more graphically put it, the judges developing
the common law proceed,

> from case to case, like the ancient Mediterranean mariners,

hugging the coast from point to point and avoiding the danger of the open sea of system and science.[182]

CONSEQUENTIALISM AND POLYCENTRIC PROBLEMS

I have said enough by now, I hope, for the reader to discern that Lord Reid's guidelines served a dual function. To the extent that they represented or reflected the dominant orthodoxy amongst the Law Lords in the early 1970s and beyond as to the appropriate limits for judicial law-making, to that extent they also doubled as arguments with which a Law Lord could justify his activism or restraint in particular cases. Perhaps nowhere can the dual nature of the guidelines be seen more clearly than in the case of Lord Reid's final criterion - that the Law Lords should eschew activist solutions to appeals involving complex or polycentric issues, on the grounds that it was impracticable for the Law Lords to gauge the consequences of tampering with the existing legal provisions. This criterion demonstrates the importance which some Law Lords attach to consequentialist arguments - those relating to the consequences of deciding in one way as opposed to another - when providing reasons in their speeches to justify their decisions. This, of course, is just what Professor MacCormick has recently argued[183] judges in hard cases ought to do, and, he asserts, what they actually do. Indeed it is now juristic commonplace to recognise that hard cases involve not only the logic of antecedents but also the logic of consequences,[184] and that purposive reasoning and result orientation, the 'sins' of activist tribunals like the Warren Court,* are inextricably linked to consequentialist discourse.

When asked whether they considered that they ought to be concerned with the possible social and legal consequences of their decisions, ten of the eleven active Law Lords interviewed answered in the affirmative. The sole dissentient was Lord Guest who agreed with Lord Devlin's dictum that, 'a healthy judiciary is a judiciary that is not concerned with where the law leads to'.[186]

Several of them specifically related their answers to the limits of law-making. Thus Lord Pearson replied,

---

*For a critique of the US Supreme Court for being insufficiently consequentialist in its outlook, see D. L. Horowitz, *The Courts and Social Policy*.[185]

Oh, I think yes, as far as we can. But you see, we are not a Royal Commission; we do`not have the sort of evidence that a Royal Commission would have, and therefore we are a bit shy of bringing in policy considerations to that extent.

Lord Hailsham commented,

Obviously they must be concerned. Equally obviously their concern cannot, or should not convert them into legislators ....
All judges should be aware of the facts of modern life, and apply legal principles in the light of them.

and a third added,

I think you've got to relate ... the way you deal with common law subjects to the new structure of the State and the way it is built up economically .... But I think broadly speaking most of us would realise that changes to meet social requirements cannot normally be made by judges because they haven't got the research facilities in order to get a proper basis for doing it.

Undoubtedly the most vociferous champion of this limit on judicial creativity in recent times has been Lord Simon of Glaisdale. His caustic remarks in *Miliangos*[187] (aimed at his colleagues who were prepared to overrule an earlier decision in the House) were merely a high point in an extended series.

'I am not trained to see the distant scene: one step enough for me' should be the motto on the wall opposite the judge's desk. It is, I concede, a less spectacular method of progression than somersaults and cartwheels; but it is the one best suited to the capacity and resources of a judge ... the very nature of the problem makes this a most unsuitable case for a revolutionary change in the law to be undertaken by judges.[188]

However, Lords Reid and Simon did not stand alone. A majority of the fifteen active Law Lords endorsed this guideline (including Lords Cross,[189] Diplock,[190] Dilhorne,[191] Hailsham,[192] Kilbrandon,[193] Pearson,[194] Reid, Salmon,[195] Simon and Wilberforce[196]) and three of the six Law Lords appointed between 1973-80 (Lords Fraser,[197] Russell[198] and Scarman[199]) have also done so. While this criterion has not infrequently figured in the course of dissenting speeches it has been explicitly relied on by a majority of Law Lords in at least two recent hard cases - *Morgans* v. *Launchbury*[200] and *Lim Poh Choo* v. *Area Health Authority* - as a ground for refusing to develop the law.

As in the case of the criteria for the use of the 1966 Practice Statement, the guidelines in relation to the limits of judicial law-making were, and are, of different weights. Those suggested by Lord Reid were, it would appear, either 'pivotal' or 'relevant' expectations in the role of the Law Lord in the early 1970s. There were, however, subjective variations amongst the Law Lords both as to the weight of the criteria, and as to their application. This was particularly so in the realm of consequentialist discourse. In the words of MacCormick,

> [The] *consequentialist* mode of argument ... is in part at least *subjective*. Judges evaluating consequences of rival possible rulings may give different weight to different criteria of evaluation, differ as to the degree of perceived injustice, or of predicted inconvenience which will arise from adoption or rejection of a given ruling .... At this point we reach the bedrock of the value preferences which inform our reasoning but which are not demonstrable by it. At this level there can simply be irresoluble differences of opinion between people of goodwill and reason.[201]

Moreover, although the Law Lords may be agreed that, in general, consequentialist arguments are 'relevant' to their role, they may attach 'pivotal' or 'peripheral' importance to particular versions of such arguments. Thus the 'floodgates' argument - if the court makes a particular ruling it will create a flood of litigation - is a well-known consequentialist assertion, yet the consensus amongst counsel[202] that it carries little weight with the Law Lords seems to be correct. Although the argument (or one similar to it) has occasionally been put forward by counsel, it does not feature in Law Lords' speeches with any frequency. Even when it has appeared, as for example it did in the *Jones*[203] case, in *Gouriet* v. *Union of Post Office Workers*[204] and in *Fitzleet* v. *Cherry*[205] it has either been dismissed or treated as a 'peripheral' (or possibly 'relevant') argument.

PARLIAMENTARY INACTIVITY

A study of reported appeals to the House from 1966-80 reveals
that the Law Lords deployed a variety of other criteria relating to
the limits of judicial law-making in addition to those advocated by
Lord Reid. The available evidence suggests, however, that few if
any of them were more than 'peripheral' to the role of the Law
Lord during this period. Foremost amongst these additional
criteria, at least in terms of frequency of invocation, was the
argument from 'parliamentary inactivity'. In fact, there are two
principal (and contradictory) versions of this argument. In its best-
known form the argument runs,

> This is an area of law where Parliament has legislated in the
> recent past. It did not alter the existing judge-made law,
> therefore it must be taken to have endorsed it, accordingly it
> would be wrong for the courts now to change the law.[206]

Were one to proceed solely on the basis of the frequency with
which this proposition found favour in a Law Lord's speech, one
might well conclude that this criterion formed part of the Law
Lord's role during this period. At least eight Law Lords (Lords
Diplock,[207] Donovan,[208] Fraser,[209] Kilbrandon,[210] Morris,[211]
Reid,[212] Simon[213] and Wilberforce[214]) used it in a variety of cases
and a further three (Lords Gardiner, Guest and MacDermott)
indicated in their interviews that they could envisage situations
where such an argument would be valid. Yet a closer examination
of the cases reveals that not infrequently the argument was
rejected, sometimes in the same cases by other Law Lords (*e.g.*
Birmingham Corporation v. *West Midland Baptist (Trust) Association*,[215]
Herrington,[216] *Knuller*[217] and *Taylor* v. *Provan*[218]) and sometimes by
the same Law Lords in other cases (*e.g.* Lords Diplock,[219] Reid[220]
and Wilberforce[221]). The explanation of this apparent dissensus
and inconsistency amongst the Law Lords emerged from the
interviews. We saw earlier that the majority of counsel
interviewed did not attach great weight to the argument.[222]
Although a response on the issue was elicited only from ten of the
Law Lords interviewed, the clear picture to emerge from their
answers was that they agreed with counsel. Lord Reid disliked the
argument. 'It's too expedient', he said. Lord Gardiner thought it
'improper', MacDermott thought it 'weak', Pearson thought it

'unreliable' and Salmon thought it 'illegitimate'. Even those more sympathetic to the argument only accorded it 'peripheral' status. As one of them observed,

> You may sometimes be faced with a situation in which Parliament having had an opportunity of acting, has not acted, and then you ask yourself the question ... Parliament having abstained, is it right for us to take action? Sometimes, yes, sometimes, no; if Parliament has said the law has not to be changed or doesn't want to change it for the moment, who are we to change it? It's an argument.

Lord Denning on the other hand, said,

> Well, we use it when it suits our book ... I use it if I don't want it altered, but, on the other hand if it doesn't suit our book, I can say, 'Oh, well, Parliament can't notice everything and doesn't notice everything and they haven't got time to do it.'

Lord Radcliffe was equally candid,

> People will use these points in order to support something which they want to decide anyway. You'd be fantastic, I think, to argue that because Parliament hasn't moved, therefore the legislature agrees with you .... It's a sort of bad point thrown in.

The second version of the argument, though couched in similar terms to the first, leads to exactly the opposite conclusion. As such, it has from time to time been coupled with an express rejection of the first argument.[223] It runs,

> Parliament over the years has not legislated in this particular field, therefore they must be satisfied with the way the Courts have been developing the common law, therefore we may continue to develop the law in this field.

In some respects this is very similar to Lord Reid's assertion that the Law Lords have a greater freedom to develop the law in the area of lawyers' law. At any rate it received support from the same quarters, *i.e.* Lords Diplock,[224] Edmund-Davies, Guest, Morris, Pearce,[225] Reid, Simon and Wilberforce. However, it is in its strongest form that this argument is most interesting. 'The legislature has had a chance to act, hasn't done so, therefore an obligation to reform the law falls upon the courts.' This highlights what Judge Friendly once called, 'The Gap in Law-making' or 'Judges who can't and Legislators who won't'.[226] Although more frequently voiced in the US Supreme Court, the argument has occasionally been heard in the House of Lords. The intriguing point about it is that it appears to envisage that there are situations where the House would be justified in stepping outside the normal limits of judicial law-making. Thus Lord Reid having twice[227] expressed his dissatisfaction with the state of English law on third party rights in contracts, to no avail, was provoked into asserting in *Beswick* v. *Beswick*[228] that,

> if one had to contemplate a further long period of Parliamentary procrastination this House might find it necessary to deal with this matter. But if legislation is probable at an early date I would not deal with it in a case where that is not essential.

This threat did not have the desired effect. Twelve years later in *Woodar* v. *Wimpey* Lord Scarman was to be found repeating Lord Reid's words, adding 'Certainly the crude proposition for which [the appellant] contends ... calls for review, and now, not 40 years on.'[229] The Law Lords have not always been so patient. Lord Reid himself appeared to act on the argument in *Herrington*[230] - using it to justify 'usurping the functions of Parliament', as did Lord Wilberforce in *Miliangos*.[231] Even Lord Devlin was prepared to invoke it - at least in his lecture on 'Judges and Lawmakers',

> The strongest argument for judicial activism is not that it is the best method of law reform but that, as things stand, it is in a large area of the law the only method. The judges who made the common law must not abrogate altogether their responsibility for keeping it abreast of the times. Of course they can protest, as they frequently do, that it is for Parliament to change the law. But these protestations ring hollow when Parliament has said, as loudly as total silence can say it, that it intends to do nothing at all.[232]

Lord Devlin, in fact, had a strong preference for law-making through the Law Commission, and at least six Law Lords (including Lords Cross, Elwyn-Jones,[233] Kilbrandon, Russell,[234] and Simon[235]) seemed to agree with him that the creation of the Law Commissions had reduced the need for the Law Lords actively to develop the common law. There were, however, at least six other Law Lords of the opposite persuasion numbering in their ranks Lord Gardiner, the founder of the Law Commissions, as well as Lords Denning, Hailsham, Pearson, Reid and Salmon. As Lord Pearson remarked, 'It's our job to come to a decision: it's slightly cowardly to leave it to the Law Commission, except in a very suitable case.'

In sum, Lord Reid's criteria for fixing the limits of judicial law-making, whether established by his innovative activities or merely empathically identified from his colleagues, were important elements in the role of the Law Lord in the early 1970s (and probably remain so, still), though the additional criteria we have looked at, were not. The latter seem at best to have played a supportive role - functioning in a cumulative fashion (though all the criteria did this)[236] or as makeweight rationalisations to justify a Law Lord's chosen outcome.

LORD REID: LEADERSHIP AND MULTIPLE JUDGEMENTS

Lord Reid attempted to influence his colleagues on one further issue which he considered to be inextricably bound up with judicial law-making - that of multiple judgements. For the past decade and more there has been a body of opinion amongst academics and the Bar to the effect that the freedom of each Law Lord to contribute a separate speech in appeals to the House has led to undesirable consequences. The central thrust of the criticism[237] is that a multiplicity of assenting speeches tends to obscure the principle on which the court is acting and thus causes unnecessary difficulties for lower courts and the profession. To quote the authors of *Final Appeal*,

not infrequently [assenting judgements] serve only to fudge the areas of real agreement, and sometimes in the interstices of an apparent assent there lurk all the signs of partial dissent .... As such, they are insidious to ... clarity and certainty in the law.[238]

The Law Lords and counsel whom I interviewed were very conscious of the criticism - they had thought more about this topic than any other which I discussed with them. For some of the Law Lords it had caused much heart-searching, for most of them it continued to pose problems.

Opinion, both at the Bar and in the House, was divided. A clear majority of the counsel expressed a dislike for multiple judgements but were themselves divided as to the situations where it was more or less desirable to have a single opinion of the court. However, a sizeable minority (at least a third) favoured the existing practice. Amongst the Law Lords the lead, as so often before, came from Lord Reid. He was strongly in favour of multiple judgements. First, because he found that where the Law Lords gave only one judgement then there was a tendency for the lower courts to approach that judgement as if it were an Act of Parliament.[239] The single speech in *DPP* v. *Smith*[240] on objective intention in murder, was, he considered, a 'disaster' which might have been mitigated had there been more than one judgement.* Secondly, because in his view,

... it is often not possible to reach a final solution of a difficult problem all at once. It is better to put up with some uncertainty - confusion if you like - for a time, than to reach a final solution prematurely.[241]

As he told me,

I take the view that when you have got a case like *Indyka*, where you are breaking new ground, you don't know what your successors are going to do and you have got to leave a certain number of options open, and if you are going to try and define everything you'll do it wrong, it can't be done with one bite. You are far better, I think, to put down your own views, having

*As we saw earlier, in the *Smith* case the Lord Chancellor and the Lord Chief Justice were very insistent that there should be only one judgement to prevent confusion in the lower courts. Lord Denning, who took part in the case, told me,
I tried to get one or two modifications in it, but not with much success and I've regretted that ever since. It would have been much better if I had expressed my own views in my own words. It's a case we rushed through, the case was heard in June and we thought we ought to get the thing out by the end of the summer term in July.

read the other man's (if they think their own views are sufficiently different they put them down for themselves), and then leave it to the next generation to pick out what they like best. The law develops very slowly you know, and we can't do it, not satisfactorily, by making a sort of final pronouncement on a new point. It would never do ... and get us into far more trouble than the way we do it now.

Even Lord Radcliffe who strongly disagreed with Lord Reid on the desirability of multiple opinions, was at one with him on this point. As he put it,

I believe in the law as an inter-woven system and I do not believe in these great formative single decisions .... It's the infinite number of cases which are influenced by a House of Lords case one way or the other that really make the law.[242]

Whether, and to what extent, Lord Reid's oft-repeated views on this topic influenced his colleagues is very difficult to judge. They were certainly aware of the stance he took on the matter. Lord Pearce, for instance, remarked,

Scott Reid has always been in favour of separate judgements as against a joint judgement ... he is very much against forcing everybody's point of view into one judgement, because he thinks you get weakness, and he has got a point.[243]

At any rate, once again he was to be found in the majority group, as can be seen from Table 7.2.

The table does, it must be admitted, represent somewhat of an oversimplification. Thus, although in non-criminal common law cases only two active Law Lords generally favoured a single judgement, in criminal appeals on a point of statutory construction, probably a majority of the active Law Lords favoured that approach. Nevertheless in the general run of cases in the late 1960s and early 1970s Lord Reid's position was clearly in the ascendant. As one of his 'opponents' conceded,

If you can agree on a single judgement with precision then I think it's got big advantages. If you can only agree on it by blurring legal distinctions, it's got disadvantages. The advan-

TABLE 7.2 *Attitudes to multiple judgements (1972–3)[a]*

	Generally favourable	Mixed	Not in favour
Active Law Lords	Cross Diplock[b] Hailsham[c] MacDermott Pearson Reid Salmon[d]	Guest[g] Wilberforce[h]	Gardiner
Non-Active Law Lords	Denning[e] Devlin[f]	Pearce	Radcliffe

NOTES TO TABLE 7.2

a. Unless otherwise stated the classification of individual Law Lords was made in accordance with their responses to questions in my interview with them. The views of four active Law Lords were not ascertained.

b. Implied in 'The Courts as Legislators', at p.14; *Cassell* v. *Broome* at p.1129 H. In *Final Appeal*, p.94 it is stated that he favoured single judgements in cases turning on statutory construction. See also *D.* v. *NSPCC* at p.220F-G.

c. Interview; implied in *Cassell* v. *Broome* at p.1068A-B.

d. Interview; *Pickett* v. *British Rail Engineering Ltd* at p.157G. See also Lord Scarman at p.166G.

e. Lord Denning remarked, 'You can't get out of them so easily if it's one judgement, whereas if there were three or four then other people can pick out the bits they want.'

f. In view of *Rookes* v. *Barnard* it is rather ironic that Lord Devlin should tell me that he broadly favoured multiple judgements because they gave greater flexibility to the lower courts. But he added that he thought it was a good thing to have only one judgement in a case like *Rookes* where a new line was being taken.

g. His preference for single judgements related primarily to criminal appeals.

h. See his dicta in *BRB* v. *Herrington* at p.912C-D, *The Atlantic Star* at p.464G, and *Pickett* v. *BRE* at p.147F; his suggestion in 'La Chambre des Lords', p.96 that there should be fewer multiple speech appeals in the future; and his actions in cases such as *London Borough of Lewisham* v. *Lewisham Juvenile Court Justices* (where he withdrew his opinion to prevent duplication) and *Heatons Transport* v. *TGWU* and *Johnson* v. *Agnew* (where he appears to have insisted on a single judgement of the Court).

tage of a number of people putting their own viewpoint, even slightly disparately, with precision is that you get growing points in the law.

It has only been in the years since Lord Reid's death in 1975 that the evidence of the report cases has begun to suggest that the pendulum is swinging more strongly against multiple judgements.

CONCLUSION

In the penultimate chapter of *The Politics of the Judiciary* Professor Griffith observes,

> What is lacking ... is any clear and consistent relationship between the general pronouncement of judges on [the] matter of creativity and the way they conduct themselves in court ....
> The public position adopted by judges in the controversy about creativity is not consistently reflected in their judgements ... more important are their reactions to the moral, political and social issues in the cases that come before them.[244]

Julius Stone in a similar vein, concluded in *Social Dimensions of Law and Justice*,

> The doctrine [of judicial restraint] gives no clear guidance as to when and why a particular court should proceed creatively to adapt the pre-existing law to the case before it, and when and why it is duty bound to leave inadequacies for the legislature's attention .... Twist as we may, no coherence can be given to the growth of the common law, whether in America or elsewhere, in terms centred on judicial self-denying ordinances.[245]

Thirdly, as we saw in Chapter 6, Robert Seidman has claimed that, 'there are no commonly accepted norms defining the judge's role in deciding hard cases'.

Yet, when applied to the House of Lords (in the past twenty-five years), it is I hope clear from this and the previous chapter that each of these statements is false. Commonly accepted norms defining the role of the Law Lord in hard cases have existed throughout the period in question. The problem has been that some of the norms conflict with each other, for example the obligation to foster certainty in the law and the obligation to produce a just and fair decision. Moreover, some of them, for example the expectation that Law Lords should not usurp the functions of the legislature, have at times been lacking in specific content. The dominant response of the House to these conflicts in the mid-1950s involved a ranking of the competing expectations - dubbed by Stevens as substantive formalism. By 1962 the predominant mode was 'Dissimulation'. While it might seem that the dominance of the 'facade' approach at this time proves Griffith's point, in fact the inconsistency involved in this tactic was not between the general pronouncements of the Law Lords on creativity and what they did in court (which were quite compatible) but between what they said in their speeches and what they actually did. There was, and is, no incompatibility between the 'facade' approach and judicial restraint, as the activities of some of the Law Lords in the 1970s proved; the problem in the late 1950s and early 1960s was the combination of the facade approach with an insufficiently defined prohibition on judicial legislation. It was this lack of content in a 'pivotal' expectation in a Law Lord's role (identified by Stone in his comments on judicial restraint), which made it easier for some of the Law Lords to implement their value preferences in cases such as *Shaw* v. *DPP*.

The period from 1962 to 1966 was an era of significant change - in part attributable to the innovatory response of Lord Reid to role conflict - the end product being the 1966 Practice Statement on Precedent. Thereafter, the ban on judicial legislation was rescued from the realm of rhetoric by the emergence of norms governing the exercise of the Practice Statement and (*pace* Stone) of general guidelines as to the parameters of legitimate judicial law-making. Contrary to Griffith's thesis, we have seen that the perceptions elicited from the Law Lords in interviews, from their publications and speeches, of these norms and guidelines (*i.e.* their perceptions of their role) were highly consistent, both *inter se*, and with their performance in actual cases. Thanks in large measure to Lord Reid, by these means judicial restraint was imposed on the flexibility of response open to a Law Lord in a hard case when confronted with the conflict between justice and certainty.[246]

This did not mean, of course, the end of judicial individualism. There were dissenting voices as to the scope and even the existence of the norms and guidelines. The norms and guidelines were also, as MacCormick's comments on consequentialist reasoning showed, open to different interpretations. Occasionally the self-imposed fetters were cast off. Lord Reid would not have wished it any different. In the words of Lord Scarman (with which Lord Reid would undoubtedly have agreed),

Judicially indicated guidelines should not be treated as though they [are] a rule of law. They are to be followed unless the particular circumstances of a case ... indicate that they would be inappropriate.[247]

8 The Final Curtain?

REFLECTIONS

The fuller implications of the findings set out in the previous chapters for such fields as Social Psychology, Political Science, Legal Philosophy and the Sociology of Law cannot be pursued in detail here. Nevertheless, notwithstanding the spatial constraints of a concluding chapter, some, at least, require elaboration.

THE FREEDOM TO CHOOSE

First, freedom of choice. Much of the discussion in the two foregoing chapters was predicated on the assumption that in hard cases the Law Lords have, and often perceive themselves as having, a certain room for choice between the various alternative solutions to the legal problems confronting them in such cases. This assumption, if true, has considerable implications for the Hart/Dworkin debate in Jurisprudence.

On the one hand Ronald Dworkin asserts that even in hard cases judges are so constrained by existing legal standards that no significant element of choice is left open to them.[1] Even in such cases, he maintains, there is a single correct solution to be derived from the existing legal rules and principles. Reasonable lawyers, Dworkin concedes, may very well disagree as to what this solution actually is (as dissenting opinions testify), but this, he argues, merely points to the practical difficulties of identifying the solution. It does not refute the proposition that a right answer in law to which a litigant is entitled, does exist in hard cases.[2]

H. L. A. Hart, on the other hand, considers that in hard cases judges have a certain room for choice since, in his analysis, such cases are not determined by the mandatory sources of law. This is not to say that they have a licence to make arbitrary choices. Hart makes it clear that, in his view, judges are under an obligation to search conscientiously for the best available solution to a case. Moreover in reaching a decision by 'informed, impartial choice',[3] they must deploy an acceptable general principle, *i.e.* one derived from a persuasive or permissive source of law.[4] Finally, for Hart,[5] (and indeed for Llewellyn,[6] MacCormick[7] and Cross[8]) hard cases do not necessarily have a single correct answer on the basis of the existing law. In such cases no litigant is legally entitled to demand that the judge choose in one rather than another permissible way.

I asked the Law Lords several questions on these issues. The first ran,

> In the context of Appellate Court decisions, Lord Macmillan said 'In almost every case, it would be possible to decide the issue either way with reasonable legal justification.'[9] Cardozo, however, felt that 90 percent of such cases could only be decided one way.[10] What is your opinion?*

Ranking the Law Lords on this produced three groups,

1. *Those who generally agreed with Lord Macmillan*
Only Lords Cross and Radcliffe came in this group.

2. *Those who took a middle line*
As Lord Guest put it,

> Well, I think there is a middle line. I don't think that a majority of cases *must* be decided one way. On the other hand, I don't altogether agree with Macmillan that you can *always* decide every case either way. I think that there are a great number of cases where it is a question of impression and it might be decided the other way, but I don't agree with every case. I think that Cardozo is probably wrong in saying a majority.

Lords Hailsham, Kilbrandon, Denning, Devlin and Pearce held similar views.

---

*Llewellyn estimated that only 20 per cent of cases were worth appealing, but failed to develop the point in *The Common Law Tradition*.[11] A recent survey of US Federal Circuit Judges found that in less than a tenth of their cases did they consider that they had an 'opportunity to fashion new legal rules'.[12]

3. *Those who thought a third or less cases could go either way*
At least six active Law Lords came within this group, including
Lords Diplock,[13] MacDermott, Morris[14] and Reid. Lord Reid
replied,

> Where we are unanimous it really wouldn't, in nine cases out of
> ten, be possible to decide the case the other way. But ... you
> can't play about with a thing as much as that, you know, ... I
> think that two thirds of the cases ... could only go one way.

and Lord MacDermott added,

> It depends on the field of enquiry. There are a number of
> borderline cases but Lord Macmillan puts it too high. I would
> say that more than 50 per cent of cases have a plainly right
> solution.

Thus it can be seen that although divided over exact percentages,
all the Law Lords whose views on this matter could be discerned,
considered that in at least 20 per cent of the cases coming to the
Lords, the decision could go either way with reasonable legal
justification. This finding is not conclusive however, since some of
the Law Lords might have agreed (as Lord Pearson did) with
Lord Salmon's response,

> A case doesn't often get to the House of Lords unless it is a very
> evenly balanced case. There is obviously a great deal to be said
> on either side, but I don't agree that that means that if the
> judgement went the other way it would be just as good as it is in
> the way in which it does go.

To resolve this problem I asked a further question,

> Do you think that there is always one correct solution to a
> House of Lords case on the basis of the existing legal rules and
> principles, or are there some cases where the Law Lords have a
> choice about which way the law is to develop?

Of the fifteen active Law Lords, three agreed that there was a right
answer to every case,

> Oh, yes. I think there must always be one solution that is better

than any other in law. But it may not be possible to perceive it at the time. (Lord Kilbrandon)[15]

I think there is one view that ought to prevail ... I don't think you would get the same result if you spun a coin. You cannot say, 'Well, that's just as good', because it is such a finely balanced thing that you cannot be sure one way or the other. (Lord Salmon)

There certainly must be some cases which could go either way. But whether you know what it ought to be or not, there has got to be a decision. You cannot say, 'This is an interesting point of law for somebody else to decide.' The function of a judge is *over et terminer*. They are both equally important. You must listen and you must decide, even if it is only a hair's breadth in favour of one side, you have got to use that hair's breadth to pin down the scale. (Lord Pearson)

But at least eight other active Law Lords (including Lords Cross, Diplock,[16] Guest, MacDermott, Morris[17] and Reid) and all four 'non-active' Law Lords considered that there were cases coming to the Lords to which there was no single correct solution on the basis of the existing legal rules and principles, and in which they had a measure of choice.

As one Law Lord replied,

No, things are very seldom as simple as that, unfortunately; in most cases there is a conflict, sometimes between the merits of a particular case and the merits of a particular rule, and whether we should change something or leave it to legislation; that is the interest here, there are many choices open.

Other comments were:

No.You have got a choice ... most cases you have got a choice into which category you put a thing, or which interpretation you adopt. [In making the choice] I go by policy and social considerations. (Lord Denning)

In each case you have a choice. Shall I just apply a simple development of the existing cases, or shall we strike out? (Lord Devlin)

Generally the pre-existing principles decide the case, but there are some cases where the decision has to reflect the fact that the law keeps a blurred edge, and of course there have to be some policy choices. (Lord MacDermott)

Some cases are on the borderline as things are. Right one way, right the other. They have to be decided. They have to be faced. I don't think the courts as a matter of policy think, we will now make a departure ... I would think that they are faced with a borderline case or a split of the ways, and realise, 'Well, we might dodge it, but let's ... be men.' (Lord Pearce)

Well, of course there isn't [a single right answer] ... otherwise we should only be computers .... You see, it's not that the legal principles cannot solve cases ... legal principles normally lead you in the same direction but sometimes they don't, and you have got to choose between them, and public policy comes in more than perhaps we would like to admit .... But you can't produce any of that sort of thing through rules and regulations, you've got to depend in the end of the day you know, on discretion, which you hope is exercised reasonably with the experience you have behind you, but you have got to depend in the end of the day on instinct. (Lord Reid)

I have quoted the Law Lords' views *in extenso* here so that the reader can make his own assessment of their implications for Jurisprudence. Inasmuch as Dworkin's theory purports to be empirical as well as normative,[18] and more particularly since Dworkin seems to rest some of his argument on what lawyers and judges say about what they do,[19] the views of the majority group of Law Lords constitute evidence against his case and in favour of Hart's, both as to 'discretion' and to the existence of 'right answers'. If it is simply a question of whose account fits the available facts better, on the crucial aspect of what the Law Lords themselves think,* the answer is clear cut. Law Lords do exercise

*The importance of this is that, as has been pointed out, 'If men define situations as real, they are real in their consequences'[20] and if the Law Lords perceive themselves as free to make choices then they are likely to act accordingly. It is possible that Dworkin acknowledges that British (as opposed to American) judges do act in this way.[21]

choices. Many cases do not have right answers which the Law Lords could divine if only they were sufficiently discerning. Their job is to make the best decision they can from the materials available - in the last analysis, Law Lords are craftsmen, not treasure hunters.

On the other hand Dworkin has recently stated that,

> Positivists and I do not dispute about details of practice that could be settled by ... framing more intelligent questionnaires for judges. We may disagree about matters of that sort, but this disagreement is not fundamental. We fundamentally disagree about what our practice comes to, that is, about which philosophical account of the practice is superior.[22]

On the basis of this comment it is far from clear to me what empirical evidence, if any, Dworkin would accept as a refutation of parts of his thesis.

LEGITIMATION

The rejection of Dworkin's characterisation of the judicial process raises once again the difficult problem of the legitimacy of judicial law-making. As Dworkin himself has argued[23] law-making by a non-elected judiciary which is not in practice responsible to society, is open to the objection that it is both undemocratic and retroactive. To put the same point in somewhat different terms: both the House of Lords and the US Supreme Court are confronted by the need to reach an accommodation between judicial independence and public accountability.[24]

How then can decisions in hard cases attain legitimacy? Certainly not from the informed consent of the public. Repeated research in America has revealed widespread public ignorance of the work of the Supreme Court.[25] These findings would undoubtedly be replicated in relation to the British public and the House of Lords. Nor can it rest on a claim that the House acts as a surrogate legislature. Dworkin rightly rejects the suggestion that judges are deputy legislators making law 'in response to evidence and arguments of the same character as would move the superior institution'.[26] This appears not only from the makeweight status of arguments from parliamentary inactivity* in the eyes of counsel and Law Lord[27] but also from the fact that the Law Lords use as a criterion for not developing the law the very fact that the methods of investigation and decision-making adopted by the legislature are not available to them.[28]

The traditional solution has been to stress the restricted confines within which judges act and the constraints on the exercise of their powers - limits imposed by institutional factors, the rule of law and the operation of judicial restraint. Institutional constraints undoubtedly reduce the scope for judicial creativity, for example the requirement of leave to appeal (or *certiorari*), of standing to sue, the ban on hypothetical or advisory rulings, the operation of the rules on mootness,[29] the dependence of the courts on clients and counsel bringing cases before them† and, as we saw earlier,[30] particularly in the House of Lords, their dependence on the arguments which counsel are prepared to run before them. But to restrict the scope of judicial creativity is not to legitimate the occasions when it does occur.

The rule of law,[31] fresh from its triumphs in the neo-Marxist camp,[32] seems to offer more hope. Whether in the guise of formal legal rationality, of principled decision-making or of the search for neutral principles of constitutional law,[33] it does engender a measure of objectivity and impartiality in the judicial process. Yet Weber failed to explain how the autonomy and neutrality of 'legal rational domination' confers democratic legitimation on judicial law-making.[34] Roberto Unger[35] has endeavoured to show how the connection can be made, though I am not sure with what success; but, Unger apart, recent attempts to legitimate judicial law-making by reference to formal legal rationality seem all too frequently to rely on an implicitly and sometimes explicitly consensus-oriented model of society.[36] It seems more likely that often there is no shared consensus of understandings and values in liberal society. Given that the bulk of the Law Lords see themselves as having to make choices in hard cases, such choices may be between competing beliefs in society. 'To this extent', comments Unger,[37] 'adjudication aggravates rather than resolves, the problem of unjustifiable power.' The rule of law in the last

---

*The somewhat similar argument from congressional deadlock as a justification for judicial activism seems to carry more weight in the Supreme Court.

†The startling spectacle of an appeal court 'correcting' one of its decisions by a practice note, see [1976] 1 W.L.R. 799, is fortunately not a common one.

analysis is only the rule of some men.[38]

Alternatively, it could be argued that the proponents of principled decision-making,[39] or even those of substantive rationality,[40] purposive reasoning[41] and result-oriented decision-making can offer a form of legitimacy, or at least objectivity, to the extent that reasoned, non-arbitrary judgements provide a rational basis for accepting decisions. By this means the public audience can be reconciled to 'the use of power which the decision authorises'.[42] There are two problems with this argument. First, the public ignorance of the work of the House of Lords and the US Supreme Court coupled with the finding that generally Law Lords' speeches are not aimed at the public,[43] suggests that in practice this legitimation device is of limited efficacy.

Secondly, there is the problem (ignored by Robert Summers in his seminal article on common-law justification[44]), of who is to decide what counts as a good reason for a judicial decision. If it is not the public, is it left to the subjectivity of each judge? If so, how can this confer any legitimacy on his decisions? One possible answer is that objectivity, if not legitimacy, comes from the practices of the legal profession as a whole. The Law Lords act as a reference group for counsel in determining what are tenable arguments[45] but are themselves influenced by the climate of legal opinion in hard cases,[46] and the reasons which they give in their speeches are ones which they think are regarded as acceptable within the legal community. As we saw in earlier chapters,[47] shared understandings do exist both amongst and between counsel and Law Lords as to the relative strengths and weaknesses of certain types of argument as a justification for judicial decisions. To the extent that lawyers and judges constitute a 'caste of experts'[48] linked by training, practice and habits of thought,[49] interaction and socialisation are likely to go some distance to ensuring the objectivity of the arguments used by British judges in the course of their judgements.

The third limiting factor in relation to judicial law-making, judicial restraint, is also derived in part from the legal community. Although examples of the operation of this doctrine can be pointed to both in the UK and America,[50] its content, seen through the eyes of US Supreme Court Justices, seems protean. This may be because the role of a Justice in a hard case particularly one involving judicial review - is in a more embryonic form than that of a Law Lord.[51] In the Lords on the other hand, as I have shown, the last twenty-five years has witnessed major shifts in the prevailing role perceptions of the Law Lords and under the aegis of Lord Reid, the emergence of guidelines demarcating the role of the Law Lords as law-makers from that of Parliament. Such role restraints have an objectivity from their acceptance by the bulk of the judicial community. Further, the Law Lords might argue that the limits to judicial law-making which they endorsed have a democratic legitimacy inasmuch as they are derived from the public and the legislature (as symbolic reference groups). Thus the Judicial Committee of the Privy Council refer in *Geelong Harbour Commissioners* v. *Gibbs Bright* to,

> the consensus of opinion of the public, of the elected legislature and of the judiciary as to the proper balance between the respective roles of the legislature and of the judiciary as law-makers[52]

as determining the frequency with which a final court of appeal ought to overrule its previous decisions.

Perhaps more realistically Lord Reid argued that the guidelines and criteria which he advocated were derived from common sense,* legal principle (which he regarded as 'organised common sense') and public policy.[53] All of these factors were, in his mind, linked to the movements of public opinion, and he regarded contact with ordinary people of all grades of society as essential for any judge in order to obtain a proper view of public opinion.

At the end of the day, however, role expectations as to the limits of judicial law-making and as to the exercise of the 1966 Practice Statement, can only impose restraints, they cannot determine behaviour. Moreover, a central theme of this book has been to stress that the concept of role is a dynamic one.

The consensus amongst Law Lords on certain role restraints is ephemeral. Law Lords disagree as to the existence of particular guidelines and as to their weight in particular cases. In the very interpretation and application of the guidelines, the subjectivity of a Law Lord has a part to play. The Law Lords' responses to role conflict, although along lines predicted from other fields of research, depend in part on their personalities. Thus when justice

---

*Lord Reid regarded himself as a 'common-sense lawyer'[54] and his reliance on common sense to assist him in identifying the limits of judicial law-making was shared by several of his colleagues, e.g. Lords Upjohn,[55] Pearce and Salmon.

and certainty conflict, some Law Lords, for example Lords Diplock,[56] Pearce, Salmon and Denning, consider that they have a tendency to favour flexibility and justice, others, for example Lords Cross, Guest, Pearson and Upjohn[57] have admitted to a tendency in the opposite direction, while the bulk of the remainder endeavour to strike a balance between the two expectations. It may be, as some have suggested,[58] that in making such choices the Law Lords are taking account of community standards of fairness and justice - though such a description would surprise some of the Law Lords. Thus Lord Morris once wrote,

> The judge is sworn to administer justice according to law .... But there is so much that is nowhere written down in black and white, and then the judge must ... [have] recourse to a personally built conception of what [he] thinks is fair.[59]

Similarly Lord Cross agreed that it was necessary in hard cases to apply certain standards, but added, 'everybody has got their own standards of what is fair and just and desirable. The trouble is that people, of course, differ very much as to what these are.' But Lord Pearson found a way to link his views with those of the wider community,

> We have a certain amount in our minds from having lived in this country for maybe sixty odd years, and having read the newspapers and talked to people. You have got to take Her Majesty's judges, I suppose, to that extent as representative of popular opinion. They do what they think is just. One hopes it coincides with what the community think just, but then the community is probably divided into sections which think different things are just.

Once it is recognised that Law Lords like the wider community differ in their attitudes to issues such as justice and certainty, it might be argued that a partial solution to the problem of the legitimacy of judicial law-making could lie in attempting to achieve a balance between judges of opposing tendencies, both in the selection of Law Lords to sit on a case and in the long-term promotion policy of judges from lower courts. Several Law Lords have made suggestions along these lines. Lord Reid considered that a 'balance of power' was required on an appeal court between

black letter lawyers, legal reformers and common-sense lawyers.[60]
Lord Hailsham in 'The English Law and its Future'[61] identified a
need for judicious mixture of 'reformer' and 'traditionalist' role
orientations amongst judges. And Lord Pearce commented,

> As far as I am concerned, I think flexibility should not be
> sabotaged for certainty, rather than some of my colleagues who
> might take a more rigid line, and it is a very good thing that we
> are a mixture. I mean if we were all too flexible or all too rigid,
> you would get nowhere.

In practice, during the period of this study, it seems that little
effort was made to achieve balance in this sense, at least in the
selection of the Law Lords to sit on the Appellate Committee,
probably because any attempt to do so would have made impossibly complex a task which was already complicated enough.[62] Yet
Lord Gardiner told me that when he was Lord Chancellor he
favoured a selection policy which aimed to achieve a good mixture
between the Law Lords. His policy in promoting judges from the
Court of Appeal also reflected his desire for balance,

> Basically you want different types ... if there are two
> outstanding lawyers, and one is rather rigid and the other is too
> flexible, well then have both and they will even things out.[63]

Since it is probable that the Law Lords cannot avoid making
law it is to be hoped that Lord Gardiner's successors will, like him,
see the need for balance in the court.[64] With respect to judicial
law-making, 'judges, never will nor should they all think alike',
said Lord Reid,[65] but there is much truth in the adage, *in medio
tutissimus ibis.**

---

*'The safest route is in the middle' (Ovid *Metamorphoses* , *ii* 137).

Appendix: Role Analysis

All the world's a stage,
And all the men and women merely players,
They have their exits and entrances;
And one man in his time plays many parts.[1]

All roles are cages, but some roles are cagier than others.
(Graffiti on a steel plant wall)[2]

THE CONCEPT OF ROLE: SOME PROBLEMS

The concept of role has been a frustrating one for social scientists. Bedevilled by indeterminate or ambiguous usage, by competing definitions and abstruse ancillary substructures,[3] its theoretical pay-off has remained problematic. This lack of consensus on the meaning of the concept was but one of the drawbacks which led some scholars to label it as a redundant notion with little explanatory potential.[4] Now even the sniping by its critics in the interactionist and the structuralist camps has been superseded (at least in the United Kingdom) by considerable indifference and neglect. In some ways this can be no bad thing. 'Role' had become a victim of its own apparent utility as an analytical device. The bridge between personality and culture, the major link between character and social structure and the interface between the individual and the collectivity, it was hailed as an heuristic panacea by sociologists, social psychologists and social anthropologists alike. Each of these scholarly communities moulded the concept of role to their own purposes. Each deployed it at a different level of explanation. Not surprisingly it proved unable to bear the weight imposed upon it.

But the failure of an acceptable successor to emerge to link the micro and macro levels of sociological analysis[5] suggests that

moves to abandon role analysis are premature. Certainly the
explanatory potential of the 'role' concept will vary with the
phenomena under scrutiny,[6] with the level of explanation at which
it is deployed and the extent to which it is allowed to form part of a
coherent theoretical framework. But this is not a justification for
rejecting the concept. Rather it points to the need to map out the
areas where the concept's potential is greatest and in which
frameworks. While this book does not attempt such an ambitious
project it does endeavour to illustrate how one particular version
of 'role' and its related conceptual structure can be used to
advantage in the study of an elite group, namely, appellate judges.

'ROLE' DEFINED

Role in this book denotes the normative expectations (subjective
and objective) concerning the behaviour and personal attributes
which are associated with the occupancy of a specific social
position. Karl Llewellyn once wrote that the,

> role of appellate judge is so peculiarly established, so clearly felt,
> so implemented and documented not only in content but in
> panoply, not only in panoply but in behaviour, that its careful
> study might well refine general role theory ... [7]

If the thesis propounded in Chapters 6 and 7, that the role of a
Law Lord in a hard case has changed during the period of my
research, is correct, then one such refinement to general role
analysis[8] is the accent on the subjective element contained in the
above definition of role. The majority usage of the term has not
contained this subjective element.[9] It is contended, however, that
a person's own expectations and perceptions as to the proper
behaviour of an individual in his social position can have a vital
part to play in the definition of his role as well as his role
performance.

Undeniably, Reference Group Theory, the study of the ways in
which a person's orientation to others influences or constrains his
behaviour, with its concentration on the role expectations of these
reference others (commonly treated as separate groups, hence
'reference groups') has been partly responsible for this failure to

define an individual as having a say in the content of his role. It did not ignore the relational aspects of role - from it we derive the notion of the *role-set*,[10] *i.e.* the collectivity of role others who typically interact with the occupant of a particular social position. Yet nowhere is it suggested that this interaction contains possibilities for the social actor to 'negotiate' with his audience not only the proper performance of his role but also its content.

Once it is recognised that a key feature of 'role' is its dynamic aspect, that a role and its performance are to a greater or lesser degree open to 'negotiation', we can see that any given role will always remain to a certain extent problematic. As Turner puts it,[11]

> Roles 'exist' in varying degrees of concreteness and consistency, while the individual confidently frames his behaviour as if they had unequivocal existence and clarity. The result is that in attempting from time to time to make aspects of the roles explicit he is creating and modifying roles as well as merely bringing them to light; the process is not only role taking but *role making*[12] .... The Actor is not the occupant of a position for which there is a neat set of rules - a culture or set of norms - but a person ... who must act in the perspective supplied in part by his relationship to others whose actions reflect roles that he must identify. Since the role of the alter can only be inferred rather than directly known by ego, testing inferences about the role of alter is a continuing element in interaction. Hence the tentative character of the individual's own role definition and performance is never wholly suspended.

Role is dynamic in a secondary sense, *i.e.* as a result of the process of social change. With the passage of time, roles are subject to shifts in emphasis. The evolution may be gradual, incremental or marked by surges and periods of retrenchment. Roles may vary because of the activities of innovatory social actors, because of group pressures, or merely as an unintended consequence of social action. Where innovation is the moving force, the 'innovant' may, at first, be seen as a 'deviant' by his colleagues.[13] But, ironically, if his views become accepted, more reactionary colleagues who have hitherto been his critics, may themselves become labelled as 'deviants'. Since 'innovants' and innovation epitomise both of the dynamic aspects of *role* they are rewarding subjects for scrutiny, as I have shown in Chapters 6 and 7.

THE DIMENSIONS OF ROLE

Role is also a dimensional concept. The three dimensions mentioned in this book are power, legitimacy and weight. Looking first at power, the ability to have a say in the definition of a role is as much a question of power as influencing actual role performances by the application or potential application of sanctions.[14] Research is required to elicit in which social situations or institutional contexts individuals possess the power to 'negotiate' their roles and within what limits. The emphasis on the subjective element in *role* in this book was prompted in part by the hypothesis that the Law Lords, because of their position in the legal hierarchy, possess a larger autonomy in the definition of their role than some lower status actors in the hierarchy, *e.g.* police constables.[15] As Howard Becker has observed, 'In any system of ranked groups, participants take it as a given fact that members of the highest group have the right to define the way things really are.'[16]

Again, reference groups have a differential ability to have their definition of a role accepted by the position incumbent. Such differences in power formed the main theme of a study by Maureen Cain of policemen in England and Wales. There she argued that,

> the identification of role-definers (those projecting expectations) is only a preliminary step. There are differences in the importance of the definition to the role definers themselves, and in the meaning of the received definitions to the actor. More important, even given equivalent definitions and interpretations, there are structural differences in the power of different role-defining individuals or groups. Some will be more effective in influencing the behaviour of the focal person than others.[17]

This influence can be the result of the exercise of positive or negative sanctions or of persuasion in the 'negotiation' with the focal person. Nor is the influence static. The relative power of the reference groups and of the focal person will develop and vary through time, as will the role expectations which they hold.

The elite status of the research subjects also influenced the definition of 'reference group' which was used in the research. Traditional usages,[18] with their emphasis on comparison groups, were rejected in favour of a broad version, namely groups who hold and articulate expectations for the individual's role performance and are used by him to evaluate his own performance.[19] Thus defined they need not be physically present, nor need they be a group of which the individual is a member. But there may be groups who project expectations concerning the behaviour of the position occupant which the latter wishes to reject. He may wish to do so either because he does not consider that it is legitimate for that group to expect (normatively) that he will act in accordance with their normative expectations, or because he rejects as illegitimate certain of the expectations which they project. In the eyes of the focal person, therefore, role expectations have a dimension of legitimacy.

Thirdly, there is the dimension of weight or functional importance. Following earlier writings,[20] the normative expectations which make up a person's role can be classified according to their centrality or importance to the role. As we saw in Chapter 1 some expectations are 'peripheral' to the role so that compliance with or possession of them might be considered optional; next are those that are sufficiently 'relevant' to the role that their absence or variation leaves it imperfect or incomplete; finally the 'pivotal' attributes are those which are absolutely fundamental to the role. 'Pivotal' expectations are more likely to be significantly affected by structural elements, e.g. the institutionalised setting for the role performance, while 'peripheral' expectations provide more scope for individual variation. Thus deviation from a 'peripheral' expectation will simply be labelled as eccentric behaviour, e.g. a Law Lord (Lord Wilberforce) reading a horse-racing magazine in a cafe in Chancery Lane.[21] But deviation from a 'pivotal' exception will provoke severe censure and criticism (serving the function of role reinforcement).[22]

ROLE CONFLICT

A key feature in much of the literature has been the notion of *role conflict* - the situation where conflicting role expectations exist. It can be either inter- or intra-role. The former refers to a situation where an individual occupies two social positions with incompatible role prescriptions, *e.g.* a father who as a local magistrate has to try a criminal case in which his son is a defendant. The latter involves inconsistencies between expectations of different reference groups or between different members of one reference group relating to a single role, *e.g.* a judge in a rape trial dealing with the problem of whether the victim's name should be published by the press. Intra-role conflict also includes differences between reference group expectations and the position incumbent's perception of his role. Role conflict is also affected by the dimensionality of role, for not only may there be a conflict between the expectations of an individual's reference groups but there may also be a difference between or within the reference groups on the comparative weight to be attached to an expectation.

The attention devoted to situations of role conflict by role analysts is in part due to the discovery that individuals respond in certain typical ways to different forms of role conflict. A possible taxonomy of these responses is set out in Figure A.1.[23] *Positive* responses are labelled such since they involve actively taking steps to eliminate or modify the conflict, not simply for the individual involved but for all who share his position. *Innovation* occurs when a person or a group of persons endeavours to negotiate a change in the definition of their role in such a way that conflict will be reduced or institutionalised. *Innovation* involving, as it does, the individual in attempting to achieve a redefinition of his role seems hitherto to have received comparatively little attention from role analysts.[24] Ironically, rather more has been made of the tactic of convening the role-set,[25] even though in many situations it is not open to individuals because of the sheer impracticality of such an undertaking. Nevertheless, the Law Lords have convened their most significant reference group (*i.e.* themselves) on several occasions, *e.g.* prior to the 1966 Practice Statement and before the Order in Council in the Privy Council on Dissents.[26]

Adaptive responses, statistically more frequent than the other two categories of response, have not surprisingly been subjected to greater academic scrutiny than the others. There are three separate *Adaptive* techniques, *Ranking*, *Evasion* and *Absorption*. In the case of the first technique the individual ranks the conflicting

FIGURE A.1   Responses to role conflict

I. POSITIVE
   (a) *Innovation*
   (b) *Convening Role-Set or Reference Groups*

II. ADAPTIVE
   (a) *Ranking* competing expectations according to
       (1) Sanctioning power
       (2) Legitimacy
       (3) Functional importance
       (4) Perceived balance of (1), (2) and (3)
   (b) *Evasion*
       (1) Segregation of Role Performances
       (2) Dissimulation
       (3) Manipulation
   (c) *Absorption*

III. WITHDRAWAL
   (a) *Psychological*
   (b) *Physical*

expectations according to his perception of (a) the strength of the sanctions attached to the expectations,[27] (b) their legitimacy,[28] or (c) their functional importance.[29] A fourth possibility arises where the individual endeavours to strike a balance within or between the first three factors.[30] One might not expect to find that in deciding hard cases the Law Lords were influenced by their perception of the comparative strengths of the sanctions attached to the competing normative expectations involved. The threat of reversal by Parliament if the Law Lords decided against them which was made by one of the litigants in *Burmah Oil* v. *The Lord Advocate* seems to have had singularly little effect on the House of Lords in the disposal of the case. However, Law Lords quite frequently adopt arguments based on the social or legal consequences of accepting one proposition rather than another and this might be seen as attaching consideration to the strength of a sanction. Similarly, the haste and manner in which their Lordships conducted *Heatons Transport Ltd* v. *TGWU*,[31] if not the actual decision itself, might well be construed as a reaction to the possibility of the sanction of a General Strike.

Evasion as a technique for coping with role conflict has three principal forms, 'Segregation', 'Dissimulation' and 'Manipulation'. 'Segregation' of roles is such an obvious way of

avoiding inter-role conflict that it frequently becomes institutionalised, *e.g.* where a judge is forbidden also to be a member of the
House of Commons,[32] or where a judge is expected to decline to sit
in a case in which he has an interest. In such cases 'Segregation'
may amount to repudiation of one role. 'Segregation' of role
performances, *i.e.* insulating them from the observation of more
than one of the competing reference groups at the same time, is a
technique employed both in cases of inter- and intra-role
conflict.[33] It is not, however, in the nature of things, a ploy that
can be successfully invoked by a Law Lord deciding a hard case.
'Dissimulation,'[34] on the other hand, can be (see Chapters 6 and
7). This response rejects the notion that social stability depends on
the accuracy with which roles are perceived. Its proponents argue
that 'social relations may often be designed around or benefit from
inaccuracies of role perception'[35] or ignorance or dissimulation.
The essence of 'Dissimulation' is the pretence that there is no
conflict and that therefore the role performer can comply with both
expectations or sets of expectations. 'Segregation' of audiences
where intra-role conflict is involved can be seen as a form of
'Dissimulation' but Goffman suggests that there are two other
main forms. The first involves a ranking of expectations according
to the criteria above mentioned and then the violating of the lower
ranked expectation. The focal person however endeavours to
conceal the breach and thus to maintain the myth that the
expectations are compatible. The other form of 'Dissimulation'
occurs when the individual violates the expectation whose
violation he can conceal the most easily. This again maintains the
legitimacy of both ideals.[36] 'Dissimulation' as expounded by
Goffman accords well with his argument that,

> in their capacity as performers, individuals will be concerned
> with maintaining the impression that they are living up to the
> many standards by which they and their products are judged.
> ... But, *qua* performers, individuals are concerned not with the
> moral issue of realising these standards, but with the amoral
> issue of engineering a convincing impression that these
> standards are being realised.[37]

'Manipulation', the third evasive response, involves playing off
the various conflicting reference groups against each other.[38]
   The third category of *Adaptive* response, *Absorption* or internali-

sation, in many instances could equally well be described as a failure to adapt at all.[39] Its hallmarks include vacillation and procrastination. There are limits to the amount of conflict that can be handled by such a technique and it thus tends to be a more transitory response than the others.*

The final response to role conflict is *Withdrawal*. Psychological withdrawal can be described as a loss of commitment or (sometimes) apathy. When a disjunction arises between an actor's self-concept and his perception of his role,[40] Goffman has directed our attention to one of the likely outcomes - 'role-distancing'.[41] This activity consists in the individual letting it be seen (in certain circumstances) that he, as a person, is not fully committed to his role although he continues to act in accordance with it.† The most extreme reaction to intra-role conflict is to withdraw physically from the role, *i.e.* resign.[42]

Finally, it should be stated that each mechanism need not operate independently. An individual may well adopt two or more in conjunction or vary his response in different situations. There is no necessity to postulate consistency in role performers between one situation of role conflict and another.

ROLE ANALYSIS AND JUDICIAL RESEARCH

Whatever its present status in the eyes of British sociologists, role analysis in the 1970s continued to attract the attention of American political and social scientists. Certainly this is true in the field of Judicial Research. Perhaps because of the strength of the structural-functionalist paradigm in American sociology, the versions of role which have been used have tended to be both

---

*Certainly some Law Lords have been notorious amongst their colleagues for their inability to come to a decision in a case, *e.g.* Viscount Simon. Even if this can be described as a response to role conflict there is a limit to the length of time which a Law Lord can delay making a final decision in a case.
†An amusing example of judicial 'role-distancing' was supplied by Maule J. in a case quoted in W. Andrews (ed.), *The Lawyer: In History, Literature and Humour* (London: William Andrews & Co., 1896) pp. 240-1. 'Prisoner, your counsel thinks you innocent, the prosecution thinks you innocent, and I think you innocent. But a jury of your own fellow countrymen, in the exercise of such commonsense as they possess, have found you guilty, and it remains that I should pass sentence upon you. You will be imprisoned for one day, and as that day was yesterday, you are free to go about your business.'

consensus-oriented and static. Judicial reference groups have received little study[43] - a fact which may go some way to explaining some of the competing findings of researchers in the field. Role conflict has been virtually ignored as an explanatory concept, and 'the judicial role' has tended to be seen as an independent rather than as a dependent variable.[44] With the growth in empirical studies, however, this last assumption, that there is only one judicial role whose existence may be taken as read and used to explain judicial behaviour, has come under attack because a lack of congruence between the role perceptions of judges in different courts has been revealed.[45]

Although judicial role studies have produced interesting and valuable data on the self-conceptions of judges in particular courts, certain problems have arisen in the attempt to apply role analysis to judges. First, the findings have tended to be concrete, highly specific and frequently non-comparable. Little headway has been made in the search for generalisations of a more abstract, theoretical nature. In part this is due to a failure by some researchers to take role analysis seriously. Attracted by the common language usage of role as an all-purpose conceptual peg upon which to hang a set of facts and opinions, or dismayed by the inchoate status of role analysis with its plethora of competing definitions, most researchers have settled for an emasculated and anaemic version of role with little related conceptual structure.

The exceptional studies which have applied role analysis in a more sophisticated form, *e.g.* Dorothy James's study of Supreme Court Justices,[46] Beverly Blair Cook's research on Federal District Judges[47] and Kenneth Vines and Robert Glick's investigation of the role perceptions of the judges in four State Supreme Courts,[48] have demonstrated the improved insights to be gained by such an approach. This is hardly surprising since any theoretical structure is likely to fail to fulfil its explanatory potential if it is poorly developed.

Secondly, there have been difficulties in the classification and categorisation of judicial roles. Some researchers[49] have distinguished between a purposive sector and a decision-making sector in the judicial role, or between different role types, *e.g.* lawmaker, pragmatist, administrator, *etc.* Since these classifications are not related to any theoretical structure but simply to armchair speculation or empirical groupings, every researcher produces different classifications[50] and interpretations.

Finally, although it is a fundamental premiss of role analysis that it can explain certain behaviour because individuals are influenced by role expectations, few attempts[51] have been made to link the role perceptions elucidated from the judges with their actual behaviour. Until studies of this kind are undertaken the value of role analysis in judicial research will be restricted.

In the United Kingdom, judicial role studies are still in their infancy. Since the publication of Robert Seidman's seminal paper in 1969[52] several books and articles have discussed role analysis and judges.[53] However, they reflect the same problems as their transatlantic precursors. With the exception of Seidman and Palley,[54] the writers' treatment of *role* has been incidental or ancillary to other concerns and has added little to their arguments.

The foregoing comments must, however, be balanced against the potential advantages of applying role analysis to the judicial process. All research projects are located explicitly or implicitly within a particular frame of reference and there are indications that the heuristic potential of role analysis in an appropriate framework can be considerable when applied to judges. Regularities in the behaviour of individual judges can be set in an institutional context. Judicial self-concepts and motivations can be derived from semi-structured interviews with judges. A judge's role perceptions can act as a restraint to the implementation of his value preferences in a particular decision. Thus it has been argued that the reason that a judge like Lord Uthwatt, whose personal sympathies favoured the advancement of the interests of workers, frequently made decisions which had the contrary effect was that he perceived that such alterations in the law of employment were the province of Parliament, and not the judges.[55] Those who assert that Justice Frankfurter had civil libertarian sympathies account for his votes in civil liberties cases by pointing to the emphasis which he placed on judicial self-restraint in his interpretation of the judicial role.[56] Again Robert Cover in *Justice Accused*[57] has argued that the reason why so many American judges who opposed slavery, produced decisions which bolstered up the institution was that they placed their view of their institutional duty as judges (*i.e.* their role percepton) before their own moral principles. Equally there are occasions when judges allow their personal sympathies to override their role perceptions, *e.g.* Lord Simonds in *Shaw* v. *DPP*. Judicial role studies concentrating on such variations in judicial response to these self-role conflicts and endeavouring to explain when and why the variations occur, would contribute to the refinement of role analysis in general.

Role analysis has also shown itself to be a useful tool in the study of trial courts, indeed, the great majority of judicial role studies are now made at the trial court level.[58] Finally, when linked to an interactionist perspective, role analysis effectively focuses on the group activities of judges, their interaction with one another, and with counsel - an area of particular importance in the United Kingdom because of the tradition of oral advocacy.

CONCLUSION

In this appendix it has been argued that the value of a judicial role study depends on the extent to which it utilises a single, coherent and developed role model. The explanatory potential of that model will be affected by the appropriateness of the broader frame of reference adopted for the study of the chosen research area. The role model used in this study was located in an interactionist perspective and was designed to focus on interaction, dynamism and conflict. These features were chosen because preliminary research suggested that the role of a Law Lord in a hard case during the period 1957-73 involved marked role conflict and dynamism and because of a desire to focus on the group activities of judges. The research also endeavoured to examine the consistency of the Law Lords' role perceptions, as elicited from interviews, with their role performances in hard cases.

Notes and References

LIST OF ABBREVIATIONS USED

A.B.A.J.	*American Bar Association Journal*
Austr. L.J.	*Australian Law Journal*
A.J.C.L.	*American Journal of Comparative Law*
A.R.S.P.	*Archiv fur Rechts-und Sozialphilosophie*
B.J.L.S.	*British Journal of Law and Society*
Can. B. Rev.	*Canadian Bar Review*
C.L.P.	*Current Legal Problems*
C.L.J.	*Cambridge Law Journal*
Harv. L.R.	*Harvard Law Review*
I.C.L.Q.	*International and Comparative Law Quarterly*
J. of Pol.	*Journal of Politics*
J.S.P.T.L.	*Journal of the Society of Public Teachers of Law*
Law and Soc. Rev.	*Law and Society Review*
L.Q.R.	*Law Quarterly Review*
M.L.R.	*Modern Law Review*
N.I.L.Q.	*Northern Ireland Legal Quarterly*
Rev. Int. Dr. Comparé	*Revue Internationale de Droit Comparé*
U.C.L.A.L. Rev.	*University of California Los Angeles Law Review*

Except where otherwise indicated the abbreviations *L.J.*, *L.Q.* and *L.R.* have been used for *Law Journal*, *Law Quarterly* and *Law Review* respectively.

CHAPTER 1: INTRODUCTION

1. W. J. M. Mackenzie, *Politics and Social Science* (Harmondsworth: Penguin, 1967) p. 286.
2. 9 *J.S.P.T.L.* (1967) 335 at p. 341.
3. See L. Blom-Cooper and G. Drewry, *Final Appeal* (Oxford University Press, 1972) pp. 4-5 and R. Stevens, *Law and Politics* (London: Weidenfeld and Nicolson, 1979) pp. xv-xviii.
4. This applies as much to *Final Appeal* as to the case notes which appear in the *M.L.R.* and the *L.Q.R.*.
5. *cf.* Lord Reid in 'The Judge as Law Maker', 12 *J.S.P.T.L.* (1972) 22.

'[W]e do not believe in fairy tales any more.'

6.   *Labour and the Law* (London: Stevens, 1972) p. 60.

7.   For a fuller definition of such cases see p. 127-8 above.

8.   *In Search of Justice* (London: Allen Lane, The Penguin Press, 1968) p. 186.

9.   [1966] 1 W.L.R. 1234.

10.   John Griffith, *The Politics of the Judiciary* (London: Fontana, 1977) pp. 180-1.

11.   Although much of this work is of direct relevance to these jurisprudential debates (see particularly Chapter 8) it should be stated that my primary concern was to describe and explain the working of the appellate courts (and the House of Lords in particular), not to analyse or criticise the positions of those who have taken part in these debates.

12.   See C. M. Campbell, 'Legal Thought and Juristic Values', 1 *B.J.L.S.* (1974) 13 at p. 24 and J. Gibbs, 'Definitions of Law and Empirical Questions', 2 *Law and Soc. Rev.* (1968) 429.

13.   Interestingly, Professor Dworkin in a lecture delivered at Oxford University on 28 October 1970 confirmed what he had previously told me in an interview, namely, that in his opinion many of the differences between himself and Hart were susceptible to an empirical solution, *i.e.* that in the end it was a question of which theory fitted the facts best. Hart, by referring to *The Concept of Law* as 'an essay in descriptive sociology' in its preface, would appear to be in agreement with Dworkin on this point.

14.   Gibbs, *loc. cit.*, p. 446.

15.   Although there are many schools of thought in the interactionist camp most of them share three basic premises. These are that: (1) human beings act towards things on the basis of the meanings that the things have for them; (2) these meanings are a product of social interaction in human society; and (3) these meanings are modified through an interpretive process that is used by each person in dealing with the things he encounters. In short, human beings, in this perspective, are seen as constructing their realities in a process of interaction with other human beings. (This account is taken from B. N. Meltzer, J. W. Petras and L. T. Reynolds, *Symbolic Interactionism* (London: Routledge and Kegan Paul, 1975) p. 54.)

16.   *The Common Law Tradition* (Boston: Little, Brown, 1960) p. 46.

17.   *Law and the Social Sciences* (Minneapolis: University of Minnesota Press, 1966) p. 7.

18.   'The Bad Man Revisited', 58 *Cornell L.R.* (1973) 275 at p. 291.

19.   See D. McBarnet, 'False Dichotomies in Criminal Justice Research' in J. Baldwin and A. K. Bottomley (eds), *Criminal Justice* (London: Martin Robertson, 1978) p. 23.

20.   This is a difficult concept to pin down. It refers to the incumbent's perception that certain expectations are derived from groups who have a more legitimate interest in his role (because, for example, they are more closely involved or directly affected) than others. Similarly, he will consider some expectations to be more legitimate than others because they are more 'reasonable' or more 'worthy of respect'.

21. Because of spatial constraints, the methodology adopted in this research cannot be set out at great length. Nor can the list of 'hard' cases be included in the book (although the great majority of common law appeals to the Lords are 'hard' cases). The list, and further details of the methodology, can be obtained by writing to the author at Edinburgh University Law Faculty.

22. It might be argued that these cases do not form a coherent universe and that all cases coming to the Lords during the relevant period should have been included. In fact, I am not sure that this would have improved the coherence of the data base. There is a strongly biased case distribution in statutory construction appeals to the Lords (a high percentage of them are Revenue cases). Secondly, it cannot be assumed that the Law Lord's role in common law cases is the same as his role in statutory cases. Several Law Lords (including Lords Devlin, Diplock and Reid) have stated that the roles are separate and, as we shall see, the majority of their colleagues in their words and their deeds, *e.g.* on the question whether there should be a single opinion of the court or multiple speeches as at present, or in relation to the exercise of the 1966 Practice Statement on Precedent, have endorsed this point of view.

23. Using several approaches has the advantage of providing cross checks to the validity of the findings derived from the interviews.

24. The term 'Law Lord' encompasses the existing and retired Lords of Appeal, the Lord Chancellor, the Lord Chief Justice, the Master of the Rolls and all peers who have held high judicial office for two years or more.

25. A Law Lord was treated as 'active' if he had sat or was considered by the Judicial Office as able and willing to sit in the House during the calendar year 1972-3. The list of active Law Lords consisted of Lord Hailsham LC, Lords Reid, MacDermott, Morris of Borth-y-Gest, Hodson, Guest, Dilhorne, Wilberforce, Gardiner, Pearson, Diplock, Simon, Cross, Kilbrandon and Salmon.

26. Robert Wilson's doctoral research (1967-71) at LSE, on the English High Court judiciary (see Appendix), was intended to be based on interviews with the judges. After seventeen had been completed, several events led the judges to re-think their policy of co-operation. Brian Abel-Smith in the same period planned to interview 20 per cent of the practising barristers in England and Wales but the project was aborted when the Bar Council withdrew its support. See B. Abel-Smith and R. Stevens, *In Search of Justice* (London: Allen Lane, The Penguin Press, 1968) p. 13. Jenny Brock's M.Phil. research in 1970, at Bedford College (London), on the social background of the English judiciary encountered resistance which led her to abandon her attempt to send questionnaires to the judges. Again, in 1973 Maureen Cain was refused permission by the Bar Council to study their records to obtain social background information on the junior Bar. The most publicised failures by researchers to obtain the co-operation of the Bar or the Judiciary were John Baldwin and Michael McConville's research (1974-8) on plea bargaining and on jury trials in Brimingham Crown Court. See *Negotiated Justice* (London: Martin Robertson, 1977) pp. 8-9 and *Jury*

Trials (Oxford University Press, 1979). But in the latter research, at least, individual judges and solicitors (though not members of the Bar) responded helpfully to the researchers' approaches.

But these failures provide only half of the story. Robert Stevens interviewed several Law Lords as part of his research on the House of Lords (now published as *Law and Politics*) and Louis Blom-Cooper and Gavin Drewry also received assistance from several Law Lords in their study of the House (published as *Final Appeal*). Shimon Shetreet successfully issued a questionnaire to a number of judges in his research on the English judiciary. See *Judges on Trial* (Amsterdam: North-Holland Publishing, 1976). As Thomas Marvell has shown, there have now been over 100 studies on appellate judges in America using interviews or questionnaires, and the judges by and large have been very co-operative. See Bibliography D, *Appellate Courts and Lawyers* (Westport: Greenwood Press, 1978).

27.   'To tape or not to tape' is a question over which elite interviewers are divided. On the one hand, taping provides an accurate report of the interview, whilst at the same time freeing the interviewer to concentrate on the job in hand. On the other hand, it is said to introduce distortions and inhibitions into the interviews. See Jack Douglas, *Investigative Social Research* (Beverly Hills: Sage Publications, 1976) p. 33. Thus, James Eisenstein found that tape recording his interviews with US attorneys hindered the development of rapport and inhibited the respondents' answers on sensitive topics. See *Counsel for the United States* (Baltimore: Johns Hopkins University Press, 1978) p. 215. Yet, neither John Donnell in *The Corporate Counsel* (Indiana University, Bloomington: Bureau of Business Research, 1970) p. 19 nor Thomas Marvell, in *Appellate Courts and Lawyers*, p. 241, encountered significant problems in taping their interviews. Nor did I. It was not my experience that respondents who refused to be taped were noticeably more forthcoming than those who were recorded. In any event, it was always possible to switch the recorder off, if an interviewee wished to discuss matters which he considered to be particularly sensitive.

28.   Copies of these interview schedules for counsel and the Law Lords can be obtained from the author. The questions were partly factual and partly designed to elicit the role perceptions of the respondents. I benefitted greatly from the questions used in previous role research on judges (see Appendix).

29.   On elite interviewing I found L. Dexter, *Elite and Specialised Interviewing* (Evanston: Northwestern University Press, 1970) much the most helpful guide, although Hunt, Crane and Wahlke, 'Interviewing Political Elites', LXX *American Journal of Sociology* (1964) 59-68 and A. Cicourel, *Methods and Measurement in Sociology* (New York: Free Press, 1964) pp. 73-104 were also of some assistance.

30.   The confidentiality aspect of my research has caused considerable problems. Almost all my interviews were obtained on the basis of a guarantee of confidentiality on my part. This has meant that my doctoral thesis (for which the research was originally carried out) is not available for consultation. It has also meant that I have had to go back to

most of the respondents in order to obtain permission to publish material from their interviews, and (if permitted), to identify the source of the quotation or the information presented. On the general problem of confidentiality in judicial research see S. Ulmer, 'Bricolage and Assorted Thoughts on Working in the Papers of Supreme Court Justices', 35 *J. of Pol.* (1973) 286.

31. My discussion in these three chapters seems to me to be applicable to all appeals going to the House, not just to common law 'hard' cases. I know of no reason why the interchanges which I describe in these chapters should vary as between common law and statutory cases. The Law Lords in their interviews treated my questions on the Bar/Bench exchanges as relating to all appeals. So too did counsel. Although the primary barrister sample was not representative of all counsel who had appeared before the Lords in my period (but only of those who had appeared in common law 'hard' cases) most of them had argued statutory cases before the Lords. So too had most of the secondary sample of counsel. None of them referred to a difference *in the interaction process* as between statutory and common law cases.

CHAPTER 2: WHO INFLUENCES LAW LORDS?

1. Ch. Perelman and L. Olbrechts-Tyteca, *The New Rhetoric* (Indiana: University of Notre Dame Press, 1969).
2. *The Styles of Appellate Judicial Opinions* (Leyden: A. W. Sythoff, 1960) p. 72.
3. *Judges and Biographers* (Inaugural Lecture, Southampton University, 1967) p. 23.
4. 'Characteristics of Judicial Style in France, Britain and the U.S.A.', 24 *A.J.C.L.* (1976) 43.
5. 'Courts and Codes in England, France and Soviet Russia', 48 *Tulane L. R.* (1974) 1010.
6. 'Judicial Reasoning in the Common Law and Code Law Systems', LXIV *A.R.S.P.* (1978) 417 at p. 420.
7. 'La Cour Judicaire Suprême', 30 *Rev. Int. Dr. Comparé* (1978) at p. 71. For empirical evidence on the audiences perceived by American judges, see T. Marvell, *Appellate Courts and Lawyers* (Connecticut: Greenwood Press, 1978) pp. 110-11.
8. For a convenient description of the ceremony, see L. Blom-Cooper and G. Drewry, *Final Appeal* (Oxford: Clarendon Press, 1972) p. 102.
9. Up until 1971 it was the practice to state that a decision of the House was the outcome of the votes cast on the motion handed down. Thus, if a Law Lord died after writing his opinion, but before the date set for the judgement to be delivered, his speech and vote were disregarded as far as the outcome of the appeal was concerned. Attempts were made to incorporate the speeches with those of another Law Lord voting the same way, but such a policy would only work provided the deceased Law Lord was not in a minority of one. However, when Lord Donovan died on 12 December 1971 four days before judgement was due to be

delivered in *Ealing London Borough Council* v. *Race Relations Board*, Lord Dilhorne, the presiding judge, delivered Lord Donovan's speech separately from his own. Although this change in practice can be seen as a logical extension of permitting Law Lords' speeches to be read out in absentia and their votes cast by proxy, it is understood that Lord Dilhorne's action caused disquiet amongst some of his fellow Law Lords. The change of practice was adhered to on Lord Dilhorne's own death. See *British Steel Corp.* v. *Granada Television Ltd.*

10. At p. 1054 B-E, where he rebuked the Court of Appeal for refusing to follow a precedent of the House of Lords. For a more recent example see the leading speech in *R.* v. *Lawrence*.

11. Lord Reid made a similar comment in his address 'The Judge as Law Maker', 12 J.S.P.T.L. (1972) 22 at p. 25. In *Gibson* v. *Manchester City Council* Lord Edmund-Davies revealed (at p. 980) that he had written his speech with the losing respondent (and other members of the public in his position) in mind. Similarly, Sir Robert Megarry in 'Temptations of the Bench', 154 *Austr. L.J.* (1980) 61 at p. 64 comments 'the most important person in court is the litigant who is going to lose'.

12. Removal is arguably the severest sanction for judicial 'deviance' but it has never formally occurred in the case of a Law Lord. The distasteful episode in which Lord Atkinson was 'requested' to resign in 1927 (see R. F. V. Heuston, *Lives of the Lord Chancellors 1885-1945* (London: Oxford University Press, 1964) pp. 303-4) involved not so much the application of sanctions for deviance as the sensitivity demonstrated by successive governments to issues involving appeals to the Privy Council. It was Australian criticism which eventually led to the publication of dissents in the Privy Council in 1966, ensured that five judges sat on Australian Appeals and that they were normally presided over by Lord Reid or Lord Wilberforce during the latter years of my period. It also helped to make the Privy Council reluctant to grant leave to appeal in an Australian case.

13. See Heuston, *Lives*, p. 531.

14. This has changed a little in the past three years because of Hugo Young's success in persuading a number of judges to discuss legal matters on his BBC Radio 4 series, 'Talking Law'. Lord Denning has given numerous television, radio and newspaper interviews in the past ten years. Amongst the most revealing of these appeared in the *Sunday Times* on 17 and 24 June 1973 (Hugo Young was again the interviewer). Lords Radcliffe and Devlin appeared on a Thames Television programme on 'The Judges' broadcast on ITV on 12 October 1971 but they were both retired at the time. Lord Reid appears to have given an informal interview to Marcel Berlins, *The Times* law correspondent on the eve of his retirement, see *The Times*, 14 January 1975.

Responses by Law Lords in the media, to criticisms of their or their colleagues' decisions, have been few and far between. Lord Davey wrote a letter to *The Times* (published on 26 September 1904) in defence of his judgement in the Lords in the celebrated Scots Free Church appeal and does not seem to have been criticised for so doing. But Lord Maugham attracted considerable criticism for having written to *The Times* in 1941 in reply to Lord Atkin's forceful dissent in *Liversidge* v. *Anderson* (see R. F. V. Heuston '*Liversidge* v. *Anderson* in Retrospect', 86 *L.Q.R.* (1970) 33). Yet, more recently, neither Viscount Dilhorne's letter to *The Times* (published on 8 April 1975) objecting to an interpretation given in a *Times* leader to his speech in *Broome* v. *DPP*, nor Lord Scarman's letter to *The Times* (published on 31 July 1980) in defence of his colleagues' decision in the *British Steel* v. *Granada* (1980) case, seem to have been regarded as reprehensible actions. On the English Judiciary and the media in general, see S. Shetreet, *Judges on Trial* (Amsterdam: North-Holland Publishing, 1976) pp. 341-5.

15. For an example of parliamentary criticism, see H. C. Deb. vol. 781, col. 432-54 (2 April 1969).

16. There is certainly a considerable amount of *ad hoc* interaction between Law Lords and legal academics apart from dinners at the Inns of Court or 'Gaudies' in the Oxbridge Colleges. First, through occasional lectures and addresses to law faculties and university law societies, *e.g.* the Holdsworth lectures, or presiding at Moots. Secondly, through the conferences of various institutions, *e.g.* SPTL, IJA and the Ford Foundation Legal Workshops held by the Institute of Advanced Legal Studies and thirdly, through membership of various Law Reform Committees, Departmental Committees and Royal Commissions. However, not all the Law Lords take part in such exercises and some take part with much greater frequency than others. Similarly the opportunities to interact with the Law Lords on such occasions are usually restricted to a few prestigious academics.

17. In 1972-3 there were eighteen such academics.

18. Lord Devlin once or twice discussed difficult problems with academics and Viscount Simon is reputed to have done the same with some frequency. For evidence on the consultation of academics by American judges, see Marvell, *op. cit.*, pp. 98-9.

19. See *e.g.* 24 *Alabama L.R.* (1971) at p. 12 and M. Berry, *Stability Security and Continuity* (Connecticut: Greenwood Press, 1978) p. 44.

20. The one exception to this is the Lord Chancellor who frequently receives complaints about particular judges and decisions because of his position in the legal hierarchy. Few of these complaints seem to relate to decisions by the House of Lords. See Lord Hailsham, *The Door Wherein I Went* (London: Collins, 1975) p. 257.

21. For examples of critical and sympathetic letters from other judges and congratulatory letters from academics and others, see Heuston, '*Liversidge* v. *Anderson* in Retrospect', on the response to Lord Atkin's speech in that case.

22. *E.g.* R. Megarry, 'Law as Taught and Law as Practised', 9 *J.S.P.T.L.* (1966) 176 at p. 182; Lord Wilberforce, 'Educating the Judges', 10 *J.S.P.T.L.* (1968) 254 at p. 264; Lord Gardiner, 'Law Reform and Teachers of Law', 9 *J.S.P.T.L.* (1966) 190 at p. 190; Lord Reid, 'The Judge as Law Maker', 12 *J.S.P.T.L.* (1972) 22 at p. 22; Lord President Cooper (see T. B. Smith, 'Authors and Authority', 12 *J.S.P.T.L.* (1972) 3 at p. 6) and Lord Simon in his speech in *DPP* v. *Majewski*.

23. Frequent interaction with a Law Lord does not necessarily elevate a

group to the status of a reference group for a Law Lord. Thus I found little evidence to suggest that the Law Lords' wives and families or the civil servants whom they meet frequently, *e.g.* the Principal Clerk of the Judicial Office, the Lord Chancellor's Permanent Secretary, and the Law Lords' personal assistant, had much impact on the Law Lords' decisions. For an instance where civil servants did try to influence the Law Lords, see A. Lowe and J. Young, 'An Executive Attempt to Re-write a Judgement', 94 *L.Q.R.* (1978) 255.

24. On such occasions Parliament and the general public could be said to be acting as symbolic reference groups for the Law Lords.

25. See his tribute to A. L. Goodhart in 91 *L.Q.R.* (1975) 457.

26. The reading habits of Lords Dilhorne, Hodson and Morris were not ascertained.

27. See L. C. B. Gower, 'Looking Back', 14 *J.S.P.T.L.* (1978) 155. The comment in question appears in Gower, 'English Legal Training', 13 *M.L.R.* (1950) 137 at p. 198.

28. For a comment on this by a Harvard Law Professor, see W. Leach 'Revisionism in the House of Lords', 80 *Harv. L.R.* (1966) 797 at p. 801. No academic has been raised to the Bench in recent times in England despite the success of Cardozo, Douglas, Frank, Frankfurter and Holmes in the United States. There was one attempt in the 1930s when Harold Laski on Lord Chorley's suggestion attempted to persuade the then Lord Chancellor (Lord Sankey) to appoint Professor Gutteridge to the Bench. This was opposed by the senior judges and the proposal was dropped. See Heuston, *Lives*, p. 423.

29. See J. C. Smith, 'An Academic Lawyer and Law Reform' *Legal Studies* (1981) 119 and G. Bale, 'Comment' 59 *Can. B. Rev.* (1981) 164. For a discussion of the increasing influence of articles in legal periodicals on the United States Supreme Court, see H. Abraham, *The Judicial Process* (New York: Oxford University Press, 1975) pp. 231-3; and T. Becker (ed.), *The Impact of Supreme Court Decisions* (New York: Oxford University Press, 1969) pp. 13-14. See also J. W. Peltason, *Federal Courts in the Political Process* (New York: Random House, 1955) pp. 27-8.

30. An attitude which is not very surprising if *Hill* v. *Hill* is any guide. There a strong line-up of seven Law Lords was convened to reconsider the long-standing Court of Appeal decision in *Hyam* v. *Stuart King* which had been much criticised by textbook writers. Despite this, Salmon KC's attempt to cite an article of Dicey's was met by a trenchant rejoinder from Lord Jowitt LC on the Woolsack - 'What have the views of Professor Dicey to do with us? Is he an authority?' None of the Law Lords referred to academic writers in their speeches. The incident is recorded in N. Faulks, *No Mitigating Circumstances* (London: William Kimber, 1977) p. 113.

31. At p. 374. The 'certain writings' were a lecture delivered to the Law Society and subsequently published. See the note by P. V. Baker, 91 *L.Q.R.* (1975) 463 at p. 465. Counsel did not have an opportunity of commenting on the lecture in their arguments.

32. See the comments in 'Appeals from Overseas to the Privy Council', 26 *M.L.R.* (1963) 311.

33. *E.g.* G. Gardiner QC in *Rookes* v. *Barnard* at p. 1155.

34. *E.g. DPP* v. *Lynch* and *DPP* v. *Morgan*.

35. F. A. Mann, 'The Present Validity of Nazi Nationality Laws', 89 *L.Q.R.* (1973) 194. For its influence, see *Oppenheimer* v. *Cattermole* at p. 268.

36. See 'The Judge as Law Maker', *loc. cit.*, p. 22. Lord Reid's position as a presiding Law Lord throughout most of the period 1962-73 gave him added influence in the interchange with counsel and his sympathy for the change must have been of considerable importance.

37. 'A.L.G.: A Judge's View', 91 *L.Q.R.* (1975) 457 at p. 459. This statement is revealing in that it is not only a clear articulation of a 'relevant' role expectation for counsel but also because the expectation's content is diametrically opposed to the 'relevant' role expectation in the recent past that barristers should not cite living authors.

38. See also his unenthusiastic reaction to 'distinguished academic writers' and their impractical and 'esoteric classifications' in certain areas of criminal law in *DPP* v. *Stonehouse* at p. 78E.

39. 'La Chambre des Lords' in 30 *Rev. Int. Dr. Comparé* (1978) 90 at p. 95. See too his comments in *Johnson* v. *Agnew* at p. 892b.

40. See R. Cross, *Precedent in English Law*, 2nd edn (Oxford: The Clarendon Press: 1968) p. 4.

41. *Shaw* v. *DPP*; *DPP* v. *Smith*; and *DPP* v. *Beard* respectively.

42. *E.g.* the comments in *Majewski* by Lord Elwyn-Jones LC 'impressive academic comment', Lord Salmon 'distinguished academic writers' and Lord Edmund-Davies 'increasing academic criticism ... [which] is understandable.... '. Again, Lord Hailsham in *Hyam* says of the academic attacks on *DPP* v. *Smith*: 'These are weighty criticisms by responsible persons, and, in spite of the distinction of the House ... I feel bound to examine them seriously.'

43. 'Law and Social Change: An Interview with Lord Denning', *Kings Counsel* no. 22 (1969) 6 at p. 8. Somewhat ironically several of the barristers and judges whom I interviewed mentioned a rumour that Lord Justice Cohen had taken advice from Professor Goodhart on how to counter some of the arguments used by Lord Denning in his powerful dissent, in *Candler*.

44. See H. L. A. Hart, *The Concept of Law* (Oxford: Clarendon Press, 1961) pp. 246-7.

45. See Lord Diplock, 'Judicial Development of Law in the Commonwealth', *Proceedings and Papers of the Fifth Commonwealth Law Conference* (Edinburgh: Blackwood and Sons, 1978) pp. 493-500; R. Munday, 'New Dimensions of Precedent', 14 *J.S.P.T.L.* (1978) 201; and J. Miller, 'The Law Creative Role of Appellate Courts in the Commonwealth', 27 *I.C.L.Q.* (1978) 85 at p. 109.

46. This too was confirmed by the counsel interviewed.

47. See *e.g. Australian Consolidated Press Ltd* v. *Uren*; *R.* v. *Hyam*; and *Cassell* v. *Broome*.

48. See Lord Diplock, 'A.L.G.: A Judge's View', *loc. cit.*, p. 459. 'Counsel, however, still show some natural diffidence in citing some of the current notes in the *Law Quarterly* on cases decided by judges before whom they

are appearing. These we read only privately ....'

49.   Quotation derived from my notes of the oral interaction. See also Lord Wilberforce's testimony to the influence of certain commentators writing in the academic journals, and Professor Goodhart in particular ('La Chambre des Lords').

50.   One High Court judge told me that he knew that the Law Lords 'pay tremendous attention to Goodhart. He's the one chap that matters. He's the chap everybody reveres....'

51.   91 *L.Q.R.* (1975) 457 at pp. 458 and 461. Again the importance of being a Bencher is highlighted if an academic is to influence the Law Lords. Goodhart had the additional advantage of friendship with several of the Law Lords. Yet similar friendships between Supreme Court Justices and academic lawyers in the United States seem to be a rather more frequent occurrence. William Douglas recorded that Fred Rodell of Yale used to bring his constitutional law class to Washington, for a day, arranging for the class to hear cases argued and afterwards to have thirty minutes with each of four, five or six Justices (85 *Yale L.J.* (1974) p. 2). It is doubtful whether any Oxbridge Dons have ever come so close to the Law Lords as to be able to request a similar favour.

52.   It was the exception rather than the rule for counsel to say that they had no clear view on a particular role expectation for the Law Lords. Even when they did they could usually articulate the arguments for or against a particular norm.

53.   See *e.g. British Rail* v. *Herrington* at pp. 883, 884 and 890; *Jones* v. *Secretary of State* at pp. 950, 954, 959 and 962-3; and *Knuller* v. *DPP* at p. 452. Counsel who intend to invite the House to depart from one of its own decisions must, since 1971, give the House clear warning in advance in the written documents (the printed Case). This provision was introduced following the debacle of the initial hearing of *Jones* v. *Secretary of State for Social Services*. After three days (3, 4 and 8 March 1971) it became clear that the respondent's counsel, Roger Parker QC, would have to ask the Appellate Committee to overrule *Dowling*'s case. Since the only member of the Committee sitting to hear the *Jones* case who had sat in *Dowling* (Lord Wilberforce) had been the sole dissentient in *Dowling*, the Lord Chancellor decided that there would have to be a reconvened hearing of the *Jones* case before a committee of seven Law Lords (including some of those in the majority in *Dowling*'s case). To prevent future similar disruptions a Practice Direction was then issued.

54.   *E.g.* in *Knuller* v. *DPP*; *Indyka* v. *Indyka* at p. 106; and *British Rail* v. *Herrington* at p. 897.

55.   Personal information.

56.   At p. 133.

57.   At p. 694F.

58.   At p. 449.

59.   At p. 1038. This suggestion was partly at the instigation of his instructing solicitor Dr F. A. Mann of Messrs Herbert Smith & Co. who had handled at least 20 cases in the Lords including the *Greek Bank* cases, the *Carl Zeiss* case and *Cassell* v. *Broome*. Dr Mann felt that the Practice Statement was contrary to law and had written an article to this effect

but failed to find a law journal which would publish it. On the other hand Parker shared Mann's views on this topic to the extent of feeling that the change, if done at all, should have been by statute and accordingly was in the position of putting forward an argument which mirrored his role expectation.

60. Although Albery was not in my primary group of counsel I have quoted his response because it cogently summarises the dominant consensus amongst counsel who were in that group.

61. 'Stable Tips', 25 *GLIM* (1959) at p. 36.

62. *E.g.* counsel's submission in *Hedley Byrne* v. *Heller* at p. 474 that if the Law Lords decided the case in favour of the appellants that they would be opening the floodgates to a tidal wave of litigation against professional men. The respondent's counsel put forward a 'floodgates' argument in *Rondel* v. *Worsley* at p. 220 as did the appellant's counsel in *Home Office* v. *Dorset Yacht Co.* at p. 1012.

63. Legal biographers have often revealed examples of counsel who were so upset at decisions against them and their clients that they continued to argue the case in other arenas after the final appeal was over, and occasionally after many years were able to change the law to what they thought it ought to be. In my interview with Lord Pearce he told me that he had been losing counsel in *Duncan* v. *Cammell, Laird & Co.* and that he had been waiting for a chance to reconsider the case when *Conway* v. *Rimmer* came to the Lords. It was also my impression in interviewing one or two barristers who had lost important hard cases in the Lords *e.g.* *British Rail* v. *Herrington* and *Carl-Zeiss Stiftung* v. *Rayner and Keeler Ltd* that they had been hampered in their arguments by a lack of belief in the merits of their clients' case.

64. James Boswell, *A Journal of a Tour to the Hebrides*, ed. L. F. Powell (London: J. M. Dent, 1958) p. 10. See also for a similar viewpoint, Lord Macmillan in 'The Ethics of Advocacy' in *Law and Other Things* (Cambridge University Press, 1937) pp. 171-99; and Denning LJ in *Tombling* v. *Universal Bulb Co.* at p. 297.

65. E.C. 7-4.

66. ABA Opinion 28 (1949).

67. This can place counsel in a difficult position. For example, in *D.* v. *NSPCC*, David Hirst QC was required to argue that a Law Reform Committee report signed by himself, two Law Lords and four Lord Justices had inaccurately represented the state of the existing law. Perhaps not surprisingly at least one Law Lord found the suggestion 'incredible' (per Lord Hailsham at p. 227F).

68. See Rudden, *op. cit.,* p. 1018.

69. R. Nader, 'Law Schools and Law Firms', *The New Republic* (11 October 1969); Teschner, 'Lawyer Morality', 38 *George Washington Law Review* (1970) 789; and J. S. Auerbach, *Unequal Justice* (New York: Oxford University Press, 1976) p. 278. There are dangers in this argument as the difficulty in obtaining representation for terrorists in West Germany has shown in recent times.

70. G. Bellow and J. Kettleson, 'The Mirror of Public Interest Ethics' (1977) unpublished paper; W. Simon, 'The Ideology of Advocacy:

Procedural Justice and Professional Ethics', *Wisconsin L.R.* (1978) 29.

71.   At p. 176D-E.

72.   At the time of my survey 24 of the 30 'counsel' to be interviewed were
       Benchers at their Inns, but since this figure takes no account of counsel's
       status at the time of arguing the hard cases before the Lords it inevitably
       exaggerates the proportion of Benchers to non-Benchers who appear
       before the Lords in such cases.

73.   It is not entirely surprising to find such diffidence amongst counsel. As
       'court regulars' (see A. S. Blumberg, 'The Practice of Law as a
       Confidence Game', 1 *Law and Soc. Rev.* (1967) 15) and 'repeat players'
       (see M. Galanter, 'Why the "Haves" Come Out Ahead', 9 *Law and Soc.
       Rev.* (1974) 95) they have got to take their future clients' positions into
       account - they will not appreciate starting at a disadvantage in an appeal
       because their counsel has antagonised some of the Law Lords earlier in
       his career. Also some barristers consider it bad taste to criticise a fellow
       Bencher on his performance of his job.

74.   See p. 12 above, on the geographical problems of interaction with the
       Law Lords. Non-federal State judges have sometimes been known to
       criticise Supreme Court Justices of the United States in very explicit
       terms. In *Salt Lake City* v. *Piepenburg*, Elliot CJ of the Utah Supreme
       Court rejected the obscenity test supported by certain Justices of the
       Supreme Court of the United States, stating that State judges who took
       the same view should resign or be impeached. He continued, 'Judges
       who seek to find technical excuses to permit such pictures to be shown
       under the pretence of finding some intrinsic value to it are reminiscent
       of a dog that returns to his vomit in search of some morsel in that filth
       which may have some redeeming value to his own taste.' Quoted in 52
       Austr. L.J. 11978) at p. 480.

75.   *E.g.* Lord Hailsham and several of his colleagues rebuking the Court of
       Appeal in *Cassell* v. *Broome*. See also *Farrell* v. *Alexander* at pp. 91-2 per
       Lord Simon and p. 105 per Lord Russell; *Davis* v. *Johnson* at p. 326 per
       Lord Diplock; and *Miliangos* v. *George Frank Ltd* at p. 496 per Lord
       Cross. In a similar fashion in April 1978 the US Supreme Court was to
       be found rebuking the Court of Appeals for the District of Columbia for
       alleged judicial legislation stating that its reasoning bordered 'on the
       Kafkaesque' and that their actions were 'judicial intervention run riot'.
       Vermont Yankee Nuclear Power Corporation v. *NRDC* 435 U.S. 519, 557.

76.   At. p. 1026G. Lord Denning agreed that professional opinion could
       have an effect but pointed out the difficulties facing a judge in
       ascertaining whether, and amongst which groups (*e.g.* Benchers,
       academics, barristers or solicitors) a consensus on a point exists.

77.   Lord Simon's remarks on this point are very much in line with
       Dworkin's arguments on the role of a judge in a hard case. The other
       judges quoted tend, on this point, to favour Hart's model for they do not
       argue that the Law Lords are *bound* to take account of the consensus of
       professional opinion but only that they may do so if they feel so inclined.
       In terms of role analysis, the 'obligation' to pay heed to a consensus of
       professional opinion is one that the judges (excluding Lord Simon)
       define as 'peripheral' to their role.

78.   Sir Kenneth Diplock, 'The Civil Courts in Contemporary Society', 12 *GLIM* (1964).

79.   Of course not every Law Lord has the time or the inclination to read the judgements in a case in which he has not sat. But they will often do so if the case is of particular importance or is in a field in which they have an interest.

80.   At p. 398.

81.   At pp. 467-8.

82.   At p. 275.

CHAPTER 3: COURTROOM INTERACTION: THE BAR'S PERSPECTIVE

1.   K. Llewellyn, *The Bramble Bush* (New York: Oceana Publications, 1951) p. 147.

2.   F. Frankfurter, 'Mr Justice Jackson', 68 *Harv. L.R.* (1955) 937 at p. 939.

3.   The role of the advocate receives only cursory treatment in Blom-Cooper and Drewry's, *Final Appeal* (Oxford: Clarendon Press, 1972) and none at all in Robert Stevens', *Law and Politics* (London: Weidenfeld and Nicolson, 1979). (For a similar criticism of *Final Appeal* see Viscount Radcliffe's review in 36 *M.L.R.* (1973) 559 at p. 561.) To be fair, much the same can be said of most of the articles and case notes written about the work of the Lords. One honourable exception is Neil MacCormick's *Legal Reasoning and Legal Theory* (Oxford: Clarendon Press, 1978).

4.   See on oral argument in the Supreme Court, H. Abraham, *The Judicial Process*, 3rd edn (New York: Oxford University Press, 1975) pp. 190-3, and B. Woodward and S. Armstrong, *The Brethren* (New York: Simon and Schuster, 1979) pp. 269, 302, 304 and 305. For a recent dissenting voice on the disappearance of oral argument in US Appellate Courts, see P. D. Carrington, 'Ceremony and Realism', 66 *A.B.A.J.* (1980) 860.

5.   Although 74 per cent of English civil appeals between 1952 and 1968 occupied four days or less in the Lords, some lasted for many days. *Carl-Zeiss Stiftung* v. *Rayner and Keeler Ltd* occupied twenty-six days before the Lords. See *Final Appeal*, p. 235.

6.   Neither court hears oral argument on a Friday.

7.   See E. Re, *Brief Writing and Oral Argument*, 4th edn (New York: Oceana Publications, 1974) pp. 174-5.

8.   *E.g.* 'The Special Skills of Advocacy', 42 *Fordham L.R.* (1973) 227. See also Burger's appointment of the Devitt Committee to Consider Standards for Admission to Practice in the Federal Courts in 1976.

9.   This is confirmed in *The Brethren*. Frankfurter was one of the few Justices recently who made a great deal of use of the limited discussion permitted in the Supreme Court. One Law Lord told me that Frankfurter 'never read the briefs before going into Court, so that he had a completely open

mind, with the result that he wasted everyone's time by asking questions that were answered in the briefs'. An interesting account of the oral interchange in the Supreme Court can be found in W. F. Murphy and C. H. Pritchet (eds), *Courts, Judges and Politics*, 2nd edn (New York: Random House, 1974) pp. 493 and 501-4. For a complete record of the oral argument in *Brown* v. *Board of Education* 1952-55 see L. Friedman (ed.), *Argument* (New York: Chelsea House Publishers, 1969). The frequency of Frankfurter's interventions is graphically illustrated in this volume especially at pp. 43-9.

10. T. Marshall, 'The Federal Appeal' in Charpentier (ed.), *Counsel on Appeal* (New York: McGraw-Hill, 1968) p. 146.

11. Six of the active Law Lords at the time of my study, including Lords Cross, Guest, Kilbrandon, Salmon and Reid, considered the oral arguments to be very much more important than the written ones, and a further four, including Lords Gardiner, MacDermott and Pearson derived considerably more from the oral arguments than the written ones. Only one Law Lord relied more on the written materials and found the debate unimportant. Off the bench comments by the Law Lords and Supreme Court Justices indicate that the restriction of oral argument is the main *raison d'être* for Law Clerks in the Supreme Court and that in England the Law Lords rely on counsel for the research that the Law Clerks do in America.

12. *E.g.* Lords Dunedin, Morton of Henryton: see his 'Address', 32 *Proceedings of the Canadian Bar Association* (1949) 107 at pp. 114-15; and Lord Parmoor, *A Retrospect* (London: Heinemann, 1936) p. 71.

13. *Lawyer and Litigant* (London: Stevens, 1962) p. 170. Since 1 October 1976 all petitions for leave to appeal have to be read in advance by an Appeal Committee before an oral hearing can be obtained. Practice Direction issued on 18 May 1976 (amended 6 March 1979).

14. R. Cross, *Precedent in English Law*, 2nd edn (Oxford: Clarendon Press, 1968) p. 30.

15. Counsel interviewed in the main did not object to a judge taking advice from other judges or academics or doing his own research on the authorities and discovering cases not cited by counsel. But they considered that a judge who did this and relied heavily on the information gained, without reconvening the court and giving counsel the opportunity to consider it, was not 'playing the game' fairly.

16. Lord Justice Scrutton was capable of prefacing a judgement by saying, 'counsel will be surprised and possibly pained to find that the judgement that I am giving will not relate in any way to the arguments that have been put forward, but I have no doubt that the right way to decide this case is as follows....' I am indebted to Robert Megarry QC, *Miscellany-at-Law* (London: Stevens, 1955) p. 48 for the citation of a case in which Scrutton said just this: *Smith* v. *Smith* [1923] P 191 at p. 202.

17. At pp. 423-4.

18. At p. 398.

19. Information derived from interviews with Lord Denning; see also *Goldsmith* v. *Sperrings Ltd* [1977] 2 All E.R. 566 at p. 572a.

20. Lord Devlin voiced the expectation in my interview with him. Judged

on his comments on this matter in *Boardman* v. *Phipps* at pp. 131E and 132E Lord Upjohn, who became a Lord of Appeal in 1963, would appear to share the expectation also. This impression was confirmed for me in a conversation with a friend of Lord Upjohn's.

21. Lord Reid can, I think, fairly be placed in this school. First, because of his concurrence with Viscount Simonds' remarks in *Rahimtoola* v. *Nizam of Hyderabad* and secondly, because of his speech in *The Tojo Maru*.

22. Fittingly this group contained the two active Law Lords who admitted to writing to an academic after the oral argument in an appeal was complete.

23. For an example of Lord Kilbrandon putting these views into practice see *Alexander Ward & Co.* v. *Samyang Navigation Co.*

24. In his review of Lord Denning's *The Discipline of Law*, Lord Hailsham indicated that although private researches by judges were 'by no means necessarily to be deprecated, they are occasionally apt to produce one-sided results'. 76 *Guardian Gazette* 28 February, 1979 p. 193. See also his adherence to the norm in *National Bank of Greece* v. *Westminster Bank*.

25. *Miliangos* v. *George Frank Ltd* at p. 478C. See also his comments in *In re D* at p. 641C.

26. At p. 1037d. See also his observations in *Sovmots Investments Ltd* v. *Secretary of State* at p. 391.

27. 30 *Rev. Int. Dr. Comparé* (1978) 90 at p. 95.

28. At p. 773E-F.

29. Lord Edmund-Davies seems to be in the group which accepts the norm. He has upheld it not only in *Abbott* v. *The Queen* but also in *Gleaves* v. *Deakin* at p. 506e and *Jobling* v. *Associate Dairies Ltd* at p. 759h. Lord Scarman also seems to be in this camp. See *Lim Poh Choo* v. *Camden Area Health Authority* at p. 183D.

30. At p. 312d-e.

31. At p. 1131G. Lord Diplock's comments highlight the fact that the expectation is not as restrictive as it might at first appear. A bold judge, *e.g.* Lord Atkin in *Donoghue* v. *Stevenson* or Lord Devlin in *Rookes* v. *Barnard, provided all the relevant authorities have been cited to the court*, can distil from them a legal principle which was not argued for by counsel, and yet not infringe the expectation. In fairness, though, it should be said that Lord Denning perceives Lord Devlin's exegesis as a breach of the expectation.

32. At p. 495g.

33. At p. 573G. See also *Lambert* v. *Lewis* at p. 1192c.

34. For Lord Bridge it appears to be a pivotal role expectation for he rebuked his colleague Lord Denning in *Goldsmith* v. *Sperrings Ltd* at p. 590b-d for acting in breach of the rule of natural justice, *audi alteram partem*, when he relied on a point in his judgement which counsel had not had an opportunity to be heard on. See also *Jobling* v. *Associated Dairies Ltd* at p. 768h.

35. *Lawyer and Litigant in England*, pp. 172-3. For a recent illustration of the Court of Appeal adopting Megarry's solution see *Box Parish Council* v. *Lacey* [1979] 1 All E.R. 113 at p. 117.

36. At p. 98A.

37.   At p. 478C-D.

38.   At p. 502E. Lord Fraser only mentioned the case because it was a decision in point by the House of Lords and he expressly states that the case did not affect his decision of the appeal.

39.   At p. 23D.

40.   At p. 58F.

41.   For an interesting discussion of the expectation and the support for it amongst counsel and judges in the United States, see T. Marvell, *Appellate Courts and Lawyers* (Connecticut: Greenwood Press, 1978) pp. 121-5; and *The Brethren*, pp. 229 and 416.

42.   It should be remembered that the Law Lords are dependent for their raw material on obstinate (and wealthy) clients or counsel recommending an appeal to the Lords. As Professor Twining pointed out in 1971 (87 *L.Q.R.* at p. 400) it is a moot point as to who is the bolder spirit, the litigant or lawyer who challenges accepted notions or the judges who respond to the challenge. If the decision to fight cases to the Lords is largely controlled by the Bar then they have further powers for limiting the judicial role performance.

43.   The failure of counsel to take a point even when requested so to do by a judge can cause problems long after the case is over. In *Dann* v. *Hamilton* Asquith J. rejected the defence of '*violenti non fit injuria*' on the facts of the case. Twice in ten years it was stated in the Law Quarterly Review that the judge was at fault for not upholding an alternative defence of contributory negligence. This provoked the longsuffering Lord Asquith (as he had by then become) to retort in a note in 69 *L.Q.R.* (1953) 317 that contributory negligence had not been pleaded despite the fact that he had suggested it to counsel for the defence.

44.   At pp. 312e and 315-16 respectively.

45.   At p. 17.

46.   At p. 1081F and 1094B, per Lord Diplock.

47.   *Walker* v. *Lovell* per Lord Edmund-Davies at p. 133e. See also Lord Hailsham at p. 127c.

48.   *Ibid.*, Lord Diplock at p. 111g.

49.   Viscount Dilhorne at p. 119h; Lord Hailsham at p. 127c; Lord Kilbrandon at p. 130f, and Lord Diplock at pp. 112a-d. Lord Diplock's comments are of interest in view of his denial of the existence of the expectation in *Cassell* v. *Broome*. His restraint in *Walker* v. *Lovell* can apparently be accounted for by his feeling that,

> In a criminal appeal it would not be ... appropriate for your Lordships of your own motion to take a point of law against the accused on which the prosecution itself is not willing to rely. *It would be otherwise if the point to be taken were in favour of the accused* (emphasis added).

50.   *Ibid.*, p. 133e-f.

51.   *E.g. Farrell* v. *Alexander* per Lord Simon at p. 92 C-F and Lord Russell at p. 105B; *Liverpool City Council* v. *Irwin* per Lord Wilberforce at p. 257D, Lord Cross at p. 257G, Lord Salmon at p. 262B and Lord Edmund-Davies at p. 265G; *Nothman* v. *London Borough of Barnet* per Lord Russell at p. 151c; and *B.* v. *W.* per Viscount Dilhorne at p. 90h, Lord

Edmund-Davies at p. 92h, and Lord Keith at p. 94g.

52.   At p. 320C.

53.   *Final Appeal*, p. 247.

54.   The 'rule' is particularly strong in Scottish Appeals in view of the somewhat stricter forms of pleading which prevail in that country. See *South of Scotland Electricity Board* v. *British Oxygen Co. Ltd*; and *Demetriades* v. *Glasgow Corporation*.

55.   Procedural Direction 14(i)(a) says, '[If the parties] intend to apply in the course of the hearing for leave to introduce a new point not taken below, this should be intimated in their Case.'

56.   At p. 124.

57.   Recent cases in which the normal practice has been followed include *Blathwayt* v. *Baron Cawley*; *Wearing* v. *Pirelli*; and *Mardorf Peach & Co. Ltd* v. *Attica Sea Carriers*.

58.   See Lord Reid at p. 1178 and Lord Devlin at p. 1231.

59.   There have been occasional cases where counsel have been permitted to raise a new point which in the end of the day the Law Lords have rejected. Such cases do not necessarily invalidate the remarks of Lords Cross and Reid for they might be cases where the judges have changed their minds on further reflection as to the value of the new argument or where they are divided on the point (as they were in *Town Investments Ltd* v. *Department of the Environment*).

60.   See *Town Investments Ltd* v. *Department of the Environment*.

61.   See *e.g. Beecham Foods* v. *Customs & Excise* at p. 252H; and *Jones* v. *Wrotham Park Settled Estates* at p. 293b.

62.   *E.g. Shiloh Spinners* v. *Harding* at p. 699; and counsel's comments on the case in *Blatwayt* v. *Baron Cawley*.

63.   *E.g. Anns* v. *Merton London Borough Council*.

64.   In addition to the cases mentioned in the three preceding footnotes see also *Daymond* v. *South West Water Authority* at p. 631H; and *Federal Steam Navigation Co.* v. *The Department of Trade and Industry* at pp. 510C and 526G. *British Railways Board* v. *Liptrot* is an aberrant case for although the concession there was recognised by the Law Lords as covering the real question in the appeal they refused to allow it to be withdrawn. The refusal was apparently influenced by the Law Lords' distaste for the appellant's motive in making the original concession. See Lord Guest at p. 163.

65.   *Orloff* v. *Willoughby* at p. 87.

66.   The dissenting minority (at pp. 673-4) objected strongly to the way in which the majority took up the minor issue to the exclusion of the obscenity issue which had dominated the case lower down and which was the basis upon which *certiorari* had been granted.

67.   See D. McBarnet 'Pre-trial Procedures and the Construction of Conviction' and the studies she cites at p. 174, in P. Carlen (ed.), *The Sociology of Law* (University of Keele: Sociological Review Monograph 23, 1976) p. 172; and Z. Bankowski and G. Mungham, *Images of Law* (London: Routledge and Kegan Paul, 1976) p. 118.

68.   See P. Carlen 'Remedial Routines for the Maintenance of Control in Magistrates' Courts', 1 *B.J.L.S.* (1974) 101 at p. 104.

69.   See McBarnet, 'Pre-trial Procedures' at pp. 174-5.

70.   As *e.g.* in *Vandervell Trustees* v. *White* at p. 944H; *National Westminster Bank* v. *Halesowen* at p. 808A; and *R.* v. *Taylor* at p. 986E. The concentration on the Law Lords comes about because the Law Lords alone possess the power to decide between the competing definitions, and more importantly, the power to have their decision accepted as the operant definition of the symbolic order (until reversed by Parliament) irrespective of its historical antecedents. See Paterson, 'Judges: A Political Elite?', 1 *B.J.L.S.* (1974) 118.

71.   This characterisation was volunteered by a Law Lord.

72.   This portrait of English appeals appears in Gates, 'Hot Bench or Cold Bench' in Charpentier (ed.), *Counsel on Appeal*, 109 at p. 121.

73.   See Rudden, *loc. cit.*, pp. 1014-15.

74.   Very little interruption of one's opponent is permitted in the House. In many respects the debate could proceed without the other side being present at all.

75.   'The Argument of an Appeal', 26 *A.B.A.J.* (1940) 895.

76.   Lord Justice Karminski in *Paxton* v. *Allsopp*.

77.   A caveat should perhaps be lodged at this stage. Hitherto I have argued that counsel perceive their role in the Lords in terms of putting forward submissions which will win the case for the client, with no regard to the development of the law. This is not always the case. Sometimes an appeal will be taken, even if there is little hope of victory in the Lords, in the hope that the Law Lords will produce a statement of the law which is more favourable to the appellants than the one which was laid down by the Court of Appeal. This motive lay behind the appeals in *Bolton* v. *Stone* (see Lord Birkenhead, *Walter Monckton* (London: Weidenfeld and Nicolson, 1969) p. 266) and *Home Office* v. *Dorset Yacht Co.* (information derived from an interview with Crown counsel).

78.   At p. 34. (For a further example of this phenomenon see Roskill LJ in *Congreve* v. *Home Office* at p. 713e.)

79.   One recent exception is R. A. B. Lunk and B. D. Sales 'Persuasion during the Voir Dire' in B. D. Sales (ed.), *Psychology in the Legal Process* (New York: Spectrum Publications, 1977) p. 39.

80.   At the commencement of *In re National Federation of Newsagents* counsel instead of beginning with the facts, launched immediately into the details of the Restrictive Trade Practices Acts. Lord Reid after two minutes or so said 'These statutes are unfamiliar to some of the Law Lords. It would be easier for us if you could start with the facts and give us something to bite on before turning to unfamiliar statutes.'

81.   K. Llewellyn, *The Common Law Tradition* (Boston: Little, Brown & Co., 1960) p. 238.

82.   John Davis, *loc. cit.*, at p. 896.

83.   In a book review of *Final Appeal* in 36 *M.L.R.* (1973) 559 at p. 562.

84.   E. Cockburn Millar, 'Some Memories of Lord Atkin', 23 *GLIM* (1957) 13 at p. 15. I am indebted to W. Twining and D. Miers, *How To Do Things With Rules* (London: Weidenfeld and Nicolson, 1976) for the quotations from Davis and Lord Atkin's daughter.

85.   *The Common Law Tradition*, p. 239 fn. 238.

86.   'A Lecture on Appellate Advocacy', 29 *University of Chicago L.R.* (1962) 627 at p. 639.

87.   *The Common Law Tradition*, p. 240.

88.   'A Lecture on Appellate Advocacy', p. 630. *cf.* Piero Calamandrei's comment that 'A lawyer should be able to suggest the arguments that will win his case so subtly to the judge that the latter believes that he has thought of them himself', cited in Sir Robert Megarry, 'Temptations of the Bench', 54 *Austr. L.J.* (1980) 61 at p. 63.

89.   See Charpentier (ed.), *Counsel on Appeal*, p. 128. Llewellyn in the writings referred to on p. 53 above quotes several American examples of issue framing and issue capture although his first two, 'the finest that he knew', are taken from the New Testament. The first concerned the question 'Is it lawful to give tribute unto Caesar?' and Jesus's use of the coin (Matthew 22) and the second related to the woman taken in adultery and the riposte 'He that is without sin amongst you, let him first cast a stone' (John 8).

90.   See H. Moulton, *The Life of Lord Moulton* (London: Nisbet, 1922) p. 54.

91.   Lord Macmillan, *A Man of Law's Tale* (London: Macmillan, 1952) p. 120. The Law Lords' judgements contain several emotive remarks of this character and yet the Lord Ordinary had held that there was sufficient evidence to support a finding of recklessness (which in *Derry* v. *Peek* had been held to amount to fraud in certain circumstances).

92.   'Advocacy before the United States Supreme Court', 37 *Cornell L.Q.* (1951) 1 at p. 6.

93.   At p. 422.

94.   *Ibid.*, pp. 432 and 442 respectively.

95.   *Ibid.*, p. 431 *cf.* N. MacCormick's discussion of the case in *Legal Reasoning and Legal Theory*, pp. 169-73.

96.   In fact, as we shall see, the second analogy (if not the first) emanated from the question of a Law Lord (Lord Reid) during the interaction between Bar and Bench.

97.   Local authorities and squatters appear in Lord Reid's speech at p. 296 B-C and Lord Cross's at p. 325G-H. The Shylock analogy appears in Lord Reid's speech at pp. 295G-296A, Lord Diplock's at p. 313D and Lord Simon's at p. 315D.

98.   L. Walker, J. Thibaut and V. Andreoli, 'Order of Presentation at Trial', 82 *Yale L.J.* (1972) 216.

99.   The quotations are taken from responses made by counsel. Several counsel referred to anecdotes of famous advocates in the past who had 'run for a fall' in the Court of Appeal in order to have the advantage of opening in the Lords. One or two counsel considered that having the right to speak last or the right to speak twice gave the appellant an advantage.

100.   Viscount Haldane, *Richard Burdon Haldane* (London: Hodder and Stoughton, 1929) p. 53.

101.   Address by Lord Morton of Henryton, 32 *Proceedings of the Canadian Bar Association* (1949) 107 at pp. 114-15. *cf.* Frankfurter's question to counsel in one case,

        'Is that all there is to this case?'

'No, sir', said the lawyer. 'There's a heap to this case.'

'As you state it', the justice came back, 'It's so simple that I'm suspicious .... What is the milk in the coconut?' Quoted in Murphy and Pritchett (eds), *Courts, Judges and Politics* (New York: Random House, 1961) p. 481.

102.   The phrase is Davis's, *loc. cit.*, p. 897.

103.   Adherents of this position included Justice Harlan, 'What Part does Oral Argument Play in the Conduct of an Appeal', 41 *Cornell L.Q.* (1955) 6 and Justice Jackson, *loc. cit.*, p. 5.

104.   See also MacDermott, 'The Quality of Judgement', 21 *N.I.L.Q.* (1970) 178 at p. 186.

105.   'Advocacy', 9 *Cambrian L.R.* (1978) 50 at p. 52.

106.   *Cases in Court* (London: Pan Books Ltd, 1953) p. 252.

107.   Lord Birkenhead, *Walter Monckton*, p. 74.

108.   Sir John Foster QC, my informant.

109.   'The Role of Advocacy', 16 *Journal of the Law Society of Scotland* (1971) 169 at p. 171.

110.   Quoted in Gilbert Paull QC, 'On Advocacy', 25 *GLIM* (1959) at p. 32. One High Court judge told me that when he was counsel he had on occasions adopted the technique of underplaying his case in order that the judge would take charge.

111.   To be fair the policy probably emanates from the Lord Chancellor's Office. The officials of the Judicial Office could not satisfactorily explain to me the reason for the policy and the Permanent Secretary declined to do so. Almost every counsel interviewed would have liked to know his court in advance, but although the Law Lords generally have three weeks warning of their schedule the earliest experienced counsel could discover the composition of the Committee was the evening before the commencement of the case.

112.   Lord Birkenhead, *Walter Monckton*, p. 74. John Davis had a similar piece of advice for advocates, 'Change places, in your imagination of course, with the Court', *loc. cit.*, p. 896.

113.   See Llewellyn, *The Common Law Tradition*, pp. 268 *et seq.*

114.   Sydney Templeman QC, however, told me,

   I think the whole of our profession is really concerned with 'judge management'. Most of the cases are terribly difficult and very nicely poised and they nearly all turn on about ten minutes of the argument.

115.   Haldane, *Haldane*, p. 52.

116.   At p. 118 A-B.

117.   At p. 419.

118.   At p. 445.

119.   See pp. 1033F and 1090B.

120.   Llewellyn, *The Common Law Tradition*, p. 241.

121.   Sir Owen Dixon CJ expressed somewhat similar views in *Jesting Pilate* (Melbourne: The Law Book Company, 1965) pp. 250-1. For examples of 'borrowing' in the United States Supreme Court see Re, *Brief Writing and Oral Argument*, 4th edn, p. 98 fn. 60.

122.   *Lim Poh Choo* v. *Camden and Islington Area Health Authority* at p. 183C-D.

123. *Styles of Appellate Judicial Opinions* (Leyden: A. W. Sythoff, 1960) p. 72.
124. One notable exception is Professor Neil MacCormick's *Legal Reasoning and Legal Theory*. See pp. 119 *et seq*.
125. Sydney Templeman QC hinted at such a consensus when he described the role of counsel in the Lords in our interview. 'What you are trying to do is to produce an argument that convinces them, usually it coincides with what convinces you, because you've all been trained in the same way.'
126. See p. 29 above.

CHAPTER 4: COURTROOM INTERACTION: THE LAW LORDS' PERSPECTIVE

1. For the somewhat complex rules for determining which Law Lord is entitled to preside over an Appellate Committee, see Blom-Cooper and Drewry, *Final Appeal*, p. 179.
2. Lord Campbell, *Lives of the Lord Chancellors*, 2nd Series (London: John Murray, 1846) vol. V, p. 664.
3. *Law, Class and Society* (London: Lawrence and Wishart, 1971) Book II at pp. 56-7.
4. *Cf.* Lord Denning on Lord Goddard in *The Discipline of Law* (London: Butterworth, 1979) p. 70. 'Now Lord Goddard was a great Judge, but he had one fault. He was too quick. He jumped too soon. And his colleagues sometimes were not bold enough to say "Stop".' See also Lord Hailsham reviewing F. Bresler, *Lord Goddard* in *The Listener*, 5 May 1977, p. 595. 'Goddard was a just judge. He was, of course, a good deal too hasty, and he interrupted too often and too soon.'
5. In Radcliffe's review of *Final Appeal* in 36 *M.L.R.* (1973) 559 at p. 562.
6. One senior Law Lord at the time was so polite and so predelicted to raising red herrings (thus greatly prolonging the duration of appeals) that he was the despair of the administrative staff in the Lords and the Privy Council who were charged with compiling the schedules of these courts.
7. On the drawbacks of silent judges from counsel's point of view, see Megarry, *Lawyer and Litigant*, p. 142.
8. See 'Divers Scraps, Shreds and Shards', 16 *U.C.L.A. L.Rev.* (1969) 704 at pp. 705-6. For a similar interchange between Chief Justice White and Justice Holmes see Davis, 'The Argument of an Appeal', p. 898.
9. Blom-Cooper and Drewry, *Final Appeal*, pp. 177 and 179.
10. Review, 36 *M.L.R.* (1973) at p. 561.
11. Wilberforce, *'La Chambre des Lords'*, p. 93.
12. For a discussion of the use made by appellate judges in the United States of the oral arguments see Marvell, *Appellate Courts and Lawyers*, pp. 76-7, 307-8 and N. D. McFeeley and R. J. Ault, 'Supreme Court Oral Argument', 20 *Jurimetrics* (1979) 52 (an interesting application of content analysis to oral interchanges in the Supreme Court).
13. At p. 873.

14. *Final Appeal* at p. 250. For a recent example of this, see *Orapko* v. *Manson Investments Ltd*. In earlier times there were more hopeless cases. Between 1866-71 22 per cent of appeals were dismissed without a reply being required from the respondent: Blom-Cooper and Drewry, *Final Appeal*, p. 27.

15. At p. 449. Curiously the appellant did not interpret this interaction to mean that he had lost on count 1 and he remained optimistic until the date of the judgement.

16. At p. 481. Other cases where the respondent has been restricted in his argument include *Betty's Cafes Ltd* v. *Phillips Furnishing Stores* at p. 28; *In Re Kirkwood* at p. 534; *Fawcett Properties* v. *Buckingham County Council* at p. 650; *Argyle Motors* v. *Birkenhead Corporation* at p. 120; *Howard* v. *Borneman* (no. 2) at p. 305; *Miliangos* v. *George Frank Ltd* at p. 452; *Aldebaran* v. *Aussenhandel A. G. Zurich* at p. 161; *Hobbs* v. *Marlowe* at p. 30 and *Birkett* v. *James* at p. 309.

17. See *e.g. Avais* v. *Hertford Workingmen's Social Club* and *Canaris S.A.* v. *Aseguradara* at p. 878.

18. Examples include *Rahimtoola* v. *Nizam of Hyderabad* at p. 391; *Branwhite* v. *Worcester Works Co.* at p. 562; *DPP* v. *Withers* at p. 854C; *Baker* v. *Willoughby* at p. 489A; *Ealing London Borough Council* v. *Race Relations Board* at p. 350, and *DPP* v. *Humphrys* at p. 12.

19. See *e.g. DPP* v. *Ping Lin* at p. 593A.

20. See p. 44 above.

21. My account of the interaction in this case is derived from personal observation and interviews with the counsel and Law Lords involved.

22. Lord Denning in *The Discipline of Law*, p. 311 admits that he invited Hirst to attack *Rookes* v. *Barnard* in *Broome* v. *Cassell & Co. Ltd*.

23. Lord Denning commented on the penalty, 'This gives me much cause for regret: for it was really my fault that the issue was raised and argued. Neither Captain Broome nor his legal advisers were at fault' (*The Discipline of Law*, p. 311).

24. Quoted in *The Sunday Times* report, *The Thalidomide Children and the Law* (London: Andre Deutsch, 1973) p. 106. The interruption does not appear in the Law Reports.

25. Something of Lord Reid's *modus operandi* can also be seen in the report of counsel's submissions in *Mobil Oil Australia Ltd* v. *Commissioner for Taxation*. See also *The Thalidomide Children and the Law*, pp. 106-12.

26. American judges confessed to Marvell, *Appellate Courts and Lawyers*, p. 77, that on occasion they or their colleagues asked improper questions during hearings.

27. Information derived from Lord Justice Russell. The answer he provided next day was 'Yes, but not necessarily in the way the person praying hoped for.' None of this interaction appears in the Law Reports.

28. At p. 339.

29. At pp. 59-60.

30. At p. 61.

31. Sir Neville Faulks, *A Law unto Myself* (London: William Kimber, 1978) p. 87.

32. See p. 22n. above.

3.   At p. 990.

.   At p. 1147. See also *Regis Property Co.* v. *Dudley* at p. 384 and *Oppenheimer* v. *Cattermole* at p. 268.

.   The United States Supreme Court exercises this power not infrequently. It was used in the case of *Brown* v. *Board of Education* under the pretext of obtaining argument on some questions drafted by Frankfurter and his clerk Alexander Bickel. In reality the re-argument was a delaying tactic exercised in the hope that time might bring some unanimity to the Court. It did. See Kluger, *Simple Justice*.

5.   'Advocacy before the US Supreme Court', 37 *Cornell L. Q.* (1951) 1 at p. 12.

7.   Quotation derived from my notes of the oral debate. The phrase has now been adopted by academic writers. See G. Williams and B. Hepple, *Foundations of the Law of Tort* (London: Butterworths, 1976) p. 69.

8.   The Judicial Office requires counsel for each side to submit estimates as to the duration of the hearing in order that a schedule of appeals can be drawn up.

9.   Patrick Neill QC my informant. *Attorney-General* v. *Times Newspapers* was another case which drastically overran its estimate because of the course taken by the oral debate. Provisionally assigned three days on the basis of counsel's estimates, it actually ran for ten days. The Judicial Office told me that such gross departures from counsel's estimates occur only once a year on average.

0.   See Lord Simon at p. 491G. The House divided 3:2 against the appellant on the point. In *Johnston* v. *Moreton* a suggestion made by one Law Lord was picked up by counsel but failed to win round the other Law Lords. See Lord Russell at p. 59g and Lord Hailsham at p. 50g.

1.   This also occurs in the US Supreme Court. In *Brown* v. *Board of Education* Douglas was willing to help counsel for NAACP who was suffering at the hands of Frankfurter. (See Kluger, *Simple Justice*, p. 567.) In another case a few years later, when Douglas again lent support to counsel, Frankfurter exclaimed 'I thought *you* were arguing this case', to the grateful counsel, who responded, 'I am, but I can use all the help I can get.' (Quoted in H. J. Abraham, *The Judicial Process*, 3rd edn (New York: Oxford University Press, 1975) p. 192.)

2.   For an example of such a clash between Lord Atkin and Lord Chief Justice Hewart in *Woolmington* v. *DPP* (1935), see J. D. Casswell, *A Lance for Liberty* (London: Harrap, 1961) p. 96.

3.   Quoted from his review of *Final Appeal*, 36 *M.L.R.* (1973) 419 at p. 561. *cf.* Cohen LJ, 'The Court of Appeal', 11 *C.L.J.* (1951) 3 at p. 13.

4.   For adverse comment on this in recent times see the Chairman of Granada Television, Sir Denis Forman's 'Journalism and the Law', *The Listener*, 4 September 1980, p. 295.

5.   Promulgated in 1954. See Erskine May, *Parliamentary Practice*, 19th edn (London: Butterworths, 1976) p. 79.

6.   According to Blom-Cooper and Drewry, *Final Appeal*, p. 249, about 71 per cent of English appeals are reported in the Appeal Cases. In about 25 per cent of those cases a year the Appeal Cases will report a judicial intervention, usually of a single line, yet it will be recalled that in *Cassell*

        v. *Broome* alone there were 99 judicial interventions on the first day.

47.   The remainder are derived from Law Lords' speeches, judicial biographies, interviews and personal observation.

48.   See Llewellyn, *The Common Law Tradition*. For a discussion of what Llewellyn meant by the phrase see Twining, *Karl Llewellyn and the Realist Movement*, pp. 219-20.

49.   See my discussion on *Heatons Transport Co.* v. *TGWU* in Paterson, 'Judges: A Political Elite?', pp. 126-7.

50.   Negative sanctions are only occasionally applied (see p. 29 above). Positive sanctions are more common. Law Lords not infrequently congratulate counsel on their arguments (and by implication, their role performance) in their speeches or at the Inns of Court or by letter. In two cases in the early 1970s, the Law Lords went even further and 'rewarded' counsel in their order on costs. In *Dingle* v. *Turner* at p. 625 the Law Lords directed that the defeated appellant's costs be paid out of the trust funds because the point decided in the case was one that the Law Lords had suggested in an earlier case 'ought to be considered by' the House. In *Gallie* v. *Lee* (No. 2) one of the reasons given by the Law Lords for awarding the successful respondents their costs from public funds was that the case had enabled the whole vexed matter of *non est factum* to be re-examined. Incentive awards of this sort have been recommended by the English Royal Commission on Legal Services, Cmnd 7648 (1979). (R. 16.4: Payment should be made from public funds to meet the costs incurred in determining a point of law of public importance.) If this suggestion were taken up it could have a significant impact on the types of case fought to the Lords and the types of argument put forward by counsel in the process.

51.   See. pp. 64 and 35 above.

52.   *E.g.* the appellants' counsel in *Conway* v. *Rimmer*, in *Hedley Byrne* v. *Heller*, in *Beecham Foods* v. *Customs & Excise* and in *Kendall* v. *Lillco*, all relied on statements made in the Court of Appeal by Lord Denning, Lord Justice Cross and Lord Justice Diplock respectively.

CHAPTER 5: LAW LORD INTERACTION AND THE PROCESS OF JUDGEMENT

1.   See 'Judicial Secrecy: A Symposium', 22 *Buffalo L.R.* (1973) pp. 797-883.

2.   B. Woodward and S. Armstrong, *The Brethren* (New York: Simon and Schuster, 1979). See also now *The Court Years, 1939 to 1975: The Autobiography of William O. Douglas* (New York: Random House, 1980).

3.   At least three detailed versions of the 'behind the scenes' story of *Brown* v. *Board of Education* have now been published. S. Ulmer, 'Earl Warren and the Brown Decision', 33 *J. of Pol.* (1971) p. 689; R. Kluger, *Simple Justice*; and M. F. Berry, *Security, Stability and Continuity* (Connecticut: Greenwood Press, 1978) pp. 123-5, 154-61, They contradict each other on a number of significant points, *e.g.* what the original division of

opinion was in the first conference on the case, why the case was continued for re-argument, what the split in the court was when Warren became Chief Justice, what part Frankfurter played in the decision-making process and the identity of the last Justice to hold out against Warren. In *The Brethren*, however, such ambiguities and conflicts in the evidence are conspicuous by their absence. Its readers are led to believe that the authors, although relying heavily on the indirect evidence of more than 170 clerks as to events which occured up to ten years prior the interviews, only once encountered a discrepancy in the evidence which they obtained. This seems unlikely.

4. See p. 12 above.

5. See *e.g. Gilmour* v. *Coats* at p. 442 per Lord Simonds; *SSEB* v. *British Oxygen Co.* at p. 1070 per Viscount Simonds; *United Marketing Co.* v. *Kara* at p. 524 per Lord Hodson; *National Bank of Greece* v. *Westminster Bank* at p. 957A per Lord Hailsham; and *General Electric Company* v. *The General Electric Company Ltd* at p. 512j per Lord Diplock.

6. See particularly Viscount Dilhorne. H.L. Debs., Vol. 297 Col. 462. A convenient summary of the debate is contained in Blom-Cooper and Drewry, *Final Appeal*, p. 150. According to Lord Denning, Lord Simonds objected strongly to the 'leap-frog' procedure for the same reason, *The Discipline of Law*, p. 300. In reinforcement of the Law Lords' views, an Appeal Committee rejected a 'leap-frog' application in *Oldendorff* v. *Tradax Export* on grounds that they wished to have the views of the Court of Appeal on issues raised in the case. See G. Drewry, 'Leap-frogging - A Lords Justices' Eye View', 89 *L.Q.R.* (1973) 260 at p. 274.

7. For a detailed account of one of the last cases where the judges were summoned to assist the Lords see Heuston, *Lives*, p. 119ff.

8. This pheneomonon is also found in the United States Supreme Court. See. R. Richardson and K. Vines, *The Politics of Federal Courts* (Boston: Little, Brown & Co., 1970) p. 130.

9. At p. 330.

10. Judgements in the Court of Appeal which are drafted with the House in mind are, as Lord Diplock's remarks indicate, primarily directed at counsel in the hope that they will pick up the point or points and run them in the House of Lords. For a recent case where this occurred see *Jones* v. *Wrotham Park Estates* at p. 293b.

11. See Lord Denning's comment in *The Discipline of Law*, p. 301.

12. Examples include *British Movietonews Ltd* v. *London and District Cinemas*; *National Provincial Bank* v. *Hastings Car Mart*; and *Morgans* v. *Launchbury*. One case where the Law Lords openly acknowledged that their discussion had been broader as a result of the judgements of the Court of Appeal was *Gallie* v. *Lee*. See Lord Reid p. 1015E and Lord Pearson p. 1032F.

13. See p. 45 above.

14. *Bremer Handelsgesellschaft mbh* v. *Mackprang*.

15. *Bremer* v. *Vanden Avenne-Izegem PVBA*.

16. *Final Appeal*, chap. vii contains a detailed discussion of the right of appeal to the Lords. The U.S. Supreme Court's control of its docket is

discussed in R. Hodder-Williams, *The Politics of the Supreme Court* (London: George Allen & Unwin, 1980) chap. 3 and in Abraham, *The Judicial Process*, chap. V.

17. Only rarely is the Appellate Committee hearing interrupted. This did, however, occur in *G.E.C.* v. *G.E.C. Ltd.*, which was interrupted by the Appeal Committee hearing in *Hubbard* v. *Vosper*.

18. Law Lords sitting in the Privy Council are usually treated as being unavailable for an Appeal Committee on the same day.

19. Lord Hailsham put these views into practice in the case of *Heaton's Transport Co.* v. *T.G.W.U.*, when he announced a week before the hearing began that a panel had been chosen so as to exclude any Law Lord with political experience.

20. See *Final Appeal*, p. 176.

21. Information derived from the Lord Chancellor's Permanent Secretary in November 1973. See also *Final Appeal*, chap. VIII.

22. New Lords of Appeal almost invariably hear their first appeal in the Privy Council.

23. Exclusions on this ground occur not infrequently, for example, there were six in 1960 and nine in 1971.

24. See p. 80 above. Counsel for each side in an appeal provides the Judicial Office with estimates of the length of hearing which the appeal will require. Where their estimates differ by more than two or three days the Judicial Office will try to get them to come to some agreed length.

25. Such declinatures are not common. One a year was the estimate given me by the Judicial Office. Lord Simon LC declined to sit in *Liversidge* v. *Anderson* because of his prior involvement with the regulation in question. (See Heuston, 'Liversidge v. Anderson in Retrospect', p. 43.) Lord Denning was apparently asked to sit in *Hedley Byrne* v. *Heller* but declined to do so because his dissent in *Candler* v. *Crane, Christmas & Co.* would come under review. (See *The Discipline of Law*, p. 245.)

26. Although written in the present tense the passages on judicial interaction in this chapter relate primarily to the practice of the Law Lords between 1957 and 1973, as they reported it to me. I found virtually no discrepancies between the accounts given by the various Law Lords. Nothing in my more recent contacts with Law Lords suggests that their practice has significantly altered since 1973.

27. Justices in the US Supreme Court also lunch together in small groups or with their clerks. Such groups are probably better indicators of those Justices who are friends or who share similar views than the groups of Law Lords are. See Berry, *Stability, Security and Continuity*, pp. 46 and 211, *The Brethren*, p. 88 and Ulmer, 'Earl Warren and the Brown Decision', p. 699.

28. In 1972 the Law Lords acquired, for the first time, a Conference Room, and it may be that this is now used in preference to the corridor.

29. On occasion, a Law Lord will meet one of his colleagues, whether sitting on the same case or not, in the evening or while travelling to work. In such situations they may discuss their current cases, particularly if one of them is sitting on a difficult case.

30. See Lord Morton, 'Address', pp. 115-16.

31. See Lord Wilberforce, 'La Chambre des Lords', p. 94.

32. If the conference is adjourned to a later time or to the Conference Room the clerk will not be present at the conference.

33. This can be highly disconcerting for a Law Lord who is sitting in his first case - particularly if he is unaware that this is the procedure. Members of the Judicial Committee of the Privy Council also express their views in inverse order of seniority (see Lord Morton, 'Address', pp. 115-16), but in the US Supreme Court and other appellate courts in America, opinions are expressed, first by the Chief Justice and then by his colleagues in descending order of seniority.

34. Morton, 'Address'.

35. See T. Clark. 'Internal Operation of the US Supreme Court', 43 *Judicature* (1959) 45.

36. See Burger CJ's remarks quoted in J. Schmidhauser, *Judges and Justices* (Boston: Little, Brown and Co., 1979) pp. 193-4; Berry, *Stability, Security and Continuity*, p. 73 and *The Brethren*, pp. 196, 406, 418 and 419.

37. Woodward and Armstrong, *The Brethren*, pp. 43 and 417, suggest that the formal process of voting has now been abandoned.

38. This seems to be the order preferred in many of the world's Supreme Courts. See 'La Cour Judicaire Suprême, 30 *Rev. Int. Dr. Comparé* (1978) 1.

39. In the Privy Council the presiding judge when assigning the opinion takes account of the respective workloads and expertise of the members of the Committee. At the beginning of 1959 the same five judges sat on the Judicial Committee to hear five Australian cases in a row. The 'chore' or writing the Court's opinion was rotated so that each judge ended up with only one opinion to write.

40. This is one of the repeated allegations made against Chief Justice Burger in *The Brethren*, *e.g.* pp. 64, 65, 179-80 and 418. But, as a number of scholars have observed, other Chief Justices have acted in this way without their personal integrity being attacked, see *e.g.* Hodder-Williams, *op. cit.*, p. 94 and J. Grossman in reviewing *The Brethren* in *Wisconsin L.R.* (1980) 429 at p. 434. On opinion assignment in the Supreme Court generally see S. Goldman and T. P. Jahnige, *The Federal Courts as Political System*, 2nd edn (New York: Harper & Row, 1976) pp. 187-8, and the references cited therein.

41. Lords Cross and Denning told me that in a majority of cases it is not clear who will write, yet Lord Radcliffe in his review of *Final Appeal* in 36 *M.L.R.* (1973) 559 at p. 562 states that, 'It is generally understood before writing begins who is going to prepare and deliver the major opinion on the majority side.'

42. Justice Powell 'What the Justices are saying', 62 *A.B.A.J.* (1976) 1454 at p. 1455.

43. Justice Oliver Wendell Holmes, *The Pollock-Holmes Letters*, vol. II (Cambridge University Press, 1942) p. 113.

44. Berry, *Stability, Security and Continuity*, p. 172.

45. *Final Appeal*, pp. 235-6.

46. *E.g.* Lords Diplock and Wilberforce. There is considerable

circumstantial evidence from the law reports of these Law Lords' speed of composition. Lord Diplock's ability to produce (and type) opinions under pressure has been attested to by the former senior clerk of his chambers, Sydney Aylett, in *Under the Wigs* (London: Eyre Methuen, 1978) p. 112. Lord Wilberforce produced the single opinion of the House of Lords in the difficult case of *Heaton's Transport Co.* v. *T.G.W.U.* within eight days. See Paterson, 'Judges: A Political Elite?', pp. 126-7.

47. *E.g.* Holmes, Van Devanter and Douglas. See H. Hart, 'Foreword: The Time Chart of the Judges', 73 *Harv. L.R.* (1959) 84 at p. 85 fn. 3 and G. E. White, *The American Judicial Tradition* (New York: Oxford University Press, 1976) p. 195.

48. *E.g.* Lords Cross and Pearson (information derived from interviews), and Justices Burton (Berry, *Stability, Security and Continuity*, pp. 149 and 232-3), Harlan and Blackmun (*The Brethren*, pp. 63, 172 and 224).

49. *E.g.* Justices Brandeis and Black (J. P. Frank reviewing *The Brethren* in 66 *A.B.A.J.* (1980) 161 at p. 164).

50. Similarly it is said of a former Australian Chief Justice (Owen Dixon) that, 'when he was concerned that a decision should go in a particular way, his aim was to get his own judgement out first for circulation to other members of the court.' D. I. Menzies, 'The Rt. Honourable Sir Owen Dixon' 9 *Melbourne University Law Review* (1973) at p. 3.

51. See also Lord Edmund-Davies in *Blathwayt* v. *Baron Cawley* at 437D.

52. There is also the further question, what does a judge mean by saying 'I concur'? See Sir Charles Russell, 'Behind the Appellate Curtain' Presidential Address, Holdsworth Club, University of Birmingham, 1969 at pp. 4-5, and Marvell, *op. cit.*, p. 115.

53. For recent examples of such withdrawals, see *London Borough of Lewisham* v. *Lewisham Juvenile Justices* at p. 299, *Raineri* v. *Miles* at p. 165d and *William and Glynn's Bank Ltd* v. *Boland* at p. 416e.

54. See, *e.g. Final Appeal*, pp. 90-5; and Lord Radcliffe, *loc. cit.*

55. 'The Ratio Decidendi and the plurality of speeches in the House of Lords', 93 *L.Q.R.* (1977) 378 at p. 384.

56. From 1952-68 the Law Lords produced a single judgement in 9 per cent of English and 12 per cent of Scottish appeals to the Lords (*Final Appeal*, p. 185). However, most of these were caused by the esoteric or insubstantial nature of the case rather than the policy reasons which lay behind *Heaton's* single judgement.

57. See p. 629 where Viscount Simon states,

> In framing my opinion, I have had the advantage of consultation with and contribution from the six Noble and Learned Lords who sat with me at the hearing of the appeal, and, while what I am about to say is the expression of my own view, I have reason to think it also expresses the judgement of my colleagues.

58. The Law Lords were divided over the size of the minority. See p. 186 below.

59. C. Nesson, 'Mr Justice Harlan', 85 *Harv. L.R.* (1971) 390 at p. 391.

60. W. Murphy, *Elements of Judicial Strategy* (University of Chicago Press, 1964) p. 60.

51. B. Cardozo, 'Law and Literature', 14 *Yale Review* (1925) 699 at pp. 715-16; and C. Hughes, *The Supreme Court of the United States* (New York: Columbia University Press, 1928) p. 68.

52. Where the dissent is in the Court of Appeal one alternative arena is the House of Lords. Lord Denning told me there was more point in dissenting in the Court of Appeal and thus providing the House with both points of view, than dissenting in the House of Lords itself.

63. *E.g.* Lord Hailsham '[When I dissent] I am moved by the necessity to express an honest opinion on the case before me and possibly to point a way for future legislators in the field of law reform.'

64. Only the votes cast, and by whom, are recorded in this book. It is difficult to tell how frequently written dissents were produced in the Privy Council before 1966 because they were not usually kept, their existence was not always recorded in the judgement book and in any event the judgement books for before the mid-1930s were destroyed by fire in a bombing raid in the Second World War.

65. 'The Ratio Decidendi and Plurality of Speeches in the House of Lords', *loc. cit.*, p. 383: ' ... in the interest of a coherent system of law, it is surely possible for a judge to suppress an occasional doubt rather than to give a separate speech ...'

66. J. R. Kaufman, 'Chilling Judicial Independence', 88 *Yale L.J.* (1979) 681 at p. 711.

67. Lord Diplock in several appeals has indicated that where a point of statutory construction is involved and the House is providing guidance to lower courts he considers there is no point in publishing a dissent, since this will merely confuse matters. See *e.g. Smedley's Ltd* v. *Breed* at p. 590. Lord Wilberforce has shown in a variety of appeals that he believes there is merit in giving a dubitante opinion rather than a full opinion. See *e.g. University of Strathclyde* v. *Carnegie Trs.* at p. 47. Another Law Lord told me he had dissented in a criminal case but not written an opinion. 'You see', he said, 'I saw no point if one was dissenting in a criminal case. Better to accept the majority.'

68. *Cf.* Justice Douglas, 'the right to dissent is the only thing that makes life tolerable for a judge of an appellate court'. *America Challenged* (Princeton: Princeton University Press, 1960) p. 4.

69. See *La Cour Judicaire Suprême*. See also K. Nadelmann, 'The Judicial Dissent', 8 *A.J.C.L.* (1959) 415.

70. See S. Goldman, 'Conflict and Consensus in the United States Courts of Appeals' *Wisconsin L.R.* (1968) 461 and J. W. Howard, *Courts of Appeals in the Federal Judicial System* (Princeton University Press, 1981) Chap. 7.

71. This occurred both in 1972 and in 1977. The overall rate for the Burger Court from 1970-7 was 0.92

72. As occurred in the early 1970s with Nixon's appointments to the Court.

73. D. Danelski, 'The Influence of the Chief Justice in the Decisional Process' in R. Wolfinger (ed.), *Readings in American Political Behavior* (New Jersey: Prentice-Hall, 1966) pp. 206-7. Danelski fails to explain why the dissent rate began to rise in 1938 and not in 1941 (on Stone's promotion), as his analysis would imply.

74.   Murphy, *Elements of Judicial Strategy*, pp. 47 and 61 fn.

75.   For an elaboration of the concept of social leadership see Danelski, 'Influence of the Chief Justice', pp. 200-1.

76.   E. McElwain, 'The Business of the Supreme Court as conducted by Chief Justice Hughes', 63 *Harv. L.R.* (1949) 5 at p. 19.

77.   B. Boskey, 'Chief Justice Stone', 59 *Harv. L.R.* (1946) 1200 at p. 1201.

78.   Danelski, 'Influence of the Chief Justice', pp. 202-3.

79.   R. Jackson, *The Supreme Court in the American System of Government* (Harvard University Press, 1955) p. 19.

80.   See A. Fortas, 'Chief Justice Warren: The Enigma of Leadership', 84 *Yale L.J.* (1975) 405.

81.   *Ibid.*, p. 412.

82.   All three versions of the 'behind the scenes' aspects of the *Brown* case (see p. 236 above) agree on this point.

83.   So much can be gleaned both from the private papers of Frankfurter and Burton and from Warren's comments about Harlan and the frequency with which he dissented. See 'Mr Justice Harlan' 85 *Harv. L.R.* (1971) 369 at p. 370.

84.   *Madzimbamuto* v. *Lardner-Burke*.

85.   Slesser, *Judgement Reserved* (London: Hutchinson, 1941) p. 252.

86.   Information derived from a number of Law Lords and Lords Justices and from Lord Denning himself.

87.   See *e.g.* Murphy, *Elements*, pp. 56-68; A. Bickel, *The Unpublished Opinions of Mr Justice Brandeis* (Harvard University Press, 1957); J. Howard, 'On the Fluidity of Judicial Choice', 52 *American Political Science Review* (1968) 43; P. Weiler, 'Two Models of Judicial Decision-Making', 46 *Can. B. Rev.* (1968) 406 at pp. 454-5; Abraham, *op. cit.*, pp. 212-15; Goldman and Jahnige, *op. cit.*, pp. 181-4; Berry, *op.cit.*; and *The Brethren*, *e.g.* pp. 233, 332-3 and 411.

88.   While a majority opinion of the Supreme Court is not required, its absence robs a decision of much of its precedent value. On the drawbacks of such cases, see 'Plurality Decisions and Judicial Decisionmaking', 94 *Harv. L.R.* (1981) 1127. On the value of near unanimous decisions, see 'The "Released Time" Cases Revisited', 83 *Yale L.J.* (1974) 1202 at p. 1216 fn84.

89.   One Judge of the International Court of Justice has described the situation of the majority opinion writer in that court 'as like a whale attacked by a school of killer whales which tear big chunks of flesh from its body'. Quoted in L. Prott, *The Latent Power of Culture and the International Judge* (Abingdon: Professional Books, 1979) p. 62.

90.   On bargaining in this Court, see Prott, *op. cit.*, chap. 2.

91.   The pioneer was D. Danelski in his seminal paper 'The Influence of the Chief Justice on the Decisional Process'. See also Goldman and Jahnige, *op. cit.*, pp. 178-92 and the references cited therein.

92.   *Cf.* Frankfurter's opinion that Chief Justice Hughes saw the judicial conference as 'a place where nine men do solos'. Quoted in White, *op. cit.*, p. 213.

93.   *E.g.* at the first conference.

94.   *E.g.* during some of the post-hearing discussions at the end of the day.

For a debate as to whether the US Supreme Court should be more akin to nine individuals rather than a group, see Judge Thurman Arnold, 73 *Harv. L.R.* (1960) 1298 and Dean Griswold, 74 *Harv. L.R.* (1961) 81.

5.   Some forms of interaction are hard to classify. How, for instance, should one describe situations where one Law Lord picks up a point made by a colleague in the hearing see *e.g. Devis & Sons Ltd* v. *Atkins* at p. 52g and *Attorney-General* v. *Leveller Magazine Ltd* at p. 462E, or replies in his speech to a point made by a colleague in his speech, see *e.g. Nova Knit Ltd* v. *Kammgarn Spinnerei GmbH* at pp. 469c and 476h, where Lord Wilberforce's dismissal of a Court of Appeal precedent as obscure and unnoticed by major textbook writers was countered by Lord Salmon's statement that 'Authorities of such impeccable lineage cannot lightly be swept aside. I am afraid I cannot agree that [it] should be regarded as inanimate because [modern cases and textbooks do not refer to it].' Are these (as they appear to be) merely exchanges between individuals? Does it make any difference if one Law Lord's efforts are expressly rejected by all four of his colleagues (as occurred to Lord Denning in *Rahimtoola* v. *Nizam of Hyderabad*, see p. 38 above).

96.   *Final Appeal*, pp. 184-5. The figure has gone up in recent years.

97.   *Ibid.* Judged by recent years, this figure is now on the high side.

98.   See p. 97 above.

99.   For examples, see p. 93 above.

100.   See *Final Appeal*, Table 21, p. 185.

101.   Lord Denning relies strongly on the power of the printed word as a means of persuasion. As Lord Justice Templeman recently observed (*Talking Law*, Radio 4, 16 September 1979), Denning's judicial style is that of an advocate. Like a good advocate he relies heavily on the 'picture of the facts' which he sets out at the beginning of his opinions. (See *e.g. Re Brocklehurst* and *Midland Bank Trust* v. *Green*). Lord Pearce made the same point in discussing dissenting speeches,

> If you disagree, you really want to put the whole story, because the story in a sense builds up to what you think of it. I don't say you are putting it partially, but in point of fact you are seeing it slightly differently.

102.   See Kluger, *op. cit.*, p. 602. It is said that Douglas had concluded that attempts to persuade were futile, or, even worse, counterproductive (*The Brethren*, p. 44). Douglas himself is quoted in *Time* magazine (28 January 1980, p. 40) as saying, 'I haven't been much of a proselytizer on the court.' Nevertheless there are several occasions in *The Brethren* (*e.g.* pp. 107, 175, 231 and 356) where even he is said to have lobbied his colleagues. If *The Brethren* can be relied on, Justices Harlan and Powell were similarly reluctant to lobby their colleagues.

103.   This varies with the particular Justice as numerous notes and memoranda published by ex-law clerks have shown. See on law clerks generally, Abraham, *op. cit.*, pp. 237-42. With the growth in the workload of the court and in the number of clerks, the significance of the role played by the clerks has increased. Even if we accept that *The Brethren* (because of the bias in its sources) paints an exaggerated picture of the clerks' importance as intermediaries and confidants in the modern

court, it seems clear that there is less interpersonal contact between the Justices than once was the case.

104. Justice Powell, 'What the Justices are saying', p. 1454.

105. Justice Brennan has however indicated that there are frequent exchanges between the Justices by telephone. W. Brennan, 'Working at Justice' in A. Westin (ed.), *An Autobiography of the Supreme Court* (New York: Macmillan, 1963) p. 304. Although *The Brethren* supports Brennan on this point it is probably the case that *The Brethren*, because it focuses on the most contentious cases coming before the Court, exaggerates the extent of oral interaction which takes place between the Justices in the normal course of events.

106. See *e.g.* Berry, *op. cit.*, pp. 46, 86, 88, 126, 189, 193, 203, 205, 211 and 213; H. Black, *My Father: A Remembrance* (New York: Random House, 1975) p. 237; Kluger, *Simple Justice*, p. 600; and *The Brethren*, pp. 46, 176, 215, 231, 362, 416 and 417.

107. As far as I could trace the draft judgement of the Judicial Committee of the Privy Council is circulated with a slip attached and the draft and slip returned to the opinion writer with a variety of comments from his colleagues written on them. The comments range from 'Approved', 'I agree', 'No comment' to 'I dissent and am writing a dissent' and 'I don't agree but won't write anything'.

108. Danelski, 'The Influence of the Chief Justice in the Decisional Process', and 'Conflict and its Resolution in the Supreme Court', 11 *Journal of Conflict Resolution* (1967) 71.

109. See p. 105 above. Leadership is not restricted to the Chief Justice. Burton was an effective 'social leader'. See Berry, *op. cit.*, pp. 59-60, 230-1; 83 *Yale L.J.* (1974) 1202 at p. 1214 fn 80. So too was Brennan. See *The Brethren*, *e.g.* pp. 46, 51, 295 and 326.

110. Danelski, 'Conflict and its Resolution in the Supreme Court', p. 79.

111. This need not be overt. For example, one British appellate judge has been known to wait until the presiding judge refers to ideas which he agrees with and then say, 'Yes, that's right. You seem to have put your finger on the key to the case there ...' and thus endeavour to tie the presiding judge to the point.

112. Berry, *op. cit.*

113. Berry, *ibid.*, p. 205.

114. J. Lumbard, 'J.H.', 85 *Harv. L.R.* (1971) 372 at p. 375.

115. Berry, *op. cit.*, pp. 211, 213.

116. J. Lash, *From the Diaries of Felix Frankfurter* (New York: W. Norton, 1975) pp. 78, 230.

117. E. Gerhart, *America's Advocate* (Indianapolis: Bobbs-Merrill, 1958) 262 and Berry, *op. cit.*, p. 29. *The Brethren* (*e.g.* pp. 179 and 187) suggests that relations between Douglas and Burger were strained for much of the time when they were both on the court. Antagonisms on the Bench can have advantageous side effects for counsel, since if one judge asks counsel a question the opposing judge may answer it for him. (See p. 81 above.)

118. See p. 45 above and p. 153 above. Cf. Lord Denning, *The Discipline of Law*, p. 43: 'Viscount Simon was very critical of my judgement but

wrote me a letter to soften the blow.'

119. See H. Black, 'Mr Justice Frankfurter', 78 *Harv. L.R.* (1965) 1521; J. Cooper, 'Mr Justice Hugo L. Black', 24 *Alabama L.R.* (1972) 1 at p. 5; H. Black, *My Father*, pp. 229-30, 234-5. Similarly Black and Harlan, whose opinions frequently differed, were in fact close friends. See H. Black, *My Father*, J. Harlan, 'Mr Justice Black', 81 *Harv. L.R.* (1967) 1 and *The Brethren*, pp. 45 and 91.

120. Black, 'Mr Justice Frankfurter'.

121. *New York Times*, 11 June 1946, p. 2. See also Berry, *op. cit.*, p. 29.

122. Lash, *op. cit.*, pp. 211 and 227; Berry, *op. cit.*, p. 49.

123. E. Millar, 'Some Memories of Lord Atkin', 23 *GLIM* (1957) 13 at pp. 14-15.

124. Heuston, *Lives*, p. 481. Lord Dunedin himself was said to be 'eminently open to suggestion' by his colleagues. Sir Chales Mallet, *Lord Cave* (London: John Murray, 1931) p. 226.

125. Heuston, '*Liversidge v. Anderson* in Retrospect', p. 46.

126. *The Times*, 27 June 1944 (quoted in Heuston, *ibid.*, p. 46).

127. See p. 69 above.

128. *Cf. The Brethren*, p. 176.

129. See Berry, *op. cit.*; Howard, 'On the Fluidity of Judicial Choice'; Hodder-Williams.; *op. cit.*, pp. 103 and 106; and *The Brethren*, *e.g.* pp. 69, 71, 260, 364, 403, 419 and 420.

130. At p. 771H.

131. At p. 372b.

132. At p. 1184c. See also Lords Dilhorne and Edmund-Davies in *Vestey* v. *IRC* at pp. 1187 and 1196.

133. At pp. 78-9.

134. At p. 18.

135. At p. 523.

136. At p. 716g.

137. At p. 261C-D.

138. At p. 823F.

139. At p. 728.

140. At p. 330h.

141. At p. 1192. Apart from the Law Report itself my account of the case is derived from interviews with some of the Law Lords involved and from Sir Neville Faulks, *A Law Unto Myself* (London: William Kimber, 1978) p. 103.

142. See p. 89 above.

143. See Chapters 6 and 7 below.

144. At pp. 40, 50, 78 and 79.

145. Of the ten cases involving Lord Simonds between 1958 and 1961 in which the House split 3:2, Lord Simonds ended up on the majority side in only five.

146. See C. Palley, 'Decision-making in the Area of Public Order by English Courts' in *Public Order*, II, parts 1-5 (Bletchley: Open University, 1972) p. 58.

147. This is a form of reference group behaviour. An example can be seen in Lord Hailsham's desription of Lord Atkin's effect on his colleagues. See

Heuston, *Lives*, p. 531.

148. See on this Sir Michael Kerr, 'Modern Trends in Commercial Law and Practice', 41 *M.L.R.* (1978) 1 at p. 7.

149. *Cf.* Danelski, 'Conflict and its Resolution in the Supreme Court', p. 80.

CHAPTER 6: THE ROLE OF A LAW LORD: CONFLICT AND CHANGE

1. In *Jesting Pilate* (Melbourne: The Law Book Co. 1965) at p. 157.

2. See Chapter 2 above.

3. See Prott, *loc. cit.*, and MacCormick, *op. cit.*, chap. I.

4. See Rudden, *loc. cit.*, pp. 1013-4.

5. A. W. B. Simpson, 'The Common Law and Legal Theory' in A. W. B. Simpson (ed.), *Oxford Essays in Jurisprudence*, Second Series (Oxford: Clarendon Press, 1973).

6. See R. Dworkin, 'Hard Cases', 88 *Harv. L.R.* (1975) 1057 and J. Esser, *Vorverstandnis und Methodenwahl in der Rechtsfindung* (Frankfurt: Athenaum Verlag, 1970) reviewed by L. V. Prott 'Updating the Judicial ''Hunch''', 26 *A.J.C.L.* (1978) 461.

7. R. W. M. Dias, *Jurisprudence*, 4th edn (London: Butterworths, 1976) p. 279.

8. Reported in M. Zander (ed.), *What's Wrong with the Law* (London: BBC Publications, 1970) p. 71.

9. Roscoe Pound, *An Introduction to the Philosophy of Law* (Yale University Press, 1922) p. 19. See in similar vein, W. Friedmann, 'Judges, Politics and the Law', 29 *Can. B. Rev.* (1951) 811 at p. 837.

10. J. Stone, *Legal Systems and Lawyers' Reasonings* (London: Stevens, 1964).

11. Llewellyn, *The Common Law Tradition*, pp. 62ff.

12. Lord Reid, 'The Law and the Reasonable Man', LIV *Proceedings of the British Academy* (1968) at pp. 191 and 193.

13. 'The Judge as Law Maker', 12 *J.S.P.T.L.* (1972) 22 at 26.

14. 'Judicial Activism', 28 *C.L.P.* (1975) 1 at 13.

15. Interview.

16. Interview.

17. Lord Radcliffe, *The Law and its Compass* (London: Faber and Faber, 1961) pp. 10-11.

18. In 'The Courts as Legislators' (The Holdsworth Club of the University of Birmingham, 1965) pp. 17 and 21.

19. *Conway* v. *Rimmer* at p. 958.

20. In 'Twenty Years On', 65 *Law Society's Gazette* (1968) p. 657.

21. [1966] 1 W.L.R. 1234.

22. At p. 958.

23. At pp. 966, 993 and 1015 respectively.

24. At pp. 929-30.

25. At pp. 467E and 488F.

26. At p. 326A.

27. At p. 665.

28. At p. 389.

29. Although I discussed all the topics raised in each of the expectations outlined below with some of the Law Lords and counsel, only the topics of expectations (3), (4) and (5) were discussed with all the Law Lords and counsel whom I interviewed. The evidence leaves me in no doubt that (1) and (2) are equally well founded; indeed less controversial than (5), over which there is some dissensus.

30. See p. 38 above.

31. I am not here concerned with the aetiology of the decision. The 'hunch' theory of decision-making is not necessarily inconsistent with the expectations which I have outlined. See Cross, *Precedent in English Law*, 3rd edn, pp. 51-2.

32. On the 'all or nothing' character of judicial decision-making and the contrast between a mediator and an adjudicator, see *inter alia* V. Aubert, 'Law as a Way of Resolving Conflicts' in L. Nader (ed.), *Law in Culture and Society* (Chicago Aldine Publishing Co., 1969) p. 282 and T. Eckhoff, 'The Mediator, the Judge and the Administrator in Conflict-resolution', 10 *Acta Sociologica* (1967) 148.

33. See *Donoghue* v. *Stevenson* and *Hedley Byrne* v. *Heller*.

34. *Morgans* v. *Launchbury*; *Myers* v. *DPP*; *Home Office* v. *Dorset Yacht Co.*; and *Best* v. *Samuel Fox and Co.*

35. *E.g. National Bank of Greece* v. *Metliss*; *Rondel* v. *Worsley*; *Parry* v. *Cleaver*; and *DPP* v. *Lynch*.

36. See Appendix. It should perhaps be stated that my discussion of typical modes of conflict resolution or of the typical responses to role conflict, does not involve a value judgement that role conflict is in some sense undesirable. It merely postulates that individuals will typically respond consciously or subconsciously to a role conflict in order to cope with or avoid the sanctions of the group whose expectations they have violated or intend to violate.

37. The examples of Lord Atkin in *Liversidge* v. *Anderson* and Lord Denning in numerous cases, indicate that this point should not be pressed too far.

38. *Ras Behari Lal* v. *King Emperor* at p. 2.

39. 'The Law of "Invitation"', 66 *L.Q.R.* (1950) 454 at p. 456.

40. Quoted by Frankfurter J, 'The Social Views of Mr Justice Brandeis' in E. Pollock (ed.), *The Brandeis Reader* (New York: Oceana Publications, 1956) p. 64.

41. Llewellyn, *The Common Law Tradition*.

42. 'Judicial Caution and Judicial Valour', 45 *L.Q.R.* (1929) 293.

43. In *Candler* v. *Crane, Christmas & Co.* at p. 178.

44. 'The English Law and its Future', *The Listener*, 29 August 1974, p. 265.

45. Lord Reid, 'The Judge as Law Maker', pp. 22-3.

46. See K. Vines 'The Judicial Role in the American States', J. Grossman and J. Tanenhaus (eds), *Frontiers of Judicial Research* (New York: John Wiley and Sons, 1969).

47. See Appendix.

48. Pierre J. J. Olivier, *Legal Fictions in Practice and Legal Science* (Rotterdam University Press, 1975) p. 150. See also Lon Fuller, *Legal Fictions* (Stanford University Press, 1967) p. 53.

49. E. Goffman, 'Role Distance' in *Encounters* (London: Allen Lane, The Penguin Press, 1972) p. 75.

50. See R. Cross, *Precedent in English Law*, 3rd edn (Oxford: Clarendon Press, 1977) pp. 35-7.

51. *The Growth of the Law* (Yale University Press, 1924) p. 66.

52. In E. London (ed.), *The Law as Literature* (New York: Simon and Schuster, 1960) p. 692. See also Buckley and Phillimore LJJ in *Olympia Oil* v. *Produce Brokers* at p. 750.

53. *Pocock* v. *Pickering* at p. 798.

54. For an attack on this passive response see Lord Denning, *The Road to Justice* (London: Stevens, 1955) pp. 1-2.

55. Lord Denning has made no secret of the fact that he accepted the post of Master of the Rolls because it offered him a better chance to implement his philosophy of favouring the 'be fair' as opposed to the 'be consistent' expectation.

56. Stevens, *Law and Politics*, p. 320 *et seq.* Stevens' concept of Substantive Formalism encompasses more than the consensus expounded here.

57. *Ibid.*, p. 385.

58. The phrase is taken from Stevens, 'The Role of A Final Appeal Court in a Democracy', 28 *M.L.R.* (1965) 509 at p. 519. A similar observation was made in a book review by W. Friedmann in 15 *M.L.R.* (1952) 386 at p. 389.

59. See Lord Simonds in *Jacobs* v. *LCC* at p. 373.

60. Viscount Jowitt, 25 *Austr. L.J.* (1951) at p. 296.

61. For the implications of this, see Chapter 5 above.

62. At p. 373.

63. At p. 444.

64. See *Magor & St Mellons RDC* v. *Newport Corporation* at p. 191; *British Movietonews Ltd* v. *London & District Cinemas*; *Rahimtoola* v. *Nizam of Hyderabad*; the debate on the Charities Bill in 1960 H.L. Deb. vol. 222 cols. 530 and 533; and *Scruttons Ltd* v. *Midland Silicones Ltd*. On Simonds as the High Priest of Substantive Formalism, see Stevens, *Law and Politics*, pp. 341-54.

65. Lord Cohen, 'The Court of Appeal', 11 *C.L.J.* (1951) 3 at pp. 13-14.

66. At p. 730.

67. Had the founding fathers of the common law taken the same view as Lords Cohen and Goddard it is hard to see how it could have evolved at all.

68. *Jacobs* v. *LCC*; *London Graving Dock Co.* v. *Horton*; *Best* v. *Samuel Fox & Co.*; *British Movietonews* v. *London and District Cinemas*; *Chapman* v. *Chapman*; *Smith* v. *East Elloe RDC*; and *Lister* v. *Romford*. For a strong attack on the restrictive attitude to *stare decisis* in the Lords as exemplified by *Jacobs* v. *LCC*: see Lord Wright, *loc. cit.*, pp. 455-6.

69. Thus a 'passive' approach to a precedent is one which demonstrates a preference for certainty and treating like cases alike as opposed to paying heed to the merits of the case and different social conditions. In this way an attempt to evade a precedent in order to do justice in the individual case is always activist. Similarly a preference for a flexible principle as opposed to a precedent is a creative preference. I would not

deny that I had been using the terms evaluatively; they could equally well apply to a decision to stand by a precedent. (See Palley, *op. cit.*, p. 58 and V. Radcliffe, book review 36 *M.L.R.* (1973) 559 at p. 563.)

70. In J. D. Wilson, *Milestones on the Dover Road* (London: Faber and Faber, 1969) p. 133.

71. But see Lord Radcliffe in *The Glenbank* at p. 242; *Smith* v. *East Elloe RDC* at pp. 750 and 769 might be construed as 'role-distancing', although I have some doubts on the matter.

72. See p. 148 below.

73. *Bonsor* v. *Musicians' Union* and *BTC* v. *Gourley.*

74. *Gourley* contains a few comments of this nature, *e.g.* Lord Reid at pp. 214-15 and Lord Keith (in dissent), at p. 218.

75. See the dissents of Lords Reid and MacDermott in *London Graving Dock* v. *Horton* at pp. 762, 765 and 785 and Lord Radcliffe's dissent in *Lister* v. *Romford* at pp. 591-2. See also Lord Reid's views in *Nash* v. *Tamplin & Sons* at p. 250 and in *Smith* v. *East Elloe RDC*. On Lord MacDermott's views, see Stevens, *Law and Politics*, p. 383.

76. This follows from my arguments as to the power of the Law Lords to define their own role and from my finding that the Law Lords were their own primary reference group.

77. At p. 1124. See also his dictum in *Regazzoni* v. *Sethia Ltd* at pp. 318-19.

78. At pp. 467-8.

79. At pp. 307 and 322 respectively.

80. 'The Judicial Process in Twentieth-century England', *Columbia L.R.* (1961) 761.

81. *Samples of Lawmaking* (Oxford University Press, 1962) pp. 22 and 23.

82. R. Cross, *Precedent in English Law* (Oxford: Clarendon Press, 1961) p. 17. See also p. 27.

83. 'Precedents in Divisional Courts', 64 *L.Q.R.* (1948) 40.

84. *Law in the Making*, 7th edn (Oxford: Clarendon Press, 1964) p. 357.

85. See Lord Denning, 'The Need for a New Equity' in 5 *C.L.P.* (1952) 1.

86. See *e.g. The Road to Justice* and his interview with Hugo Young reported in the *Sunday Times*, 24 June 1973.

87. At p. 247. See also Lord Reid's speech in the same case at p. 232 and in *Scruttons Ltd* v. *Midland Silicones* at pp. 476-7.

88. At p. 489.

89. At p. 388.

90. See 'The Need for a New Equity'.

91. 'The Way of an Iconoclast', 5 *J.S.P.T.L.* (1960) 77.

92. Stated in an interview with the author.

93. At p. 525.

94. Amongst the various dicta of note in this case, Lord Denning's chiding of his colleagues for not following a binding precedent of the House is of particular interest. He appears to delight in using the arguments against his colleagues which they have previously used against him. Thus in *Scruttons* he quoted the arguments which the majority in *Close* v. *Steel Co.* used against him, against his colleagues. In *London Transport Executive* v. *Betts* (at p. 247) he used against his colleagues the very argument which Lord Simonds had used against him in *Magor and St Mellons RDC* v.

Newport Corporation (viz., that the courts should not fill in gaps in legislation). Recently he has used the same ploy (in *Miliangos* v. *George Frank (Textiles) Ltd* (1975) at pp. 499, 500), in the course of a simulated 'judicial regret'. Since Lord Denning had helped to set up the rather dubious precedent in *Schorsh Meier GmbH* v. *Hennin* his ostensible acquiescence (despite numerous contrary assertions) in his colleagues' refusal to vary the rule that the Court of Appeal is bound by its own precedents, was an opportune conversion. Lord Simon obviously shares this opinion for he quoted Denning's dictum in *Miliangos* against him in *Farrell* v. *Alexander*. In each of these cases Lord Denning had purported to rank the 'be consistent' expectation higher than the 'be fair' expectation, whereas in reality he was doing exactly the reverse. As Twining and Miers point out in *How To Do Things With Rules*, p. 97 this 'Portia phenomenon' illustrates the danger of evaluating precedent orientation as passive or non-activist.

95. Lord Radcliffe, *The Law and Its Compass* (London: Faber and Faber, 1961).

96. *Ibid.*, p. 39. See also his comments in 'Law and Order', 61 *Law Society's Gazette* (1964) 821.

97. 'The Lawyer and His Times', pp. 14-15 in A. Sutherland (ed.), *The Path of the Law from 1967* (Harvard University Press, 1968).

98. Judicial authority in Lord Radcliffe's eyes appeared to rest on something akin to Max Weber's 'charismatic' domination.

99. Lord Radcliffe's approach (which I shall hereafter call the 'facade' approach) has been accused of exhibiting 'contempt for the democratic process', by Professor Palley in 'Decision-making in the Area of Public Order by English Courts', p. 67. It has also attracted criticism from Professor Jaffe in *English and American Judges as Lawmakers* (Oxford: Clarendon Press, 1969) pp. 7-8; Robert Stevens in 'The Role of a Final Appeal Court in a Democracy' pp. 535-7; and P. S. Atiyah in 'Judges and Policy', 15 *Israel L.R.* (1980) 346.

100. Allen, *Law in the Making*, pp. 345-6. Lord Reid has twice observed that the 'facade' approach creates this kind of uncertainty. See 'The Judge as Lawmaker', p. 24 and *Jones* v. *Secretary of State for Social Services* at p. 966.

101. The description is Llewellyn's. Llewellyn regarded the judicial role as one of the 'steadying factors' in appellate courts which led to reckonability of results. See *The Common Law Tradition*, pp. 45-51.

102. 'The Judicial Process Reconsidered in the Light of Role Theory', 33 *M.L.R.* (1969) 516 at p. 531.

103. I shall return to one of the clearer exceptions to this generalisation, *Myers* v. *DPP*, at a later stage.

104. But see Lord Evershed in *Haley* v. *London Electricity Board* at pp. 800-1.

105. Lord Reid in *Myers* is an exception, as is Lord Pearce's discussion of the basis of the law of negligence in *Hedley Byrne* v. *Heller*. But Lord Devlin's exposition of the law on exemplary damages in *Rookes* v. *Barnard*, which he described to me in an interview as a pure policy decision on how to rationalise the law (an assessment shared by Lords Wilberforce and Diplock: see *Cassell* v. *Broome* at pp. 1120B and 1124B) contains no such policy discussion. The Burmah Oil case, which one might have expected

to hinge on policy considerations, instead ostensibly turned on whether Civilian writings or decisions of courts in the United States were of more persuasive authority. Despite repeated assertions that the law (whatever the Law Lords eventually held it to be) to be applied in the case was the same in England and Scotland, it was possibly the Scottish origin of the appeal and the closer links of that legal system with the Civilian systems which eventually decided the issue in favour of the Civilian writings.

106. See Lord Evershed in *Haley* v. *London Electricity Board* at p. 801 and Stevens, *Law and Politics*, Part 4.

107. See Lord Devlin's and Lord Reid's speeches in *Hedley Byrne* v. *Heller* and Lord Reid's in *Gollins* v. *Gollins*. It was however a period of increasing 'role-distancing'. See the judicial regrets in *Faramus* v. *Film Artistes Association* at pp. 938 and 948; *Cartledge* v. *E. Jopling & Sons Ltd*; *National Provincial Bank* v. *Ainsworth* at pp. 1228, 1241 and 1259; and *Myers* v. *DPP*.

108. See Lord Devlin's exposition of principle restricting the previous precedents on exemplary damages, in *Rookes* v. *Barnard*; Lord Radcliffe in *Rumping* v. *DPP* at p. 837; Lord Reid in *Myers* at p. 1021; and Lord Upjohn in *Chancery Lane Co.* v. *IRC* at p. 128. *Cf.* Lord Devlin's arguments on logic and consistency in the common law in *Hedley Byrne* at p. 516 and in *West and Son* v. *Shephard* at p. 361.

109. At p. 366.

110. Professor Lloyd, *Introduction to Jurisprudence*, 2nd edn (London: Stevens & Sons, 1965) p. 377.

111. Robert Stevens, 'The Role of a Final Appeal Court in a Democracy', pp. 522 and 526.

112. C. K. Allen, 81 *L.Q.R.* (1965) pp. 36 and 37.

113. '*Stare Decisis* in Contemporary England', 82 *L.Q.R.* (1966) 203 at p. 203 (the article was published prior to the Practice Statement). See also *Precedent in English Law*, 2nd edn (1968) p. 218.

114. *Cf.* Lord Radcliffe's comments quoted at p. 142 above. Lord Salmon, although not in the Lords in 1966, considered that before 1966 an earlier decision which was considered manifestly wrong was seen as a wonderful opportunity for the exercise of ingenuity in order to distinguish it.

115. See his address, 'Twenty Years On', esp. p. 657. I find some difficulty in reconciling Lord Upjohn's views as represented in this address with his performance in the *Chancery Lane* case, and in *Conway* v. *Rimmer* where he alone of all the Law Lords felt able to evade *Duncan* v. *Cammell Laird & Co.* by describing it as having been decided *per incuriam*. (Stevens, *Law and Politics*, pp. 527ff, seems to have experienced the same difficulty.)

116. See Stevens, *Law and Politics*, pp. 403-5.

117. Reid, 'Judge as Law Maker', at pp. 26 and 25.

118. At p. 250.

119. At p. 609.

120. 1956-57, 203 H.L. Deb., col. 262.

121. At p. 232.

122. At pp. 476-7.

123.   At p. 111.

124.   I have taken the quotation out of its context in *Jones* v. *Secretary of State for Social Services* at p. 966C, but the application is, I think, a valid one.

125.   *Ibid.*, p. 966.

126.   See p. 20 above. It is perhaps not surprising that some of the more junior Law Lords whom I interviewed should stand a little in awe at a presiding Law Lord before whom they had frequently appeared as counsel. In some ways Lord Reid as an *innovant* met the criteria suggested by Lord Diplock more than Lord Denning. The latter stayed a much shorter period in the House of Lords and his open attacks on precedent and his occasional bending of the rules were less acceptable to the community of the Inns of Court, than Lord Reid's less extreme tactics. (Some of Lord Denning's critics whom I interviewed described his treatment of the rules of precedent as 'cheating'.)

127.   See 'Precedent in English and Continental Law', 50 *L.Q.R.* (1934) 40; 'Precedents in the Court of Appeal', 9 *C.L.J.* (1947) 349; and 'Precedents in Divisional Courts', 64 *L.Q.R.* (1948) 40. Several previous Law Lords (apart from Lords Reid and Denning) had indicated their dislike of the doctrine or had even asserted that it did not really exist. *E.g.*, Lord Wright, 'Precedents', 8 *C.L.J.* (1963) 144; Lord Evershed in *The Court of Appeal in England* (London: Athlone Press, 1950) pp. 17-18; and Lord Cohen in 'The Court of Appeal', 11 *C.L.J.* (1951) at p. 11. Surprisingly Lord Atkin was not in this camp (see his obituary written by Lord Wright in XXXII *Proceedings of the British Academy* (1946) 307 at pp. 316-17.

128.   *E.g.* G. Williams in the 11th edn of *Salmond on Jurisprudence* (London: Sweet & Maxwell, 1957) at pp. 175-88 and 538-9; Cross, *Precedent in English Law*, 1st edn, p. 250; R. Dias, *Jurisprudence*, 2nd edn (London: Butterworth, 1964) p. 75; G. Paton, *Jurisprudence*, 2nd edn (Oxford: Clarendon Press, 1951) pp. 162-3; and P. Fitzgerald, *Salmond on Jurisprudence*, 12th edn (London: Sweet and Maxwell, 1966) p. 144.

129.   For further details see 83 *L.Q.R.* (1967) 176-7; T. B. Smith, 'Authors and Authority', 12 *J.S.P.T.L.* (1972) 3 at p. 5; and L. Scarman 'Law Reform - Lessons from English Experience', 3 *Manitoba L.J.* (1968) 47 at p. 57.

130.   This description and certain of the details concerning events after 17 March 1966 are derived from my interview with Lord Gardiner on 20 April 1972. Owing to the passage of time certain discrepancies exist in the accounts given to me by the Law Lords. I have tried to indicate where these arise. My account is the one which I think makes most sense of all the Law Lords' recollections on the matter.

131.   See the Judicial Committee (Dissenting Opinions) Order in Council 1966. Unpublished dissents had always been permitted in the Privy Council. At the Privy Council conference memoranda were obtained from ex-Law Lords and circulated to all the Law Lords and relevant Privy Councillors. There was a strong minority view against allowing published dissents.

132.   This assertion rests on the the unsupported recollection of Lord Guest.

133.   Sir Leslie Scarman, then Chairman of the English Law Commission,

told me that he knew this as a fact.

134. Neither Lord Gardiner nor Lord Reid could recall whether the 'non-active' Law Lords had been consulted. In keeping with this, Lord Denning had no memory of being involved in the change. But he was present when the Statement was announced and he has since recorded that both he and the Lord Chief Justice (Parker) took part in the discussions prior to the announcement (*The Discipline of Law*, p. 296). On the other hand, Lord Guest indicated that the 'non-active' Law Lords had been consulted, and both Lord Devlin and Viscount Radcliffe asserted that they had attended the formal meeting despite their 'non-active' status. In the text I have treated the recollection of the latter group as conclusive.

135. 'The Changing Face of English Law', 7 *Cambrian L.R.* (1976) 54 at p. 62. *Cf.* Lord Salmon's statement 'that the announcement was made with the unanimous approval of all the Law Lords': *Davis* v. *Johnson* at p. 344D.

136. See Gardiner and Martin (eds), *Law Reform NOW* (London: Gollancz, 1963).

137. This of course was a problem which greatly exercised the commentators both before and after the Statement. See *e.g.* Julius Stone in '1966 and All That!', 69 *Columba L.R.* (1969) 1163 at p. 1168 and the Bar Council statements quoted in the *New York Times*, 27 July 1966, p. 1. As we saw earlier (see p. 22 above) counsel in *Cassell* v. *Broome* raised the question of the constitutional validity of the Practice Statement, but did not press the point.

138. Professor Goodhart in 82 *L.Q.R.* (1966) 441 at p. 444 wrote that those who contributed to the change were Sir Frederick Pollock, Lord Wright, Lord Evershed and Lord Denning. I do not deny that they may have had some influence in producing a climate receptive to the change but none of them (with the possible exception of Lord Denning) played as large a part in the events immediately prior to the change as Lord Reid did.

139. Cross, *Precedent in English Law*, 1st edn, p. 32.

140. Letter to *The Times*, 16 March 1978.

141. *Jurisprudence*, 4th edn, pp. 180-1. See also A. L. Goodhart in 85 *L.Q.R.* (1969) 171 at p. 173; Diplock LJ in *Boys* v. *Chaplin* (1968) at p. 35; and Salmon LJ in *Gallie* v. *Lee* (1969) at p. 49.

142. Cross, *op. cit.*, p. 32.

143. *E.g.* Viscount Simon in *Young* v. *Bristol Aeroplane Company* at p. 169; Lord Porter in *Bonsor* v. *Musicians' Union* at p. 128; Lord Morris in *Conway* v. *Rimmer* at p. 958; Lord Hailsham in *Cassel* v. *Broome* at p. 1055B; Lord Simon in *Miliangos* at p. 470 and in *Farrell* v. *Alexander* at p. 92D; and Lords Diplock, Dilhorne, Kilbrandon, Salmon and Scarman in *Davis* v. *Johnson* at pp. 323H, 336C-D, 340B, 343G and 349G.

144. *A-G of St Christopher* v. *Reynolds* at p. 659.

145. *Precedent in English Law*, 3rd edn, p. 111.

146. See p. 129 above.

147. See *e.g.* Lord Hailsham in *Cassell* v. *Broome* at p. 1053; Lord Simon in *Farrell* v. *Alexander* at pp. 91-2; Lord Wilberforce, Viscount Dilhorne and

Lord Russell in *Farrell* v. *Alexander* at pp. 72F, 81C and 105A; and Lord Diplock and Lord Hailsham in *The Siskina* at pp. 260C and 262B-C.

148.   At the time of my second interview with Lord Denning (on November 1972) he told me that he had been unable to win over even a majority of the Court of Appeal. See also his statement in *Tiverton Estates Ltd* v. *Wearwell* at p. 218.

149.   See Fitzgerald, *Salmond on Jurisprudence*, pp. 160-1; Dias, *Jurisprudence*, 4th edn, p. 181 fn 1; and J. Stone '1966 and All That!', 69 *Columbia L.R.* (1969) 1162 at p. 1168.

CHAPTER 7: THE LAW LORDS IN 1973 AND BEYOND

1.   Even Lord Devlin, who in 1962 had written, 'I doubt if judges will now of their own motion contribute much more to the development of the law' (see p. 136 above), was moved to comment in 1973 in the following terms, 'In the last decade there has been more judicial law-making ... than in any previous decade in the century.' See 'The Greatest Judge of Judges', *The Sunday Times*, 28 October 1973, p. 19.

2.   See *e.g. Indyka* v. *Indyka*; *Rondel* v. *Worsley*; *Esso Petrol* v. *Harper's Garage*; *Pharmaceutical Society of Great Britain* v. *Dickson*; *Boys* v. *Chaplin*; *Parry* v. *Cleaver*; *Home Office* v. *Dorset Yacht Co.*; *Cassell* v. *Broome*; *British Railways Board* v. *Herrington*; and *Morgans* v. *Launchbury*.

3.   See *e.g. Myers* v. *DPP* at p. 1021; and *Pettit* v. *Pettit* at p. 795.

4.   'The Judge as Law Maker', p. 22.

5.   Lord Reid displayed the same dislike for 'Dissimulation' as a response to the role conflict when he said,

> ... in this day and age I dislike [legal fictions] intensely. Why should we tell lies when the truth will serve our purpose equally well if only we give a little care to the formulation of our principles. ('The Law and the Reasonable Man', p. 200)

6.   'The Judge as Law Maker', p. 22; *cf.* W. Friedmann, 'The Limits of Judicial Lawmaking and Prospective Overruling', 29 *M.L.R.* (1966) 593 at p. 595.

7.   These expectations were again in part derived from the public and the legislature as symbolic reference groups. See *Geelong Harbour Trs* v. *Gibbs Bright* at p. 820G.

8.   See *Jones* v. *Secretary of State for Social Services* at p. 966.

9.   See *Ross Smith* v. *Ross Smith* at p. 303; the *West Midland Baptist Association* case; *Indyka* v. *Indyka* at p. 69; 'The Law and the Reasonable Man', pp. 194-6; and 'The Judge as Law Maker'. In my interview with him he said,

> Take the case of an old decision in the field of Contract upon which many people have relied and based many contracts on - we wouldn't dream of overruling such a case .... We shouldn't exercise the freedom in areas where certainty is required.

10.   See the *Jones* case at p. 966. His reasoning was that since such questions could frequently go either way it was difficult to say positively that one

construction was right and another was wrong. In such circumstances he implied that it was better to stick to one interpretation than to chop and change every few years as the composition of the House varied.

1. See *Steadman* v. *Steadman* at p. 542C.
2. *DPP* v. *Myers* at p. 1022; *Cassell* v. *Broome* at p. 1086F; and *Haughton* v. *Smith* at p. 500.
3. See *Knuller* v. *DPP* at p. 455. Lord Reid remarked to me in connection with that case,

> Surely no one really expected us to overrule *Shaw*'s case? It was quite the wrong type of case to depart from, far too controversial ... that was Parliament's province.

4. See the *Jones* case at p. 966; and *Oldendorff* v. *Tradax Export* at pp. 533 and 535.
5. See the *Jones* case at p. 966; and more generally his dicta in *Conway* v. *Rimmer* at p. 938; in *Indyka* v. *Indyka*; and in *British Railways Board* v. *Herrington*.
6. See *Vestey* v. *IRC* at p. 1178A.
7. See Lord Simon in *Knuller* at p. 486, citing Lord Reid's comments in the *Jones* case, at length; Lord Simon in *Miliangos* v. *George Frank* at p. 472D; Lord Cross in *Miliangos* at 496A; Lord Kilbrandon in *Dick* v. *Burgh of Falkirk* at p. 27; and Lord Edmund-Davies in 'Judicial Activism', p. 13. Lord Kilbrandon during my interview with him, said,

> I don't think you'll ever get a better exposition on when and whether to exercise it, than in Lord Reid's judgement in *Jones* v. *Secretary of State for Social Services*.

See more recently Lord Edmund-Davies in *Fitzleet Estates* v. *Cherry* at p. 1001 and *Vestey* v. *IRC* at p. 1196F; Lord Dilhorne in *Vestey* at p. 1186; Lord Keith in *Vestey* at p. 1198D; and Lord Hailsham in *R.* v. *Cunningham*.
18. *R.* v. *Sakhuja* at p. 180: 'only in exceptional cases'.
19. 'Judicial Development of Law in the Commonwealth'. Address in *Proceedings and Papers of the Fifth Commonwealth Law Conference* (Edinburgh, 1977) p. 495.
20. *Cassell* v. *Broome* at p. 1055: 'sparingly and cautiously'.
21. The *Jones* case at p. 1024: 'most sparingly'.
22. *Conway* v. *Rimmer* at p. 990: 'rarely and sparingly'.
23. *Duport Steels Ltd* v. *Sirs* at p. 548f.
24. *Vestey* v. *IRC* at p. 1198: 'rare cases'.
25. *Vestey* v. *IRC* at p. 1178: 'sparingly'.
26. See their acquiesence in Lord Salmon's dicta in *A-G of St Christopher* v. *Reynolds* at p. 660E: 'very exceptional cases'.
27. He also remarked, 'I think the business men do not so much care as to whether the court decision is ideally right. They want to have a decision so that they can base their future transactions on [it].'
28. *Lynall* v. *IRC* at p. 696 and *O'Brien* v. *Robinson* at p. 925.
29. *Lynall* v. *IRC* at p. 702.
30. *Farrell* v. *Alexander* at p. 75. He was in fact arguing the converse proposition that it is more legitimate to overrule a decision if to do so will not upset any person's legitimate expectations.

31. *Lynall* v. *IRC* at p. 703.
32. The *Jones* case at p. 1015; *O'Brien* v. *Robinson* at p. 930; and in 'Judicial Developments of Law in the Commonwealth'.
33. The *Jones* case at p. 993; *Fitzleet* v. *Cherry* at p. 1000f.
34. *Fitzleet* v. *Cherry* at p. 1002g.
35. *Lim Poh Choo* v. *Area Health Authority* at p. 189.
36. Not simply because the Law Lords as a reference group perceive it to be so, but also because they treat the public as a symbolic reference group on this matter.
37. On the topic generally, see R. Traynor, *Quo Vadis* (University of Birmingham, 1971). The issue has been discussed by the Law Lords in several cases. See the *Jones* case by Lords Simon and Diplock; in *Morgans* v. *Launchbury* by Lord Wilberforce; in *Miliangos* by Lord Simon and in *Aries Tanker Co.* v. *Total Transport* by Lords Wilberforce and Simon. Lord Diplock favoured it in 'The Courts as Legislators', pp. 17-18 as did Lord Simon in 'Some Judicial Processes in England', 1 *Liverpool L.R.* (1979) 7 at p. 17. Lord Reid, in interview and in 'The Judge as Law Maker', p. 23, was less sure and Lord Devlin deprecated it in 'Judges and Lawmakers', p. 11 (although in my interview he supported its introduction in cases on lawyer's law). Those who supported the idea (in interviews), included Lords Kilbrandon, Denning and Devlin. Those who disapproved of it (in the interviews) included Lords Guest and Cross. This was not a topic which I was able to discuss with all the Law Lords.
38. Here again *Innovation* is the response to a role conflict. There are other tactics which can achieve much the same effect as prospective overruling, *e.g.* laying down a legal principle on an issue which is not central to the case in hand. This was done by the Law Lords in *Hedley Byrne* v. *Heller*.
39. At pp. 966, 973, 995, 996, 1015 and 1024. Viscount Dilhorne who rejected the criterion at p. 993 appears to accept it in *R.* v. *Sakhuja* at pp. 180-1.
40. At pp. 216, 218 and 227.
41. At p. 90H.
42. At pp. 925 and 930.
43. At pp. 1187C, 1196G and 1176B.
44. At p. 497.
45. At p. 480. See also the *Jones* case at p. 1025B-C.
46. At pp. 695-6.
47. At p. 765G-H.
48. At pp. 541F and 544.
49. Per Lords Hailsham, Reid, Wilberforce and Kilbrandon at pp. 1083E, 1086E, 1115A and 1133D.
50. See *e.g.* Lord Wilberforce in *Miliangos* at p. 468A; Lord Scarman (his colleagues concurring) in *DPP* v. *Nock* at p. 992; Lord Wilberforce in *Hesperides* v. *Muftizade* at p. 537; Lord Scarman in *R.* v. *Lemon* at p. 658H and Lord Scarman (Lords Diplock, Dilhorne and Simon concurring) in *Lim Poh Choo* v. *Area Health Authority* at p. 189B.
51. A remark made by the Scots judge Lord Pitfour in *Sinclair* v. *Sinclair*

at p. 248.
52. Per Lord Diplock, *Geelong Harbour Trust* v. *Gibbs Bright* at p. 818G.
53. At p. 1023. Lord Morris seems to apply the criterion in *Cassell* v. *Broome* at p. 1098.
54. At pp. 463 and 486.
55. At p. 818H.
56. At pp. 496A and 472D.
57. At p. 469.
58. See *e.g. Helvering* v. *Griffith* at p. 403.
59. At pp. 480B and 486F.
60. At p. 552.
61. 'The Role and Functions of a Final Appellate Court', 7 *Cambrian L.R.* (1976) 31 at p. 32.
62. At p. 1001e.
63. At p. 552.
64. At p. 93.
65. At pp. 464F, 466D, 490B, 497E and 501D.
66. At p. 27.
67. Lord Upjohn 'Twenty Years On' p. 657.
68. At p. 537.
69. At pp. 1186, 1196 and 1198.
70. It follows that I disagree with MacCormick's assertion, *Legal Reasoning and Legal Theory*, p. 128 'that the House of Lords has failed as yet to articulate a clear and satisfactory set of justifying criteria for departing from precedents'.
71. *Knuller* v. *DPP* at p. 463B.
72. *Federal Steam Navigation Co. Ltd* v. *Dept of Trade and Industry* at p. 520.
73. *Knuller* at p. 486B.
74. *Fitzleet* v. *Cherry* at p. 1002f.
75. At pp. 281-2.
76. See *DPP* v. *Morgan* at p. 213F; *Oldendorff* v. *Tradax* at p. 533F per Lord Reid; *DPP* v. *Majewski* at p. 494H per Lord Edmund-Davies and p. 498F per Lord Russell.
77. At p. 993.
78. At p. 26. Lord Wilberforce refused to accept this proposition in *Miliangos* at p. 469H.
79. At p. 846H.
80. At pp. 476C, 465E, 497C and 503C.
81. At p. 993.
82. At pp. 1014-15.
83. At p. 938A.
84. At p. 997E.
85. See p. 180 above.
86. *DPP* v. *Nock* at p. 997E. See also Lord Reid in *Conway* v. *Rimmer* at p. 938A.
87. *Fitzleet* v. *Cherry*.
88. See *e.g. Hesperides Hotels* v. *Muftizade* at pp. 536F and 545A.
89. See p. 19 above.
90. *E.g. The Albazero* at p. 844.

91. See p. 18 above. Apart from the *Knuller, Majewski* and *Hyam* cases, see also *Hesperides Hotels* v. *Muftizade* at p. 536.

92. *Pace* Cross, 'The House of Lords and the Rules of Precedent' in P. Hacker and J. Raz (eds), *Law, Morality and Society* (Oxford: Clarendon Press, 1977) p. 159 and Stevens, *Law and Politics*, p. 217 *et seq.*, who would probably say that the correct figure in January 1980 was only four.

93. *Vestey* v. *IRC* at p. 1187F per Lord Dilhorne and p. 1196G per Lord Edmund-Davies.

94. See p. 2 above.

95. *Vestey* v. *IRC* per Lord Wilberforce at p. 1176C.

96. MacCormick, *Legal Reasoning and Legal Theory*, chap. VI.

97. *E.g.* Blom-Cooper and Drewry, *Final Appeal*, p. 38, and Stone, '1966 and All That'.

98. *E.g.* Lord Elwyn-Jones LC, 'The Role and Functions of a Final Appellate Court', p. 32; Cross, 'The House of Lords and the Rules of Precedent', pp. 158-9; Stevens, *Law and Politics*, pp. 618, 621 and 624; and *Final Appeal*, p. 38.

99. *Law and Politics*, p. 621.

100. See p. 144 above.

101. H. Ball, *Judicial Craftmanship or Fiat* (Connecticut: Greenwood Press, 1978) p. 15.

102. Sir Victor Windeyer, reviewing *Final Appeal* in 89 *L.Q.R.* (1973) 282 at p. 283. Lord Elwyn-Jones LC used an almost identical description in 'The Role and Functions of a Final Appellate Court', p. 32. See also A. L. Goodhart, 87 *L.Q.R.* (1971) at p. 456.

103. See Lord Diplock in *Herrington* at pp. 934-5; and Lord Upjohn, 'Twenty Years On', p. 657.

104. The counsel interviewed were also divided on this issue.

105. 'Judicial Activism'. *Pace* Atiyah, 'Judges and Policy', p. 358, where he argues on the basis of one phrase that Edmund-Davies is probably in the Radcliffe camp. Atiyah is strongly opposed to the 'facade', approach, see pp. 360 and 369.

106. 'Judges and Lawmakers', p. 11.

107. See his speeches in the *Jones* case at p. 1027 and *DPP* v. *Lynch* at p. 695.

108. Derived from his interview.

109. See *e.g. Myers* v. *DPP* at p. 1021 and *Pettit* v. *Pettit* at p. 795.

110. Lord Reid, 'The Judge as Law Maker'. See also *The Atlantic Star*, pp. 453-4.

111. 'The Law and the Reasonable Man', p. 193.

112. *Ibid.*

113. *Ibid.*, pp. 194-5. Even here, where he thought the need for certainty was strongest, he felt that the law had gone too far towards injustice, *e.g.* in treating as legally irrelevant matters which the layman saw as affecting the justice of the situation. Role performances by Lord Reid which are in accordance with his views on the need for certainty in property law include, *Gallie* v. *Lee* and *Pettit* v. *Pettit*. *Birmingham Corporation* v. *West Midland Baptist (Trust) Association* is not a contradictory role performance, see Lord Reid at p. 899.

114. 'The Law and the Reasonable Man', pp. 195-6. His decisions in *Scruttons* v. *Midland Silicones*; *Tsakiroglou* v. *Noblee Thorl GmbH;* and *Davis Contractors* v. *Fareham UDC* are compatible with this view. His decisions in the *Regazzoni* case and the *Esso Petrol* case do not really contradict his position for they reflect his views on public policy.

115. 'The Judge as Law Maker', p. 23.

116. See *Shaw* v. *DPP* at pp. 281-2.

117. Lord Reid, 'The Law and the Reasonable Man', p. 197.

118. *Shaw* at p. 281.

119. Lord Reid, 'The Judge as Law Maker', p. 23 and the *Birmingham Corporation* case at p. 899.

120. 'The Law and the Reasonable Man', pp. 197-203. Decisions of Lord Reid's which are in accordance with these views include *Haley* v. *London Electricity Board*; *Hedley Byrne* v. *Heller*; *Parry* v. *Cleaver*; *Home Office* v. *Dorset Yacht*; *The Tojo Maru* especially p. 268; and *British Railways Board* v. *Herrington*. Two cases which go against his views on this topic are *Rondel* v. *Worsley* and *Cassell* v. *Broome*. Again, the former case reflects his views on public policy. Lord Reid's willingness to innovate in this area of law can also be seen in his suggestion in *Taylor* v. *O'Connor* at p. 129 that inflation should be taken into account in the assessment of damages in a personal injuries claim.

121. See *e.g. Ridge* v. *Baldwin*, particularly pp. 64-5; *Conway* v. *Rimmer*; *Anisminic* v. *Foreign Compensation Commission*; *Attorney-General* v. *Nissan*; and *Rogers* v. *Home Secretary*.

122. *Pettit* v. *Pettit* at p. 795. He drew the same distinction in 'The Judge as Law Maker', p. 23. Lord Reid's distinction between 'lawyer's law' cases and those in areas of public controversy as a limiting factor for judicial law-making was endorsed by W. Friedmann in 'Judicial Law-Making in England' in R. Holland and G. Schwarzenberger (eds), *Law, Justice and Equity* (London: Pittman and Sons, 1967) p. 24, and by Lord Justice James in the 1976 Holdsworth Lecture, 'Law in Our Time' (The Holdsworth Club, Birmingham, 1976) p. 7. It was rejected, however, by M. D. A. Freeman in 'Standards of Adjudication, Judicial Law Making and Prospective Overruling', 16 *C.L.P.* (1973) 166 at pp. 190-1.

123. See *e.g. Indyka* v. *Indyka*.

124. See *Pettit* v. *Pettit* at p. 795 and 'The Judge as Law Maker', p. 23. It is difficult to understand Lord Reid's decisions in *Gollins* v. *Gollins* and *Williams* v. *Williams* in the light of this distinction.

125. See *Shaw* v. *DPP* and *Knuller* v. *DPP.*Both are consistent with Lord Reid's views on the second category.

126. Lord Reid, 'The Judge as Law Maker', p. 23.

127. At p. 1022. See also 'The Judge as Law Maker', pp. 24-5.

128. *Steadman* v. *Steadman* at p. 542C.

129. At p. 554.

130. At pp. 453-4.

131. See *e.g.* the *Suisse Atlantique* case at p. 406.

132. P. Weiler, 'Two Models of Judicial Decision-Making', 46 *Can. B. Rev.* (1968) 406 at p. 423. See also Lon Fuller, 'The Form and Limits of

Adjudicaton', 92 *Harv. L.R.* (1978) 353 at pp. 394-404. Reviews of the literature on 'justiciability' and polycentric disputes are contained in this article and in Freeman's 'Standards of Adjudication', pp. 185-6. Leflar, 'Appellate Judicial Innovation', p. 339 contains a somewhat related discussion, as does W. Friedmann, 'Judicial Law-Making', p. 24. The latter criticises the decision of *Hedley Byrne* v. *Heller* on the grounds that it displayed insufficient concern for the indirect consequences of a law-making decision.

133. Lord Devlin, 'The Greatest Judge of Judges'.

134. See his review of *The Discipline of Law* in *The Guardian Gazette*, 28 February 1979.

135. See his review of Stevens', *Law and Politics* in *New Society*, 15 November 1979, p. 384.

136. Interview and implied in *Miliangos* v. *George Frank* at p. 497.

137. 'Judges and Lawmakers', 39 *M.L.R.* (1976) 1 at p. 12.

138. 'The Courts as Legislators'; 'Judicial Development of Law in the Commonwealth'; *Cassell* v. *Broome* at p. 1127 B-D and *B.R.Bd.* v. *Herrington* at p. 941D.

139. *Myers* v. *DPP* at p. 1047.

140. Interview.

141. See his dissent in *London Graving Dock* v. *Horton* at p. 765.

142. Interview.

143. Interview, confirmed in *Herrington* at pp. 929-30.

144. Interview, confirmed in *Liverpool CC* v. *Irwin* at p. 263B; in *Morgans* v. *Launchbury* at p. 511D; and *Abbott* v. *The Queen* at p. 767.

145. *Miliangos* at p. 464 and *Herrington* at p. 921.

146. *Cassell* v. *Broome* at p. 1107D-E.

147. *DPP* v. *Lynch* at p. 700G-H. Yet in our interview he agreed that the obligation was part of a Law Lord's role.

148. *Miliangos* at p. 480 and *Knuller* v. *DPP* at p. 492.

149. 'Twenty Years On', p. 657.

150. 'Judicial Activism', p. 2.

151. Interview.

152. See Scarman's review of *Law and Politics*, *New Society*, 15 November 1979.

153. See 'Judicial Development of Law in the Commonwealth', and *Federal Commerce Co.* v. *Tradax Export* at pp. 8F and 14E.

154. *Aries Tanker Co.* v. *Total Transport* at p. 409 and *China NFTT Co.* v. *Evlogia Shipping Co.* at p. 1056f.

155. *Aries* at p. 407f.

156. *Aries* at p. 404.

157. E.g. *National Provincial Bank* v. *Ainsworth*; *Pettit* v. *Pettit*; *Gallie* v. *Lee*; *Federal Commerce Co.* v. *Tradax Export*; and the *Aries Tanker* case.

158. 'The Role and Functions of a Final Appellate Court'. The views of Lords Hailsham and Edmund-Davies appear in *R.* v. *Cunningham*. The other Law Lords' statements were made in their interviews.

159. See *Knuller* v. *DPP*.

160. 'The Role and Functions of a Final Appellate Court', at p. 34. The views of the other Law Lords were obtained in interviews.

161. Unfortunately, due to the exigencies of time and other difficulties the views of only half the Law Lords were elicited on this point.

162. In *Home Office* v. *Dorset Yacht* and 'Judicial Development of Law in the Commonwealth'.

163. In *Boys* v. *Chaplin*.

164. In *Knuller* v. *DPP* at pp. 487-8.

165. The creativity of the Law Lords in this case is in marked contrast to their reticence in *Ross Smith* v. *Ross Smith* six years before.

166. 'Judicial Development of Law in the Commonwealth', p. 449; and 'Judicial Activism'.

167. *E.g. Padfield* v. *Ministry of Agriculture*; *Conway* v. *Rimmer*; *Anisminic Ltd* v. *FCC* (a decision in marked contrast to *Smith* v. *East Elloe RDC* the decade before); *AG* v. *Nissan;* and *Rogers* v. *Home Secretary*.

168. 'Judicial Development of Law in the Commonwealth', p. 500. But see now *Bushell* v. *Sec. of State*.

169. But see now *Bushell*. These cases do reveal, however, a disagreement amongst the Law Lords as to whether the categories of public interest are closed.

170. *DPP* v. *Shannon* at pp. 765-6; and *D.* v. *NSPCC* at p. 235. But see Lord Gardiner, cited in Stevens, *Law and Politics*, p. 431.

171. *DPP* v. *Lynch* at p. 676.

172. *Miliangos* at pp. 469-70; *Herrington* at p. 921; and *Lynch* at pp. 684-5.

173. *Lynch* at p. 713.

174. *DPP* v. *Lynch* at pp. 695 and 697; and *Knuller* v. *DPP* at p. 489.

175. *Lynch* at pp. 700-1; and *Knuller* at p. 497A-B.

176. *Cf. Hesperides Hotels* v. *Muftizade* at p. 537A.

177. 'The Role and Functions of a Final Appellate Court', p. 34.

178. *Lim Poh Choo* v. *Area Health Authority* at p. 184A-B.

179. See *Cassell* v. *Broome* per Lords Hailsham, Reid, Wilberforce and Kilbrandon at pp. 1083E, 1086E, 1115A and 1133D. See also *Gammell* v. *Wilson* and the cases cited at p. 256 n50 above.

180. See Lord Wilberforce in *Indyka* v. *Indyka* at p. 103D-E and in *Miliangos* at p. 468A; Lord Diplock in *D.* v. *NSPCC* at p. 220G and *MacShannon* v. *Rockware Glass* at p. 811B-C; Lord Hailsham in *D.* v. *NSPCC* at p. 225H; and Lord Devlin in 'Judges and Lawmakers', p. 11. On the incrementalism of judicial development of the law, see generally Shapiro, 'Stability and Change in Judicial Decision-making', 2 *Law in Transition Quarterly* (1964) 134 and L. Friedman and J. Ladinsky, 'Law as an Instrument of Incremental Social Change', unpublished paper delivered to the 1967 Annual Meeting of the American Political Science Association.

181. *Indyka* at p. 66B.

182. 'The Study of Law' 54 *L.Q.R.* (1938) 185 at p. 186. Lord Wright himself took a broader view, favouring appellate judgements which surveyed a whole field of law. See Devlin, 'Judges and Lawmakers', p. 6.

183. *Legal Reasoning and Legal Theory*, chap. VI.

184. See Ch. Perelman and P. Foriers (eds), *La Motivation des Décisions de Justice* (Brussels: Bruylant, 1978).

185.   P. L. Horowitz, *The Courts and Social Policy* (Washington: The Brookings Institution, 1977) particularly chap. 7.

186.   M. Zander (ed.), *What's Wrong with the Law?* (London: BBC Publications, 1970) p. 91. In interview Lord Devlin indicated that he no longer adhered to this position.

187.   At p. 480.

188.   See the *Jones* case at p. 1025B-C; *DPP* v. *Lynch* at pp. 695-6; *DPP* v. *Shannon* at p. 765G-H; *D.* v. *NSPCC* at p. 235A-B.

189.   *Morgans* v. *Launchbury* at pp. 145-6.

190.   *Home Office* v. *Dorset Yacht Co.* at p. 1058F-G.

191.   *Hesperides Hotels* v. *Muftizade* at p. 541F.

192.   'The Independence of the Judicial Process', 13 *Israel L.R.* (1978) 1 at p. 8.

193.   *DPP* v. *Lynch* at p. 700.

194.   *Morgans* at p. 143.

195.   *Morgans* at p. 111.

196.   *Morgans* at pp. 136-7.

197.   *Hesperides* at p. 544F.

198.   *Pickett* v. *British Rail Engineering* at p. 166.

199.   *Lim Poh Choo* v. *Area Heath Authority* at p. 189B (Lords Diplock, Dilhorne and Simon concurring).

200.   For a fuller analysis of Morgans as a 'polycentric' case see Freeman, 'Standards of Adjudication', pp. 187-9.

201.   *Legal Reasoning and Legal Theory*, pp. 105-6.

202.   See p. 24 above.

203.   Where it was accepted by Lord Reid at p. 966G, Lord Wilberforce at p. 995F and Lord Simon at p. 1024B.

204.   At p. 510B where it was rejected by Lord Edmund-Davies.

205.   Where it was accepted by Lord Edmund-Davies at p. 1003b and possibly by Lords Wilberforce and Dilhorne at pp. 999d and 1000g respectively.

206.   For strong attacks on the validity of this argument by academics, see Leflar, 'Appellate Judicial Innovation', p. 341 and H. Friendly, 'The Gap in Lawmaking', 63 *Columbia L.R.* (1963) 787. The argument was supported however, by Friedmann in 'The Limits of Judicial Lawmaking and Prospective Overruling'.

207.   *O'Brien* v. *Robinson* at p. 930.

208.   *Birmingham Corporation* v. *West Midland Baptist (Trust) Association* at p. 911.

209.   *Hesperides Hotels* v. *Muftizade* at p. 545B.

210.   *Knuller* v. *DPP* at p. 496.

211.   *British Rail Board* v. *Herrington* at p. 904B and *Knuller* at pp. 464F and 466C.

212.   *Shaw* v. *DPP* at p. 275 and *Herrington* at p. 897F.

213.   *Jones* v. *Sec. of State* at p. 1025C; *Knuller* at p. 489F; *Taylor* v. *Provan* at p. 221; and *DPP* v. *Lynch* at p. 697F.

214.   *Indyka* v. *Indyka* at p. 106; *Taylor* at p. 216H; *Photo Production* v. *Securicor Transport* at p. 843. More recently Lord Edmund-Davies has used the argument in *Attorney-General* v. *BBC* at p. 311.

215. Per Lord Reid at p. 898.
216. Per Lords Wilberforce and Diplock at pp. 921B-C and 939.
217. Per Lords Reid and Diplock at pp. 455F-G and 480D-E.
218. Per Lord Salmon at p. 227B. Rather neatly disposing of Lord Wilberforce's argument on the point (in the same case) that a certain proposition had survived several revisions of the Income Tax Code and could not therefore be departed from, by observing that the Code still referred to 'travel on horseback or by horse-drawn vehicles'. Lord Pearce rejected the argument in *Owen* v. *Pook* at p. 258G-H.
219. See his speeches in *Herrington* and *Knuller*.
220. See his speeches in *West Midland* and *Knuller*.
221. See his speeches in *Herrington* and *Farrell* v. *Alexander* p. 74F-H.
222. See p. 24 above.
223. See *e.g. Herrington* per Lords Wilberforce and Diplock at pp. 921B-D and 939.
224. *Herrington* at p. 939.
225. *Indyka* at p. 85D.
226. This is the title to chapter four of his book, *Benchmarks* (University of Chicago Press, 1967).
227. *Hedley Byrne* v. *Heller* at p. 484 and *Hepburn* v. *Tomlinson* at p. 470.
228. At p. 72C-D.
229. At p. 591 Lords Salmon and Keith expressly agreed with him on the point. See pp. 583 and 589.
230. At p. 897.
231. At p. 470B.
232. Lord Devlin, 'Judges and Lawmakers', p. 12. See also Lord Upjohn, 'Twenty Years On', p. 657 and Lord Edmund-Davies, 'Judicial Activism', p. 13.
233. 'The Role and Functions of a Final Appellate Court', pp. 34-5.
234. *Pickett* v. *BRE Ltd* at p. 166D.
235. *D.* v. *NSPCC* at p. 235C.
236. See *e.g.* Lords Hailsham and Simon in *D.* v. *NSPCC* at pp. 225G-H and 235A-C; Lord Fraser in *Hesperides Hotels* v. *Muftizade* at pp. 544-5; and Lord Scarman in *Lim Poh Choo* v. *Area Health Authority* at p. 189A-C. *Cf.* the criteria as to the exercise of the 1966 Practice Statement.
237. See Cross, *Precedent in English Law*, 3rd edn, pp. 100-1 and 'The Ratio Decidendi and a Plurality of Speeches in the House of Lords'; *Final Appeal*, pp. 90-5; A. L. Goodhart, 88 *L.Q.R.* (1972) at p. 311; and Viscount Radcliffe in 30 *M.L.R.* (1973) 559 at p. 562. Goodhart was either ambivalent on this topic or he changed his mind, see 87 *L.Q.R.* (1971) 145 at p. 147.
238. At p. 93.
239. See *London Graving Dock Co. Ltd* v. *Horton* at p. 779; *Chancery Lane Safe Deposit Co.* v. *IRC* at p. 110; *Cassell* v. *Broome* at pp. 1084-5; *Gallie* v. *Lee* at p. 1015 and 'The Judge as Law Maker', pp. 28-9.
240. For Lord Reid's views on the case see 'The Judge as Law Maker', p. 29.
241. 'The Judge as Law Maker', p. 29.
242. In interview. Lords Diplock and Roskill appear to have a more rigid view of the common law. See *Lambert* v. *Lewis* at p. 1189j and *Pioneer*

Shipping v. *BTP Tioxide* at p. 1046f-j respectively.

243.   In interview.

244.   Griffith, *Politics of the Judiciary*, pp. 180-1.

245.   Julius Stone, *Social Dimensions of Law and Justice* (London: Stevens Sons, 1966) pp. 669-70.

246.   This had one curious and probably unintended consequence. highlighted the Law Lords' awareness of the role conflict between justi and certainty. In the circumstances they were forced to choose betwee 'Dissimulation' and *Withdrawal* as the only responses available to ther We might therefore predict that (certainly amongst Law Lords wh disliked the 'facade' approach) 'role-distancing' would increase aft 1966. This in fact is precisely what happened. See the *Suisse Atlantiq* case at p. 406, per Lord Reid; *Beswick* v. *Beswick* at p. 72 per Lord Rei *Knuller* v. *DPP* at p. 455 per Lord Reid; *Morgans* v. *Launchbury* at p 136-7 per Lord Wilberforce; *DPP* v. *Lynch* at p. 700A per Lor Kilbrandon; *Spicer* v. *Holt* at pp. 993G and 1008B per Lords Diplock an Edmund-Davies; *Orapko* v. *Manson Invest.* at p. 107B per Lord Diploc Simmons v. *Pizzey* at p. 61F-H per Lord Hailsham; *Tyrer* v. *Smart* at p 328C-D per Lord Scarman and *Gibson* v. *Manchester City Council* at p 976h and 980d-e per Lords Diplock and Edmund-Davies.

247.   *Cookson* v. *Knowles* at p. 579E-F.

CHAPTER 8: THE FINAL CURTAIN?

1.   For his denial of this strong sense of 'discretion' in a judge see 'Is Law System of Rules?' in R. Summers (ed.), *Essays in Legal Philosoph* (Oxford: R. Blackwell, 1970) p. 25.

2.   See 'No Right Answer' in P. Hacker and J. Raz (eds), *Law, Morality an Society* (Oxford University Press, 1977) p. 58, and 'Can Rights b Controversial?' in R. Dworkin, *Taking Rights Seriously* (Harvar Universiy Press, 1977).

3.   *The Concept of Law* (Oxford University Press, 1961) p. 200.

4.   *Ibid.*, pp. 246-7.

5.   'Law in the Perspective of Philosophy', 51 *New York University L.R.* (1976) 538 at pp. 550-1.

6.   *The Common Law Tradition*, p. 213.

7.   *Legal Reasoning and Legal Theory*, pp. 246 *et seq.*

8.   *Precedent in English Law*, 3rd edn, p. 220.

9.   *Law and Other Things*, p. 48.

10.   *The Growth of the Law*, p. 60.

11.   See Twining, *Karl Llewellyn and the Realist Movement*, pp. 249 and 254.

12.   J. W. Howard, 'Role Perceptions and Behaviour in Three US Courts of Appeals', 39 *J. of Pol.* (1977) 916 at p. 922.

13.   Implied in 'Courts as Legislators', p. 5 and in 'Judicial Development of Law in the Commonwealth'. The latter address in particular lays a heavy emphasis on the judicial room for choice.

14.   Implied in 'Natural Justice', 1973 *C.L.P.* 1 where he indicates that in

the Lords choices between two reasonable contentions of opposing parties have often to be made.

15. Lord Kilbrandon was difficult to classify because his answer is ambiguous and elsewhere in the interview he conceded that there were 'gaps' in the law which could be filled by judicial law-making.

16. See p. 264 n13 above.

17. In 'Natural Justice', p. 1.

18. See the footnote on p. 2 above.

19. See M. Mandel, 'Dworkin, Hart, and the Problem of Theoretical Perspective', 14 *Law and Soc. Rev.* (1979) 57.

20. W. Thomas, *The Child in America* (New York: Knopf, 1928) p. 584.

21. See his penultimate comment in 'Equality and the Law', *The Listener*, 6 June 1974, p. 722.

22. *Taking Rights Seriously*, pp. 351-2.

23. 'Hard Cases', p. 1061.

24. Lord Hailsham has described this as one of the neglected problems of democracy in modern times. See 'The Independence of the Judicial Process', 13 *Israel L.R.* (1978) 1 at p. 9. But see Professor Atiyah in 'Judges and Policy', 15 *Israel L.R.* (1980) 346 who argues (at p. 363) that the non-accountability of judges is essential to democracy, and adds, 'I am far from clear that there is anything undemocratic about judicial creativity.'

25. See the footnote on p. 14 above.

26. 'Hard Cases', p. 1058.

27. See p. 180 above.

28. See p. 177 above.

29. Under which cases whose real controversy has been negated by a later event are rejected by the court. See Marvell, *Appellate Courts and Lawyers*, pp. 40 *et seq*. The doctrine appears to have greater force in the US than in Britain.

30. See p. 43 above.

31. As will be seen, I am using this in a narrow sense rather than the broader Diceyan form found in constitutional law.

32. See *e.g.* E. P. Thomson, *Whigs and Hunters* (New York: Pantheon, 1975), and I. D. Balbus, *The Dialectics of Legal Repression* (New York: Russell Sage, 1973).

33. H. Weschsler, 'Towards Neutral Principles of Constitutional Law', 73 *Harv. L.R.* (1959) 1.

34. See Paterson, 'Judges: A Political Elite?', pp. 133-4.

35. *Law in Modern Society* (New York: Free Press, 1976).

36. See *e.g.* Weiler, 'Two Models of Decision-Making'; Freeman, 'Standards of Adjudication'; and Lord Devlin, 'Judges and Lawmakers'.

37. *Law in Modern Society*, p. 181.

38. For a similar argument, see J. H. Ely, *Democracy and Distrust* (Harvard University Press, 1980) chap. 3.

39. *E.g.* H. L. A. Hart.

40. *E.g.* Robert Summers, 'Two Types of Substantive Reasons', 63 *Cornell L.R.* (1978) p. 707.

41.   *E.g.* Philippe Nonet, 68 *California L.R.* (1980) 263.

42.   Prott, 'Judicial Reasoning in the Common Law and Code Law Systems', p. 418.

43.   See p. 10 above.

44.   Summers, 'Two Types of Substantive Reasons', 707.

45.   See p. 83 above.

46.   See p. 31 above.

47.   See particularly pp. 24 and 180 above.

48.   The phrase is Simpson's, see Simpson (ed.), *Oxford Essays in Jurisprudence*, p. 80.

49.   See Lord Diplock's comments on p. 20 above.

50.   See Appendix and M. Bickel, *The Morality of Consent* (Yale University Press, 1975).

51.   Thus it can be argued that there is little apparent consensus amongst the Justices or the scholarly community as to the current scope and viability of the 'strict scrutiny' standard of review, of 'rational basis' review, of the 'political question' doctrine or the 'preferred position' theory. (The gist of such an argument appears in an unpublished paper (1980) on 'Affirmative Action', by Ralph Smith, Assistant Professor, University of Pennsylvania Law School.)

52.   At pp. 820-1.

53.   'The Judge as Law Maker', p. 25.

54.   Interview.

55.   See 'Twenty Years On', p. 658.

56.   See 'The Courts as Legislators', pp. 17 and 21. The other Law Lords' preferences emerged in interviews.

57.   See 'Twenty Years On', p. 657. Lord Keith seems to be in this camp. See *Duport Steels* v. *Sirs* at p. 550. 'It is no part of the function of a court of law to form conclusions about the merits of the issue.'

58.   *E.g.* Dworkin, 'Hard Cases'; Prott, 'Updating the Judicial Hunch', p. 468; and H. Friendly, 'Reactions of a Lawyer - Newly become a Judge', 71 *Yale L.J.* (1961) 218 at p. 231.

59.   See 'Natural Justice', p. 1.

60.   'The Judge as Law Maker', pp. 22-3.

61.   Lord Hailsham, 'The English Law and Its Future', p. 265. One alternative solution put forward recently is the increased use of *amicus curiae* by interested groups or the Executive to provide more broadly based inputs into the judicial law-making process. See Lord Simon, 'Some Judicial Processes in England', 1 *Liverpool L.R.* (1979) at p. 17 and R. Dhavan, 'Judicial Decision-Making' (Mimeo, Delhi University, 1979).

62.   See p. 88 above.

63.   Interview.

64.   Lord Hailsham, however, told me that he did not promote judges from the Court of Appeal on this basis.

65.   'The Judge as Law Maker', p. 29.

APPENDIX: ROLE ANALYSIS

1. Shakespeare, *As You Like It*, Act II, Scene 7.

2. J. Banks and K. Jones (eds), *Worker Directors Speak* (Hants: Gower Press, 1977) p. 47.

3. Critical surveys emphasising these and similar points include, L. Neimon and J. Hughes, 'The Problem of the Concept of Role', 30 *Social Forces* (1950) p. 159 and B. J. Biddle, *Role Theory* (New York: Academic Press, 1979).

4. *E.g.* R. Dewey, 'The Theatrical Analogy Reconsidered', 4 *The American Sociologist* (1969) p. 309 and M. Coulson, 'Role: A Redundant Concept in Sociology?' in J. Jackson (ed.), *Role: Sociological Studies* (Cambridge University Press, 1972) pp. 107-28.

5. See P. Strong and A. Davis, 'Roles, Role Formats and Medical Encounters', 25 *The Sociological Review* (1977) pp. 775-800.

6. It is no part of the argument that all social action can usefully be perceived as role related. Role analysis is of little value for example in a situation where the actor's behaviour is the result of habit, or of prejudice, greed, indolence or other similar motives. Even in situations where there are many clear role expectations there are usually spaces leaving room for manoeuvre by the actor. To describe actions within these leeways as role performances is misleading. Some roles are more 'all embracing' than others, *e.g.* that of policeman or judge, for there is a sense in which they are never 'off duty', but not everything such individuals do can be explained in terms of role.

7. K. Llewellyn, *The Common Law Tradition* (Boston: Little, Brown & Co., 1960) p. 46.

8. The term role *theory* suggests a more highly developed body of knowledge and consensus on terminology in this field, than has hitherto emerged.

9. One or two researchers have called for an interactionist perspective in role theory which gives the social actor some scope, in conjunction with his reference groups, to define the role attached to the position which he occupies. See *e.g.* A. Cicourel, 'Basic and Normative Rules in the Negotiation of Status and Role' in D. Sudnow (ed.), *Studies in Social Interaction* (New York: Free Press, 1972) pp. 229-58 and Alan Dawe, unpublished lectures in sociology delivered at the University of York in 1968/69.

10. R. K. Merton, 'The Role-Set', *B.J.L.S.* (1957) pp. 106-20. Role others are frequently part of an actor's reference groups but the concepts are not synonymous.

11. R. H. Turner, 'Role Taking as Process versus Conformity' in A. Rose (ed.), *Human Behaviour and Social Process* (London: Routledge and Kegan Paul, 1962) pp. 22-3.

12. Emphasis added. Turner's highlighting of the links between role-taking, role-making and role performance is interesting in that one might argue from a similar standpoint that role performances can often be interpreted as a statement of what the role is or ought to be, *i.e.* that role and role performance are the product of the same 'negotiation' process.

This mirrors the argument of some legal philosophers that some norm applications of judges can also be viewed as norm creations.

13. On the distinction between 'innovants' and 'deviants', see R. K. Merton, 'Social Structure and Anomie' in *Social Theory and Social Structure* (New York: Free Press of Glencoe, 1957) pp. 141-9.

14. On the question that the ability to have one's definition of social reality accepted is an issue of power, see S. Lukes, *Power* (London: Macmillan Press, 1974).

15. See Maureen Cain, *Society and the Policeman's Role* (London: Routledge and Kegan Paul, 1973).

16. 'Whose Side are We On?', 14 *Social Problems* (1967) pp. 239-47.

17. Cain, *Society and the Policeman's Role* , at p. 5.

18. Like the term 'role', 'reference group' has had a variety of meanings ascribed to it by different researchers. A representative sample may be gleaned from H. H. Hyman and E. Singer (eds), *Readings in Reference Group Theory and Research* (London: Collier-Macmillan, 1968).

19. See *e.g.* T. Sarbin and V. Allen, 'Role Theory' in G. Lindzey and E. Aronson (eds), *The Handbook of Social Psychology* (Massachusetts: Addison-Wesley, 1968) pp. 488-576. *Cf.* A. Podgorecki, *Law and Society* (London: Routledge and Kegan Paul, 1974) p. 135.

20. See S. F. Nadel, *The Theory of Social Structure* (London: Cohen & West, 1957) pp. 31-2 and R. Dahrendorf, 'Homo Sociologicus' in *Essays in the Theory of Society* (London: Routledge and Kegan Paul, 1968). The typology employed in this research is a synthesis of these writings and therefore involves a modification of both of them.

21. See A. Sampson, *The New Anatomy of Britain* (London: Hodder and Stoughton, 1971) p. 353; *cf.* the argument of Jones *et al.*, 63 *Journal of Abnormal Social Psychology* (1961) 302-10 that minor deviations from role are the essence of individuality and personality.

22. See the House of Lords criticising the Court of Appeal in *Cassell* v. *Broome* at pp. 1054 B-E; 1084 F-G; 1113C; and 1131B-E.

23. Although the taxonomy set out in the figure has never, to the best of my knowledge, been adopted by any other role analyst, it draws on the outline suggested by G. R. Grace, *Role Conflict and the Teacher* (London: Routledge and Kegan Paul, 1972) pp. 8-11 and on the comparative Table A-1 of J. D. Donnell, *The Corporate Counsel* (Graduate School of Business, Indiana University, 1970) and has the merit of reconciling most of the previous taxonomies put forward in this area.

24. There have been occasional exceptions, *e.g.* J. Toby, 'Some Variables in Role Conflict Analysis', 30 *Social Forces* (1952) 323. It seems likely that this form of response to role conflict has been overlooked by most academics because of their insistence that position incumbents have little part to play in the definition of their roles.

25. This response appears in Merton, *op. cit.*; R. L. Kahn, D. M. Wolfe, R. Quinn, J. Snoek and R. Rosenthal, *Organisational Stress: Studies in Role Conflict and Ambiguity* (New York: J. Wiley and Sons, 1964); and R. Brown, *Social Psychology* (New York: The Free Press, 1965). W. J. Goode in 'A Theory of Role Strain', 25 *American Sociological Review* (1960) 483 seems to hint at an amalgam of these two positive strategies when he

describes attempts by the actor to tackle role conflict as 'a sequence of role bargains'.

26.   Judicial Committee (Dissenting Opinions) Order in Council 1966.

27.   See *e.g.* N. Gross, W. Mason and A. McEachern, *Explorations in Role Analysis* (New York: John Wiley and Sons, 1958); Merton, *Social Theory*; Sarbin and Allen, 'Role Theory'; and Dahrendorf, 'Homo Sociologicus'.

28.   The classical and in some ways still the best piece of research on role conflict, by Gross *et al.*, *Explorations in Role Analysis*, identifies ranking on the basis of legitimacy and sanctions as the response to role conflict which was used by the public school superintendents who were their research subjects. See also P. Kelvin, *The Bases of Social Behaviour* (London: Holt, Rinehart and Winston, 1969) pp. 157 ff.

29.   *E.g.* Nadel's typology of attributes into Pivotal, Relevant or Peripheral, *Theory of Social Structure*, and Merton, 'Role-set'.

30.   Gross *et al.*, *Explorations in Role Analysis*; D. Moment, 'Partial Performances and Total Effectiveness' unpublished paper, quoted in Donnell, *Corporate Counsel*, p. 203.

31.   On this point see my article 'Judges: A Political Elite?', 1 *B.J.L.S.* (1974) 118 pp. 126-7.

32.   *Cf.* the understanding or convention that Law Lords will refrain from speaking in House of Lords debates on highly political topics. S. Shetreet, *Judges on Trial* (Amsterdam: North-Holland Publishing Co., 1976) p. 258.

33.   On segregation of roles, see W. Burchard, 'Role Conflicts of Military Chaplains', 19 *American Sociological Review* (1954) p. 528; W. Evan and L. Levin, 'Status-Set and Role-Set Conflicts of a Stockbroker' undated, unpublished paper quoted in Donnell, *Corporate Counsel*, p. 203; and Sarbin and Allen, 'Role Theory'. On segregation of role performances, see Merton 'The Role Set' and V. Aubert, *Elements of Sociology* (London: Heinemann, 1968) chap. III.

34.   This response is hinted at by various authors but its principal exponent is Erving Goffman in his seminal work *The Presentation of Self in Everyday Life* (New York: Anchor Books, 1959).

35.   B. J. Biddle, H. A. Rosencranz, E. Tomich and J. P. Twyman, 'Shared Inaccuracies in the Role of the Teacher' in B. J. Biddle and E. J. Thomas (eds), *Role Theory* (New York: John Wiley and Sons, 1966) p. 302.

36.   Goffman, *Presentation of Self*, p. 45. The practice of 'gundecking' outlined by J. M. Johnson in chap. 9 of R. Scott and J. D. Douglas (eds), *Theoretical Perspectives on Deviance* (London: Basic Books, 1972) p. 215 seems to be an example of this form of 'Dissimulation' and can be clearly seen as a form of role conflict management.

37.   Goffman, *Presentation of Self*, p. 251. This philosophy seems to underlie the thought of those who suggest that it is more important that justice should be seen to be done than that it should actually be done.

38.   See Toby, 'Variables in Role Conflict Analysis', and Aubert, *Elements of Sociology*.

39.   See Moment, 'Partial Performances'; Burchard, 'Role Conflicts of

Military Chaplains'; and Sarbin and Allen, 'Role Theory'.

40. Otherwise known as a lack of self-role congruence.

41. E. Goffman, 'Role Distance' in *Encounters* (London: Allen Lane, The Penguin Press, 1972) p. 75.

42. *E.g.* Fielding J the Rhodesian judge who resigned when the Smith regime declared UDI, on the grounds that he could not apply the laws of an illegal regime. Resignations following inter-role conflict frequently attract publicity if not notoriety, *e.g.* the case of Abe Fortas, Associate Justice of the United States Supreme Court who resigned on 14 May 1969.

43. See V. E. Flango, L. M. Wenner and M. W. Wenner, 'The Concept of Judicial Role: A Methodological Note', XIX *American Journal of Political Science* (1975) at p. 277.

44. See J. Grossman and A. Sarat, 'Political Culture and Judicial Research' (1971) *Washington University L.Q.* 177 at p. 196.

45. *E.g.* R. Glick and K. Vines's study of the judges in four State Supreme Courts, reported in K. Vines 'The Judicial Role in the American States', chap. 14 in J. Grossman and J. Tanenhaus (eds), *Frontiers of Judicial Research* (New York: John Wiley and Sons, 1969) and R. Glick, *Supreme Courts in State Politics* (New York: Basic Books, 1971); J. W. Howard, 'Role Perceptions and Behaviour in three United States Courts of Appeal', 39 *J. of Pol.* (1977) 916.

46. 'Role Theory and the Supreme Court',30 *J. of Pol.* (1968) 160.

47. 'Perceptions of the Independent Trial Judge Role in the Seventh Circuit', 6 *Law and Soc. Rev.* (1972) 615.

48. Glick, *Supreme Courts in State Politics*.

49. Notably Vines and Glick, 'The Judicial Role', and their successors.

50. Vines and Glick exemplify this in their study of State Supreme Courts. The material derived from this study was written up by them on three occasions and in each case the sub-classification of role type (from the same data) was different. This study is suspect in its categorisation of judges in the purposive and decision-making sectors since this was done on the basis of judicial responses to two open-ended and ambiguous questions.

51. Some of these are listed in John Gibson, 'Discriminant Functions, Role Orientations and Judicial Behaviour', 39 *J. of Pol.* (1977) 984 at p. 1005. See also James Gibson, 'Environmental Constraints on the Behaviour of Judges', 14 *Law and Soc. Rev.* (1980) 343.

52. 'The Judicial Process Reconsidered in the Light of Role-Theory', 32 *M.L.R.* (1969) 156.

53. See *e.g.* R. Wilson, 'Judicial Decision-Making', unpublished Ph.D. thesis, LSE, 1971; Fred L. Morrison, *Courts and the Political Process in England* (London and California: Sage Publications, 1973); M. D. A. Freeman, 'Standards of Adjudication, Judicial Law-making and Prospective Overruling', 1973 *C.L.P.* 166; C. Palley 'Decision-making in the Area of Public Order by English Courts' in *Public Order: Decision-Making in Britain*, II, parts 1-5 (Bletchley: Open University, 1972) p. 45; and B. Baker, J. Eekelaar, C. Gibson and S. Raikes, *The Matrimonial Jurisdiction of Registrars*, SSRC Monograph (Oxford: Centre for Socio-

Legal Studies, 1977) pp. 61-7.

54. Seidman, 'Judicial Process Reconsidered'; Palley, 'Decision-making in the Area of Public Order'.

55. Claire Palley, 'Decision-making in the Area of Public Order', pp. 58-9.

56. See generally J. Grossman, 'Role-playing and the Analysis of Judicial Behaviour', 11 *Public Law* (1963) 285. Grossman's findings do not entirely substantiate the thesis but it can be argued that the role perception which he attributed to Frankfurter was excessively narrow.

57. R. Cover, *Justice Accused* (Yale University Press, 1975) pp. 119-25.

58. See G. Otte, 'Role Theory and the Judicial Process', 16 *Saint Louis University L.J.* (1972) 420; M. Galanter, F. S. Palen and J. M. Thomas, 'The Crusading Judge', 52 *Southern California L.R.* (1979) 699; and James Gibson, 'Environmental Constraints on the Behaviour of Judges'. For a notable exception, see L. Prott, *The Latent Power of Culture and the International Judge* (Abingdon: Professional Books, 1979).

Index of Cases

Subject Index